A Primer of Permutatioı

Kenneth J. Berry • Janis E. Johnston •
Paul W. Mielke, Jr.

A Primer of Permutation Statistical Methods

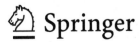 Springer

Kenneth J. Berry
Department of Sociology
Colorado State University
Fort Collins
Colorado, USA

Janis E. Johnston
Alexandria
Virginia, USA

Paul W. Mielke, Jr.
Department of Statistics
Colorado State University
Fort Collins
Colorado, USA

ISBN 978-3-030-20935-3   ISBN 978-3-030-20933-9   (eBook)
https://doi.org/10.1007/978-3-030-20933-9

Mathematics Subject Classification (2010): 62gxx, 62-07, 62-03, 01-08, 62axx

This Springer imprint is published by the registered company Springer Nature Switzerland AG.
The registered company address is: Gewerbestrasse 11, 6330 Cham, Switzerland

For our families: Nancy T. Berry,
Ellen E. Berry, and Laura B. Berry;
Lindsay A. Johnston, James B. Johnston,
Tayla, Buddy, Malia, Ollie, Cami, and Brian;
and Roberta R. Mielke, William W. Mielke,
Emily (Mielke) Spear, and Lynn (Mielke)
Basila.

Preface

A *Primer of Permutation Statistical Methods* presents exact and Monte Carlo permutation statistical methods for generating probability values and measures of effect size for a variety of tests of differences and measures of correlation and association. Throughout the monograph the emphasis is on permutation methods, although the results of permutation analyses are always compared with the results of conventional statistical analyses, with which the reader is assumed to be familiar. On this note, no statistical background other than an introductory course in basic statistics is assumed.

Included in tests of differences are one-sample tests, tests of differences for two independent samples, tests of differences for two matched samples, tests of differences for multiple independent samples, and tests of differences for multiple matched samples. Included in measures of correlation and association are simple linear correlation and regression, multiple linear correlation and regression, a number of measures of association based on Pearson's chi-squared test statistic, and a variety of measures of association designed for the analysis of contingency tables. The arrangement of the monograph follows the structure of a typical introductory textbook in statistics: introduction, central tendency and variability, one-sample tests, tests for two independent samples, tests for two matched samples, completely-randomized analysis of variance designs, randomized-blocks analysis of variance designs, simple linear regression and correlation, and the analysis of contingency tables.

Chapter 1 establishes the structure of the monograph, introduces the following ten chapters, and provides a brief overview of each chapter. The purpose of Chap. 1 is to familiarize the reader with the structure and content of the monograph and provide a brief introduction to the various permutation tests and measures presented in the following chapters.

Chapter 2 provides a brief history of the early beginnings and subsequent development of permutation statistical methods. Permutation methods are a paradox of old and new. While permutation statistical methods predate many conventional parametric statistical methods, it is only in the last 30 or so years that permutation statistical methods have become part of the mainstream discussion regarding statistical testing. Permutation statistical methods were introduced by R.A. Fisher in 1925; further developed by R.C. Geary in 1927, T. Eden and F. Yates in 1933, and H. Hotelling and M.R. Pabst in 1936, and made explicit by E.J.G. Pitman in 1937 and 1938. However, permutation statistical methods are computationally intensive, and it took the development of high-speed computing for permutation statistical methods to become practical. In the 1960s and 1970s, mainframe computers became available to academics at major research universities, and by the end of this period, desktop computers, although not common, were available to many researchers. Permutation statistical methods arrived at a level of maturity during the period between 1980 and 2000 primarily as a result of two factors: greatly improved computer clock speeds and widely available desktop computers and workstations.

Chapter 3 provides an introduction to two models of statistical inference: the population model and the permutation model. Most introductory textbooks in statistics and statistical methods present only the Neyman–Pearson population model of statistical inference. While the Neyman–Pearson population model will be familiar to most readers and needs no introduction, the Fisher–Pitman permutation model of statistical inference is less likely to be familiar. For the permutation model, exact and Monte Carlo permutation methods are described and compared. Under the Neyman–Pearson population model, squared Euclidean scaling functions are mandated, while under the Fisher–Pitman permutation model, ordinary Euclidean scaling functions are shown to provide robust alternatives to conventional squared Euclidean scaling functions.

In Chap. 3, the assumptions underlying statistical tests and measures in the Neyman–Pearson population model are explored and contrasted with the Fisher–Pitman permutation model. The permutation model does not require many of the assumptions of the population model, including random sampling, normality, and homogeneity of variance. Moreover, the null hypotheses of the two models are quite different. Under the Neyman–Pearson population model, the null hypotheses (H_0) posits a value for a population parameter or differences among values for population parameters. For example, H_0: $\mu_x = 100$ for a one-sample test or H_0: $\mu_1 - \mu_2 = 0$ for a two-sample test. By contrast, the null hypothesis under the Fisher–Pitman permutation model simply states that all possible arrangements of the observed data are equally likely, with no population parameter value specified. The primary drawback to permutation statistical methods is the sheer amount of computation required. Five computational efficiencies for permutation methods are described and evaluated in Chap. 3.

Chapter 4 provides an introduction to measures of central tendency and variability, specifically the mode, median, and mean for central tendency and the standard deviation and mean absolute deviation for variability. Special attention is paid to the mean as a minimizing function for the sum of squared deviations and to the median as a minimizing function for the sum of absolute deviations—an often neglected topic. Finally, an alternative approach to the mean, standard deviation, median, and mean absolute deviation based on paired-squared differences and paired-absolute differences between values is described.

Chapter 5 provides an introduction to the permutation analysis of one-sample tests. In general, one-sample tests attempt to invalidate a hypothesized value of a population parameter, such as a population mean. Under the Neyman–Pearson population model, Student's conventional one-sample t test is presented. Under the Fisher–Pitman permutation model, an alternative one-sample permutation test is presented. Six examples illustrate permutation statistical methods for one-sample tests. The first example utilizes a very small set of data to illustrate the calculations required for a permutation analysis of a single sample. The second example illustrates measures of effect size for one-sample tests. The measurement of effect size—the *clinical* significance in contrast to the *statistical* significance of a test— has become increasingly important in recent years, with many journals requiring measures of effect size in addition to the usual tests of statistical significance. A permutation-based, chance-corrected measure of effect size for one-sample tests is presented and compared with the two conventional measures of effect size under the Neyman–Pearson population model: Cohen's $\hat{d}$ and Pearson's r^2. The third example examines the impact of extreme values on conventional and permutation one-sample tests. The fourth example compares exact and Monte Carlo permutation statistical methods for one-sample tests. The fifth example illustrates the application of permutation statistical methods to one-sample tests of rank-score data. A one-sample permutation test for rank scores is developed and compared with Wilcoxon's signed-ranks test. The sixth example illustrates the application of permutation statistical methods to one-sample tests of multivariate data. For each of the six examples, the results obtained from the analyses conducted under the Fisher–Pitman permutation model are compared with the results obtained from the conventional analyses conducted under the Neyman–Pearson population model, when appropriate.

Chapter 6 introduces permutation-based tests of differences for two independent samples. Two-sample tests are specifically designed to test for experimental differences between two groups, such as a control group and a treatment group. Under the Neyman–Pearson population model, Student's conventional two-sample t test is described. Under the Fisher–Pitman permutation model, an alternative two-sample permutation test is presented. Six examples illustrate permutation statistical methods for two-sample tests. The first example utilizes a very small set of data to illustrate the calculations required for a permutation analysis of two independent samples. The second example illustrates measures of effect size for two-sample tests. A permutation-based, chance-corrected measure of effect size for two-sample tests is presented and compared with the four conventional measures of effect size under the Neyman–Pearson population model: Cohen's $\hat{d}$, Pearson's r^2, Kelley's ϵ^2, and Hays' $\hat{\omega}^2$. The third example examines the impact of extreme values on conventional and permutation two-sample tests. The fourth example compares exact and Monte Carlo permutation statistical methods for two-sample tests. The fifth example illustrates the application of permutation statistical methods to two-sample tests of rank-score data. A two-sample permutation test for rank-score data is developed and compared with the Wilcoxon–Mann–Whitney two-sample rank-sum test. The sixth example illustrates the application of permutation statistical methods to two-sample tests of multivariate data. A two-sample permutation test for multivariate data is developed and compared with Hotelling's two-sample T^2 test for multivariate data. For each of the six examples, the results obtained from the analyses conducted under the Fisher–Pitman permutation model are compared with the results obtained with the conventional analyses conducted under the Neyman–Pearson population model, when appropriate.

Chapter 7 introduces permutation tests of differences for two matched samples, often called matched-pairs tests. Matched-pairs tests are designed to test for experimental differences between two matched samples such as twin studies or the same sample at two time periods, that is, before-and-after research designs. Under the Neyman–Pearson population model, Student's conventional matched-pairs t test is described. Under the Fisher–Pitman permutation model, an alternative matched-pairs permutation test is presented. Six examples illustrate permutation statistical methods for matched-pairs tests. The first example utilizes a very small set of data to illustrate the calculations required for a permutation analysis of two matched samples. The second example illustrates measures of effect size for matched-pairs tests. A permutation-based, chance-corrected measure of effect size for matched-pairs is presented and compared with the two conventional measures of effect size under the Neyman–Pearson population model: Cohen's $\hat{d}$ and Pearson's r^2. The third example examines the impact of extreme values on conventional and permutation matched-pairs tests. The fourth example compares exact and Monte Carlo permutation statistical methods for matched-pairs tests. The fifth example illustrates the application of permutation statistical methods to matched-pairs tests of rank-score data. A matched-pairs permutation test for rank-score data is developed and compared with Wilcoxon's signed-ranks test and the sign test. The sixth example illustrates the application of permutation statistical methods to matched-pairs tests of multivariate data. A matched-pairs permutation test for multivariate data is developed and compared with Hotelling's matched-pairs T^2 test for multivariate data. For each of the six examples, the results obtained from the analyses conducted under the Fisher–Pitman permutation model are compared with the results obtained with the conventional analyses conducted under the Neyman–Pearson population model, when appropriate.

Chapter 8 introduces permutation-based tests of differences for multiple independent samples, often called fully or completely randomized analysis of variance designs. Completely randomized designs test for experimental differences among several treatment groups, such as color preferences or taste tests in experimental designs or political parties or religious denominations in survey designs. Under the Neyman–Pearson population model, Fisher's conventional completely randomized F test is described. Under the Fisher–Pitman permutation model, an alternative completely randomized permutation test is presented. Six examples illustrate permutation statistical methods for multiple independent samples. The first example utilizes a very small set of data to illustrate the calculations required for a permutation analysis of multiple independent samples. The second example illustrates measures of effect size for multi-sample tests. A permutation-based, chance-corrected measure of effect size for multiple independent samples is presented and compared with the four conventional measures of effect size under the Neyman–Pearson population model: Cohen's $\hat{d}$, Pearson's η^2, Kelley's $\hat{\eta}^2$, and Hays' $\hat{\omega}^2$. The third example examines the impact of extreme values on conventional and permutation completely randomized designs. The fourth example compares exact and Monte Carlo permutation statistical methods for completely randomized designs. The fifth example illustrates the application of permutation statistical methods to completely randomized tests of rank-score data. A multi-sample permutation test for rank-score data is developed and compared with the Kruskal–Wallis one-way analysis of variance for ranks test. The sixth example illustrates the application of permutation statistical methods to completely randomized tests of multivariate data. A multi-sample permutation test for multivariate data is developed and compared with the Bartlett–Nanda–Pillai trace test for multivariate data. For each of the six examples, the results obtained from the analyses conducted under the Fisher–Pitman permutation model are compared with the results obtained from the conventional analyses conducted under the Neyman–Pearson population model, when appropriate.

Chapter 9 introduces permutation-based tests of differences for multiple matched samples, often called randomized-blocks analysis of variance designs. Randomized-blocks designs test for experimental differences among the same or matched subjects over multiple treatments. Under the Neyman–Pearson population model, Fisher's conventional randomized-blocks F test is described. Under the Fisher–Pitman permutation model, an alternative permutation randomized-blocks test is presented. Six examples illustrate permutation statistical methods for multiple matched samples. The first example utilizes a very small set of data to illustrate the calculations required for a permutation analysis of multiple matched samples. The second example illustrates measures of effect size for multiple matched samples. A permutation-based, chance-corrected measure of effect size for multiple matched pairs is presented and compared with the four conventional measures of effect size under the Neyman–Pearson population model: Hays' $\hat{\omega}^2$, Pearson's η^2, Cohen's partial η^2, and Cohen's f^2. The third example examines the impact of extreme values on conventional and permutation randomized-blocks designs. The fourth example compares exact and Monte Carlo permutation statistical methods for randomized-blocks designs. The fifth example illustrates the application of permutation permutation statistical methods to randomized-blocks tests of rank-score data. A multi-sample permutation test for rank-score data is developed and compared with Friedman's two-way analysis of variance for ranks. The sixth example illustrates the application of permutation statistical methods to randomized-blocks tests of multivariate data. For each of the six examples, the results obtained from the analyses conducted under the Fisher–Pitman permutation model are compared with the results obtained from the conventional analyses conducted under the Neyman–Pearson population model, when appropriate.

Chapter 10 introduces permutation-based tests for simple linear regression and correlation. Under the Neyman–Pearson population model, Pearson's conventional product-moment correlation coefficient is described. Under the Fisher–Pitman permutation model, an alternative permutation measure of correlation is presented.

Six examples illustrate permutation statistical methods for simple correlation data. The first example utilizes a very small set of data to illustrate the calculations required for a permutation analysis of correlation data. The second example illustrates measures of effect size for correlation data. The conventional measure of effect size for correlation data is Pearson's r_{xy}^2 coefficient of determination for variables x and y. A permutation-based, chance-corrected measure of effect size is presented and compared with Pearson's conventional r_{xy}^2 measure of effect size. The third example examines the impact of extreme values on conventional and permutation correlation measures. The fourth example compares exact and Monte Carlo permutation statistical methods for simple linear correlation. The fifth example illustrates the application of permutation statistical methods to linear correlation and regression tests of rank-score data. A permutation test for rank-score correlation is developed and compared with Spearman's rank-order correlation coefficient, Kendall's rank-order correlation coefficient, and Spearman's footrule correlation coefficient. The sixth example illustrates the application of permutation statistical methods to linear correlation and regression tests of multivariate data. For each of the six examples, the results obtained from the analyses conducted under the Fisher–Pitman permutation model are compared with the results obtained from conventional analyses conducted under the Neyman–Pearson population model, when appropriate.

Chapter 11 introduces permutation statistical methods for the analysis of contingency tables. Contingency tables are commonly encountered in the research literature, and there exist a multitude of measures of association for various combinations of cross-classified variables. Six sections illustrate permutation statistical methods for analyzing contingency tables. The first section describes Pearson's familiar chi-squared goodness-of-fit test, provides a permutation alternative that generates exact probability values, and develops a new maximum-corrected measure of effect size. The second section examines contingency tables in which two nominal-level (categorical) variables have been cross-classified. Pearson's chi-squared test of independence is described, and exact alternative permutation statistical methods are presented. Cramér's V measure is described as a conventional measure of effect size, and an alternative permutation-based, chance-corrected measure of effect size is introduced. The third section examines contingency tables in which two ordinal-level (ranked) variables have been cross-classified. A permutation measure of ordinal association is developed and compared with Goodman and Kruskal's G symmetric measure of ordinal association and Somers' d_{yx} and d_{xy} asymmetric measures of ordinal association. The fourth section introduces permutation statistical methods for contingency tables in which a nominal-level variable has been cross-classified with an ordinal-level variable. A permutation measure of nominal–ordinal association is developed and compared with Freeman's θ measure of nominal–ordinal association. A permutation-based, chance-corrected measure of effect size is developed for nominal–ordinal association. The fifth section examines permutation statistical methods for contingency tables in which a nominal-level variable has been cross-classified with an interval-level variable. Pearson's point-biserial correlation coefficient is described, and an alternative permutation coefficient for nominal–ordinal association is introduced. The sixth section introduces permutation statistical methods for contingency tables in which an ordinal-level variable has been cross-classified with an interval-level variable. Jaspen's conventional measure for ordinal–interval correlation is described, and an alternative Monte Carlo permutation statistical measure is presented.

Acknowledgments The authors wish to thank the editors and staff at Springer–Verlag. For almost two decades, all of our research monographs have been published under the Springer logo because the team at Springer has been extraordinarily talented: John Kimmel who shepherded our first two monographs, Federica Corradi Dell'Acqua who guided our next two monographs, and Dr. Eva Hiripi who oversaw our last two monographs. Very special thanks to Dr. Hiripi, Statistics Editor, Springer, who guided the present project though from beginning to end. We are grateful to Roberta Mielke who read the entire manuscript. Finally, we wish to thank Steve and Linda Jones, proprietors of the Rainbow Restaurant, 212 West Laurel Street, Fort Collins, Colorado, for their gracious hospitality. Like our previous monographs, much of this monograph was written at Table 11 in their restaurant adjacent to the Colorado State University campus.

Fort Collins, CO, USA   Kenneth J. Berry
Alexandria, VA, USA   Janis E. Johnston
Fort Collins, CO, USA   Paul W. Mielke, Jr.
December 2018

Contents

Chapter 1
Introduction

Abstract This chapter provides an introduction to permutation statistical methods and an overview of the next 10 chapters. The contents of each chapter are described and summarized in considerable detail.

The primary purpose of this book is to introduce the reader to a wide variety of elementary permutation statistical methods. Most readers will be familiar with conventional statistical methods under the Neyman–Pearson population model of statistical inference, such as tests of hypotheses, confidence intervals, simple linear correlation and regression, one-way completely-randomized analysis of variance, one-way randomized-blocks analysis of variance, and chi-squared tests of goodness-of-fit and independence. However, corresponding permutation statistical tests and measures will almost certainly be less familiar to most readers. While permutation methods date back almost 100 years to the early works by R.A. Fisher and E.J.G. Pitman in the 1920s and 1930s, permutation methods are computationally-intensive methods and it took the advent of high-speed computing to make most permutation methods feasible. Thus, permutation statistical methods have emerged as a practical alternative to conventional statistical methods only in the last 30 or so years. Consequently, permutation statistical methods are seldom taught in introductory courses and there exist no introductory-level textbooks on permutation methods at this writing.[1]

Three main themes characterize the 11 chapters of this book. First, test statistic δ is introduced, defined, and detailed. Test statistic δ is the fundamental test statistic for permutation statistical methods and serves both as a replacement for many conventional statistics such as the one-sample t test, the two-sample t test, the matched-pairs t test, the complete range of completely-randomized and randomized-blocks analysis of variance F tests, and a large number of parametric

---

[1]Some introductory textbooks in statistics now include a chapter on permutation methods. For example, an introductory book by Howell titled *Statistical Methods for Psychology* contains a chapter on "Resampling and Nonparametric Approaches to Data" that includes examples of exact and Monte Carlo permutation methods as well as bootstrapping [8].

© Springer Nature Switzerland AG 2019
K. J. Berry et al., *A Primer of Permutation Statistical Methods*,
https://doi.org/10.1007/978-3-030-20933-9_1

and nonparametric tests of differences and measures of association and correlation. Moreover, test statistic δ lends itself to the development of new statistical tests and measures. As such, test statistic δ is central to the permutation analyses presented in Chaps. 5–11 and constitutes a unifying test statistic for many permutation-based statistical methods.

Second, measures of effect size have become increasingly important in the reporting of contemporary research with many journals now requiring both tests of significance and associated measures of effect size. Measures of effect size indicate the strength of a statistical difference or relationship. In brief, measures of effect size provide information pertaining to the *practical* or *clinical* significance of a result as contrasted with the *statistical* significance of a result. The two are more often than not reported in concert. Conventional measures of effect size typically belong to one of the two families: the d family or the r family. Measures of effect size in the d family typically report the effect size in standard deviation units with values between 0 and ∞, which is perfectly acceptable when comparing two or more studies but may be difficult to interpret for a single, stand-alone study. Cohen's $\hat{d}$ is probably the best-known measure of effect size in the eponymous d family. Measures of effect size in the r family report the effect size as some variety of squared correlation coefficient with values between 0 and 1. Unfortunately, under many circumstances members of the r family cannot achieve the maximum value of 1. When the maximum value is unknown, it is impossible to interpret intermediate values. Pearson's r^2 coefficient of determination is an example of a measure of effect size in the r family and is the measure from which the family gets its name.

A relatively new measure of effect size based on test statistic δ is introduced and described. Effect size measure $\mathfrak{R}$ is a permutation-based, chance-corrected measure of effect size. Chance-corrected measures have much to commend them as they provide interpretations that are easily understood by the average reader. Positive values indicate an effect size greater than expected by chance, negative values indicate an effect size less than expected by chance, and a value of zero indicates an effect size corresponding to chance. The $\mathfrak{R}$ family of measures of effect sizes serves as a replacement for both the d and r families, including Cohen's $\hat{d}$, Pearson's r^2, Kelley's ϵ^2, and Hays' $\hat{\omega}^2$. As such, effect size measure $\mathfrak{R}$ is central to the permutation analyses presented in Chaps. 5–11 and constitutes a generalized, unifying measure of effect size for many permutation-based statistical methods.

Third, conventional statistics, under the Neyman–Pearson population model of statistical inference, necessarily assume normality. The normal distribution is a two-parameter distribution in which the two parameters are the population mean denoted by μ_x and the population variance denoted by σ_x^2. For most parametric tests the population mean is estimated by the sample mean denoted by $\bar{x}$ and the population variance by the sample variance denoted by s_x^2. The sample mean is the point about which the sum of squared deviations is minimized and the sample variance is the average of the squared deviations about the sample mean. Thus, because of the assumption of normality, squared deviations among sample values are an integral and necessary component of most parametric tests under the Neyman–Pearson population model of statistical inference.

On the other hand, statistical tests and measures under the Fisher–Pitman permutation model are distribution-free, do not assume normality, and because they do not depend on squared deviations among sample values, are not limited to squared deviations about the mean. While any scaling factor can be used with permutation statistical methods, ordinary Euclidean scaling has proven to be the most justifiable. Ordinary Euclidean scaling allows permutation statistical methods to minimize, or completely eliminate, the influence of extreme values or statistical outliers, without having to trim, Winsorize, transform, or convert raw scores to ranks. Moreover, ordinary Euclidean scaling allows geometric consistency between the observation space and the analysis space. Finally, ordinary Euclidean scaling has an intuitive appeal that is absent in squared Euclidean scaling. Analyses in Chaps. 5–11 utilize both squared Euclidean scaling, on which conventional statistics rely, and ordinary Euclidean scaling, when appropriate. The squared and ordinary Euclidean scaling results are then compared and contrasted.

These three constructs, test statistic δ, effect size measure $\Re$, and ordinary Euclidean scaling, constitute the main underpinning structures of the book. Each of the substantive chapters is organized around the three constructs and each construct is compared with conventional test statistics, other measures of effect size, and squared Euclidean scaling, when appropriate.

1.1 Overviews of Chapters 2–11

This chapter provides an overview of the book and brief summaries of the following 10 chapters. The format of the book follows the conventional structure of most introductory textbooks in statistical methods with chapters on central tendency and variability, one- and two-sample tests, multi-sample tests, linear correlation and regression, and the analysis of contingency tables. No statistical background of the reader is assumed other than an introductory course in basic statistics, such as is taught in departments of statistics, mathematics, business, biology, economics, or psychology. No mathematical expertise of the reader is assumed beyond elementary algebra.

Most of the substantive chapters in this book follow the same format wherein six example analyses based on permutation statistical methods are provided. The first example in each chapter introduces the main permutation test statistic for the chapter and provides both a highly detailed exact permutation analysis and a conventional analysis; for example, a one-sample permutation test of the null hypothesis under the Fisher–Pitman model and Student's conventional one-sample t test of the null hypothesis under the Neyman–Pearson model. The second example introduces appropriate conventional measures of effect size, for example, Cohen's $\hat{d}$ or Pearson's r^2, and provides a permutation-based, chance-corrected alternative measure of effect size. Because conventional statistical methods under the Neyman–Pearson population model assume random sampling from a normally distributed population, squared deviations about the mean are necessary. Statistical methods under the Fisher–Pitman permutation model do not assume normality; thus, the third example compares permutation analyses based on ordinary and squared Euclidean scaling functions. The inclusion of one or more extreme values demonstrates the advantages of ordinary Euclidean scaling.

The fourth example introduces Monte Carlo permutation statistical methods wherein a large random sample of all possible permutations is generated and analyzed, in contrast to exact permutation methods wherein all possible permutations are generated and analyzed. Both exact and Monte Carlo permutation analyses are compared with each other and with a conventional statistical analysis. The fifth example applies permutation statistical methods to rank-score data, comparing a permutation statistical analysis to a conventional statistical analysis; for example, a permutation test for two sets of rank scores and the Wilcoxon–Mann–Whitney rank-sum test. The sixth example applies permutation statistical methods to multivariate data, comparing a permutation statistical analysis with a conventional statistical analysis; for example, a permutation test of multivariate matched pairs and Hotelling's multivariate T^2 test for two matched samples.

1.2   Chapter 2

The second chapter provides a brief history of the origins and subsequent development of permutation statistical methods. Permutation statistical methods are a paradox of old and new. While permutation methods predate many conventional parametric statistical methods, only recently have permutation methods become part of the mainstream discussion regarding statistical testing. Permutation statistical methods were introduced by R.A. Fisher in 1925 by calculating an exact probability value using the binomial probability distribution [4]. In 1927 R.C. Geary used an exact permutation analysis to demonstrate the utility of asymptotic approaches for data analysis in an investigation of the properties of linear correlation and regression in finite populations [6].

In 1933 T. Eden and F. Yates examined height measurements of wheat shoots grown in eight blocks. Simulated and theoretical probabilities based on the normality assumption were compared and found to be in close agreement, supporting the assumption of normality [3]. In 1936 H. Hotelling and M.R. Pabst used permutation statistical methods to calculate exact probability values for small samples of ranked data in an examination of correlation methods [7]. In 1937 and 1938 E.J.G. Pitman contributed three seminal papers on permutation statistical methods. The first paper utilized permutation statistical methods in an analysis of two independent samples, the second paper utilized permutation statistical methods in an analysis of linear correlation, and the third paper utilized permutation statistical methods in an analysis of randomized-blocks analysis of variance designs [14–16].

The 1940s and 1950s witnessed a proliferation of nonparametric rank tests. For example, Wilcoxon's two-sample rank-sum test in 1945 [17], Mann and Whitney's two-sample rank-sum test in 1947 [11], Kendall's book on *Rank Correlation*

Methods in 1948 [9], Freeman and Halton's exact methods for analyzing two-way and three-way contingency tables in 1951 [5], Kruskal and Wallis' C-sample ranksum test in 1952 [10], Box and Andersen's promotion of permutation methods in the derivation of robust criteria in 1955 [1], and Dwass's rigorous investigation into the precision of Monte Carlo permutation methods in 1957 [2]. In many of these papers, permutation methods were employed to generate tables of exact probability values for small samples.

In the 1960s and 1970s mainframe computers became available to researchers at major universities and by the end of the period desktop computers and workstations, although not common, were available to many investigators. In addition, the speed of computing increased greatly between 1970 and 1980. Permutation statistical methods arrived at a level of maturity during the period 1980–2000 primarily as a result of two factors: greatly improved computer clock speeds and widely-available desktop computers and workstations. By the early 2000s, computing power had advanced enough that permutation statistical methods were providing exact probability values in an efficient manner for a wide variety of statistical tests and measures [12, 13].

1.3   Chapter 3

The third chapter opens with a description of two models of statistical inference: the well-known and widely-taught Neyman–Pearson population model and the lesser-known and seldom-taught Fisher–Pitman permutation model. Under the permutation model, three types of permutation methods are described: exact permutation methods yielding precise probability values, Monte Carlo permutation methods yielding approximate but highly accurate probability values, and permutation methods based on moment approximations yielding exact moments and approximate probability values. In this chapter the Neyman–Pearson population model and Fisher–Pitman permutation model are compared and contrasted and the advantages of permutation statistical methods are described.

Because permutation methods are computationally intensive methods, often requiring millions of calculations, five computational efficiencies are described in Chap. 3. First, high-speed computing and, in the case of Monte Carlo permutation methods, efficient pseudo-random number generators. Second, the examination of all combinations instead of all permutations of the observed data. Third, the use of mathematical recursion. Fourth, calculation of only the variable portion of the selected test statistic. Fifth, in the case of multiple arrays of data, holding one array of the observed data constant. Where appropriate, each efficiency is described and illustrated with a small set of data and an example permutation analysis.

1.4   Chapter 4

The fourth chapter provides a general introduction to measures of central tendency and variability, two concepts that are central to conventional statistical analysis and inference. The sample mode, mean, and median are described and illustrated with small example data sets. The sample mode is simply the score or category with the largest frequency. Two example analyses illustrate the mode, one employing scores and the other employing categories.

Next, the sample mean is considered. The sample mean is the point about which the sum of deviations is zero and, more importantly, the point about which the sum of squared deviations is minimized. These properties are illustrated with two example analyses. Moreover, the sample mean is central to the sample standard deviation, denoted by s_x, and the sample variance, denoted by s_x^2—a point that is illustrated with a small set of example data.

The sample median is usually defined as the point below which half the ordered values fall or the 50th percentile. More importantly, the median is the point about which the sum of absolute deviations is minimized. A detailed example analysis illustrates this property. The sample median is central to the mean absolute deviation (MAD), which is illustrated with a small set of example data.

Finally, the mean, median, and mode are compared with each other and an alternative approach to the mean and median based on paired differences is presented and illustrated. The paired-differences approach to the mean and median is central to the Fisher–Pitman permutation model of statistical inference.

1.5   Chapter 5

The fifth chapter provides a general introduction to permutation analyses of one-sample tests of hypotheses. One-sample tests are the simplest of a large family of tests. For this reason, Chap. 5 is the first chapter dealing with the more technical aspects of permutation statistical methods, serves as an introduction to the basic concepts and varieties of permutation statistical methods, and lays a conceptual foundation for subsequent chapters.

First, Chap. 5 defines permutation test statistic δ for one-sample tests, establishes the relationship between test statistic δ and Student's conventional one-sample t test statistic, and describes the permutation procedures for determining exact probability values under the Fisher–Pitman null hypothesis. An example analysis with a small set of data details the required calculations for an exact test of the null hypothesis under the Fisher–Pitman permutation model of statistical inference.

Second, Chap. 5 introduces the concept of effect sizes: indices to the magnitudes of treatment effects and the practical—in contrast to the statistical—significance of the research. The development and publication of measures of effect size has become increasingly important in recent years and a number of journals now require measures of effect size prior to publication. Three types of measures of effect size are described in Chap. 5. The first type of measure of effect size, designated the d family, is based on measurements of the differences among treatment groups or levels of an independent variable. As noted previously, Cohen's $\hat{d}$ is the most prominent member of the d family, which typically measures effect size by the number of standard deviations separating the means of treatment groups. Thus Cohen's $\hat{d}$ can potentially vary from 0 to ∞.

The second type of measure of effect size, designated the r family, represents some sort of relationship among variables. Measures of effect size in the r family are typically measures of correlation or association, the most familiar being Pearson's squared product-moment correlation coefficient, denoted by r^2. The principle advantage of r measures of effect size is that they are usually bounded by the probability limits 0 and 1, making them easily interpretable.

The third type of measure of effect size, designated the $\mathfrak{R}$ family, represents chance-corrected measures of effect size. Chance-corrected measures are easily understood by the average reader, where positive values indicate an effect size greater than expected by chance, negative values indicate an effect size less than expected by chance, and a value of zero indicates an effect size corresponding to chance. The interrelationships among Student's one-sample t test, Cohen's $\hat{d}$ measure of effect size, Pearson's r^2 measure of effect size, and Mielke and Berry's $\mathfrak{R}$ chance-corrected measure of effect size are explored and illustrated with a small example set of data.

Third, six illustrative examples are provided in Chap. 5, demonstrating permutation statistical methods for one-sample tests of hypotheses. The first example utilizes a small set of data to describe the calculations required for test statistic δ and an exact permutation analysis of a one-sample test under the Fisher–Pitman null hypothesis. Permutation test statistic δ is developed for the analysis of a single sample and compared with Student's conventional one-sample t test.

The second example details measures of effect size for one-sample tests. Specifically, Cohen's $\hat{d}$ and Pearson's r^2 measures of effect size are detailed and $\mathfrak{R}$, an alternative permutation-based, chance-corrected measure of effect size is described for one-sample tests. The differences among the three measures of effect size and their interrelationships are explored and illustrated with a small set of data.

The third example is designed to illustrate the differences between permutation analyses based on ordinary and squared Euclidean scaling functions. Unlike conventional statistical tests that assume normality and are therefore limited to squared Euclidean scaling functions, permutation statistical tests do not assume normality, are extremely flexible, and can accommodate a variety of scaling functions. Inclusion of extreme values illustrates the impact of extreme values on the two scaling functions, on Student's t test statistic, on test statistic δ, on the $\mathfrak{R}$ measure of effect size, and on exact and asymptotic probability values.

The fourth example compares and contrasts exact and Monte Carlo permutation statistical methods. When sample sizes are large, exact permutation tests become impractical and Monte Carlo permutation tests become necessary. While exact permutation tests examine all possible arrangements of the observed data, Monte

Carlo permutation tests examine only a random sample of all possible arrangements of the observed data. Monte Carlo sample sizes can be increased to yield probability values to any desired accuracy, at the expense of computation time.

The fifth example illustrates permutation statistical methods applied to univariate rank-score data. The conventional one-sample tests for rank-score data under the Neyman–Pearson population model are Wilcoxon's signed-rank test and the simple sign test. Wilcoxon's signed-rank test and the sign test are described and compared with permutation-based alternatives. The permutation analyses incorporate both ordinary and squared Euclidean scaling functions. Test statistic δ is defined for rank-score data, the exact probability of δ is generated, and the $\Re$ measure of effect size is described for univariate rank-score data.

The sixth example illustrates permutation statistical methods applied to multivariate data. Multivariate tests have become very popular in recent years as they preserve the relationship among variables, instead of combining the variables into an index and then employing a univariate one-sample test. Like the previous examples, the multivariate permutation analysis incorporates both ordinary and squared Euclidean scaling functions. Test statistic δ is defined for multivariate data, the exact probability of δ is generated, and the $\Re$ measure of effect size is described for multivariate one-sample tests.

1.6   Chapter 6

The sixth chapter provides a general introduction to two-sample tests of hypotheses. Tests of experimental differences for two independent samples are ubiquitous in the research literature and are the tests of choice for comparing control and treatment groups in experimental designs and for comparing two unrelated groups of subjects in survey research.

First, Chap. 6 defines permutation test statistic δ for two independent samples, establishes the relationship between test statistic δ and Student's conventional t test statistic for two independent samples, and describes the permutation procedures for determining exact probability values under the Fisher–Pitman null hypothesis. A small example analysis details the calculations required for an exact test of the null hypothesis under the Fisher–Pitman permutation model of statistical inference.

Second, Chap. 6 describes five measures of effect size for two independent samples. Specifically, Cohen's $\hat{d}$, Pearson's r^2, Kelley's ϵ^2, Hays' $\hat{\omega}^2$, and Mielke and Berry's $\Re$ measures of effect size are described and the interrelationships among t, $\hat{d}$, r^2, ϵ^2, $\hat{\omega}^2$, and $\Re$ are explored and illustrated with a small set of data.

Third, six illustrative examples are provided in Chap. 6, demonstrating permutation statistical methods for tests of two independent samples. The first example utilizes a small data set to detail the calculations required for test statistic δ and an exact permutation test for two independent samples under the Fisher–Pitman null hypothesis. Permutation test statistic δ is developed for the analysis of two independent samples and compared with Student's conventional two-sample t test.

The second example illustrates measures of effect size for two-sample tests. Four conventional measures of effect size are described: Cohen's $\hat{d}$, Pearson's r^2, Kelley's ϵ^2, and Hays' $\hat{\omega}^2$. The four measures are compared and contrasted with Mielke and Berry's $\mathfrak{R}$ chance-corrected measure of effect size.

The third example illustrates the differences between permutation analyses based on ordinary and squared Euclidean scaling functions. The inclusion of extreme values illustrates the impact of extreme values on the two scaling functions, on Student's t test statistic for two independent samples, on test statistic δ, on the $\mathfrak{R}$ measure of effect size, and on exact and asymptotic probability values.

The fourth example compares and contrasts exact and Monte Carlo permutation statistical methods for tests of two independent samples. Both ordinary and squared Euclidean scaling functions are included and evaluated. Finally, the chance-corrected effect size measure $\mathfrak{R}$ is compared with Cohen's $\hat{d}$, Pearson's r^2, Kelley's ϵ^2, and Hays' $\hat{\omega}^2$ measures of effect size.

The fifth example illustrates permutation statistical methods applied to univariate rank-score data. The conventional two-sample test for rank scores under the Neyman–Pearson population model is the Wilcoxon–Mann–Whitney (WMW) two-sample rank-sum test. The WMW test is described and compared with alternative tests under the Fisher–Pitman permutation model. The permutation analyses incorporate both ordinary and squared Euclidean scaling functions. Test statistic δ is defined for rank-score data, the exact and Monte Carlo probability values for δ are developed, and the $\mathfrak{R}$ measure of effect size is described for univariate rank-score data.

The sixth example illustrates permutation statistical methods applied to multivariate data. The results of a permutation statistical analysis are compared with the results from Hotelling's multivariate T^2 test for two independent samples. Mielke and Berry's $\mathfrak{R}$ chance-corrected measure of effect size is described and illustrated for multivariate data.

1.7   Chapter 7

The seventh chapter provides a general introduction to matched-pairs tests of hypotheses. Tests of experimental differences between two matched samples are the simplest of a very large family of tests. In general, matched-pairs tests generally possess more power than tests for two independent samples with the same number of subjects or the same power with fewer subjects. In addition, matched-pairs tests are always balanced with the same number of subjects in each treatment group, a decided advantage over conventional tests for two independent samples, where the two samples may be markedly different in size.

First, Chap. 7 introduces permutation test statistic δ for matched-pairs tests, establishes the relationship between test statistic δ and Student's matched-pairs t test statistic, and describes the permutation procedures required for determining exact probability values under the Fisher–Pitman null hypothesis. Permutation test statistic, δ, is developed for the analysis of two matched samples and compared with Student's conventional matched-pairs t test.

Second, Chap. 7 describes measures of effect size for matched-pairs tests. Specifically, Student's t test for matched pairs, Cohen's $\hat{d}$, Pearson's r^2, and Mielke and Berry's $\mathfrak{R}$ measure of effect size are presented and the interrelationships among t, $\hat{d}$, r^2, and $\mathfrak{R}$ are explored and illustrated with a small example set of data.

Third, six illustrative examples are provided in Chap. 7, demonstrating permutation statistical methods for matched-pairs tests. The first example utilizes a small set of data to detail the calculations required for test statistic δ and an exact permutation test for matched pairs under the Fisher–Pitman null hypothesis. Permutation test statistic δ is developed for the analysis of matched pairs and compared with Student's conventional matched-pairs t test statistic.

The second example describes measures of effect size for matched-pairs tests. Cohen's $\hat{d}$ and Pearson's r^2 measures of effect size are described and Mielke and Berry's chance-corrected measure of effect size, $\mathfrak{R}$, is developed for matched-pairs analyses and compared with Cohen's $\hat{d}$ and Pearson's r^2 conventional measures of effect size.

The third example illustrates the differences between analyses based on ordinary and squared Euclidean scaling functions. Inclusion of extreme values underscores the impact of extreme values on the two scaling functions, on Student's t test statistic for two matched samples, on test statistic δ, on the $\mathfrak{R}$ measure of effect size, and on the accuracy of exact and asymptotic probability values.

The fourth example compares and contrasts exact and Monte Carlo permutation analyses for matched-pairs tests. A matched-pairs test with a large data set is utilized to generate exact and Monte Carlo permutation tests for both ordinary and squared Euclidean scaling functions. The example confirms that Monte Carlo permutation tests are a suitable and efficient substitute for exact permutation tests, provided the Monte Carlo random sample arrangement of the observed data is sufficiently large. Finally, the $\mathfrak{R}$ measure of effect size is described for matched-pairs tests and compared with Cohen's $\hat{d}$ and Pearson's r^2 conventional measures of effect size.

The fifth example illustrates permutation statistical methods applied to univariate rank-score data, comparing permutation statistical methods to Wilcoxon's conventional signed-ranks test and the sign test. A large matched-pairs data set is utilized to generate both exact and Monte Carlo permutation tests for both ordinary and squared Euclidean scaling functions. Finally, the $\mathfrak{R}$ measure of effect size is described and illustrated for univariate rank-score data.

The sixth example illustrates permutation statistical methods applied to multivariate matched-pairs data. Test statistic δ is shown to be related to Hotelling's conventional T^2 test for matched pairs with a squared Euclidean scaling function. The results for test statistics δ and T^2 are compared. Finally, Mielke and Berry's $\mathfrak{R}$ measure of effect size is described and illustrated for multivariate data.

1.8 Chapter 8

The eighth chapter presents permutation statistical methods for analyzing experimental differences among three or more independent samples, commonly called completely-randomized designs under the Neyman–Pearson population model. Multi-sample tests are of two types: tests for differences among three or more independent samples (completely-randomized designs) and tests for differences among three or more related samples (randomized-blocks designs). Permutation statistical tests for multiple independent samples are described in Chap. 8 and permutation statistical tests for multiple related samples are described in Chap. 9.

Six example analyses illustrate permutation statistical methods for multi-sample tests. The first example utilizes a small set of data to illustrate the calculations required for test statistic δ and an exact permutation test for multiple independent samples under the Fisher–Pitman null hypothesis. Permutation test statistic, δ, is developed for the analysis of multiple independent samples and compared with Fisher's conventional F-ratio test statistic for completely-randomized designs.

The second example develops the $\Re$ measure of effect size as a chance-corrected alternative to the four conventional measures of effect size for multi-sample tests: Cohen's $\hat{d}$, Pearson's η^2, Kelley's $\hat{\eta}^2$, and Hays' $\hat{\omega}^2$.

The third example compares permutation statistical methods based on ordinary Euclidean scaling functions with permutation methods based on squared Euclidean scaling functions. Inclusion of one or more extreme scores underscores the impact of extreme values on the two scaling functions, on Fisher's F-ratio test statistic for completely-randomized designs, on the permutation test statistic δ, on the $\Re$ measure of effect size, and on the accuracy of exact and asymptotic probability values.

The fourth example compares and contrasts exact and Monte Carlo permutation methods for multiple independent samples. Both ordinary and squared Euclidean scaling functions are evaluated. Finally, the $\Re$ measure of effect size is compared with the four conventional effect size measures for multi-sample tests: Cohen's $\hat{d}$, Pearson's η^2, Kelley's $\hat{\eta}^2$, and Hays' $\hat{\omega}^2$.

The fifth example illustrates the application of permutation statistical methods to univariate rank-score data, comparing a permutation analysis of example data to the conventional Kruskal–Wallis one-way analysis of variance for ranks test. Both exact and Monte Carlo permutation analyses are utilized and compared. Mielke and Berry's chance-corrected $\Re$ measure of effect size is described and illustrated for univariate rank-score data.

The sixth example illustrates the application of permutation statistical methods to multivariate data, comparing a permutation analysis of example data to the conventional Bartlett–Nanda–Pillai trace test for multivariate data. Mielke and Berry's chance-corrected $\Re$ measure of effect size is described for multivariate data and compared with η^2, the conventional measure of effect size for multivariate data.

1.9   Chapter 9

The ninth chapter presents permutation statistical methods for analyzing experimental differences among three or more matched samples, commonly called randomized-blocks designs under the Neyman–Pearson population model. Randomized-blocks constitute important research designs in many fields. In recent years randomized-blocks designs have become increasingly important in fields such as horticulture, animal science, and agronomy as it has become easier to produce matched subjects through embryo transplants, cloning, genetic engineering, and selective breeding.

Six example analyses illustrate the application of permutation statistical methods to randomized-blocks designs. The first example utilizes a small set of data to detail the calculations required for test statistic δ and an exact permutation test for multiple matched samples under the Fisher–Pitman null hypothesis. Permutation test statistic, δ, is developed for the analysis of multiple matched samples and compared with Fisher's conventional F-ratio test for randomized-blocks designs.

The second example develops the $\mathfrak{R}$ measure of effect size as a chance-corrected alternative to the four conventional measures of effect size for randomized-blocks designs: Hays' $\hat{\omega}^2$, Pearson's η^2, Cohen's partial η^2, and Cohen's f^2.

The third example compares permutation statistical methods based on ordinary and squared Euclidean scaling functions. Inclusion of one or more extreme scores underscores the impact of extreme values on the two scaling functions, on Fisher's F-ratio test statistic for randomized-blocks designs, on the permutation test statistic δ, on the $\mathfrak{R}$ measure of effect size, and on the accuracy of exact and asymptotic probability values. It is demonstrated that extreme blocks of data yield the same results with both scaling functions, but extreme values within a block can yield considerable differences.

The fourth example utilizes a larger data set to compare and contrast exact and Monte Carlo permutation statistical methods for randomized-blocks designs. Both ordinary and squared Euclidean scaling functions are evaluated. The chance-corrected measure of effect size $\mathfrak{R}$ is developed for randomized-blocks designs and compared with Hays' $\hat{\omega}^2$, Pearson's η^2, Cohen's partial η^2, and Cohen's f^2 conventional measures of effect size.

The fifth example illustrates the application of permutation statistical methods to univariate rank-score data, comparing permutation statistical methods to Friedman's conventional two-way analysis of variance for ranks. The permutation test statistic, δ, and Mielke and Berry's $\mathfrak{R}$ measure of effect size are described and illustrated for univariate rank-score data.

The sixth example illustrates the application of permutation statistical methods to multivariate randomized-blocks designs. Both the permutation test statistic δ and Mielke and Berry's chance-corrected $\mathfrak{R}$ measure of effect size are described and illustrated for multivariate randomized-blocks designs.

1.10   Chapter 10

The tenth chapter presents permutation statistical methods for measures of linear correlation and regression. Measures of linear correlation and regression are ubiquitous in the research literature and constitute the backbone of many more advanced statistical methods, such as factor analysis, principal components analysis, path analysis, network analysis, neural network analysis, multi-level (hierarchical) modeling, and structural equation modeling.

Six example analyses illustrate the application of permutation statistical methods to linear correlation and regression. The first example utilizes a small set of bivariate observations to illustrate the calculations required for test statistic δ and an exact permutation test for measures of linear correlation under the Fisher–Pitman null hypothesis. Permutation test statistic, δ, is developed for the analysis of correlation and compared with Pearson's conventional squared product-moment correlation coefficient.

The second example develops the $\Re$ measure of effect size as a chance-corrected alternative to Pearson's squared product-moment correlation coefficient. The two measures of effect size are illustrated and compared using a small set of data.

The third example compares permutation statistical methods based on ordinary and squared Euclidean scaling functions, with an emphasis on the analysis of data containing one or more extreme values. Ordinary least squares (OLS) regression based on squared Euclidean scaling and least absolute deviation (LAD) regression based on ordinary Euclidean scaling are described and compared.

The fourth example compares exact and Monte Carlo permutation statistical methods for linear correlation and regression. Both ordinary Euclidean scaling and squared Euclidean scaling functions are evaluated. The chance-corrected effect-size measure $\Re$ is developed for correlation methods and compared with Pearson's squared product-moment correlation coefficient.

The fifth example illustrates the application of permutation statistical methods to univariate rank-score data, comparing permutation statistical methods with Spearman's rank-order correlation coefficient, Kendall's rank-order correlation coefficient, and Spearman's footrule correlation coefficient. The permutation test statistic δ and Mielke and Berry's $\Re$ measure of effect size are described and illustrated for univariate rank-score data.

The sixth example illustrates the application of permutation statistical methods to multivariate linear correlation and regression. Both OLS and LAD multivariate linear regression are described and compared for multivariate observations. Permutation test statistic δ and the $\Re$ measure of effect size are described and illustrated for multivariate linear regression data.

1.11   Chapter 11

The last chapter provides a general introduction to permutation measures of association for contingency tables. Measures of association for contingency tables constitute a variety of types. One type measures the association in a cross-classification of two nominal-level (categorical) variables and the measure can be either symmetric or asymmetric. A second type measures the association in a cross-classification of two ordinal-level (ranked) variables and the measure can be either symmetric or asymmetric. A third type measures the association in a cross-classification of a nominal-level variable and an ordinal-level variable. A fourth type measures the association in a cross-classification of a nominal-level variable and an interval-level variable. And a fifth type measures the association in a cross-classification of an ordinal-level variable and an interval-level variable. These mixed-level measures are typically asymmetric with the lower-level variable serving as the independent variable and the higher-level variable serving as the dependent variable.

Six sections of Chap. 11 illustrate permutation statistical methods for the analysis of contingency tables. The first section considers permutation statistical methods applied to conventional goodness-of-fit tests; for example, Pearson's chi-squared goodness-of-fit test. Two examples illustrate permutation goodness-of-fit tests and a new maximum-corrected measure of effect size is developed for chi-squared goodness-of-fit tests.

The second section considers permutation statistical methods for analyzing contingency tables in which two nominal-level variables have been cross-classified. Cramér's V test statistic illustrates a conventional symmetrical measure of nominal association and Goodman and Kruskal's t_a and t_b illustrate conventional asymmetrical measures of nominal association.

The third section utilizes permutation statistical methods for analyzing contingency tables in which two ordinal-level variables have been cross-classified. Goodman and Kruskal's G test statistic illustrates a conventional symmetrical measure of ordinal association and Somers' d_{yx} and d_{xy} test statistics illustrate conventional asymmetrical measures of ordinal association.

The fourth section utilizes permutation statistical methods for analyzing contingency tables in which one nominal-level variable and one ordinal-level variable have been cross-classified. Freeman's θ test statistic illustrates a conventional measure of nominal-ordinal association.

The fifth section utilizes permutation statistical methods for analyzing contingency tables in which one nominal-level variable and one interval-level variable have been cross-classified. Pearson's point-biserial correlation coefficient illustrates a conventional measure of nominal-interval association.

The sixth section utilizes permutation statistical methods for analyzing contingency tables in which one ordinal-level variable and one interval-level variable have been cross-classified. Jaspen's $r_{Y\bar{Z}}$ correlation coefficient illustrates a conventional measure of ordinal-interval association.

1.12 Summary

This chapter provided an introduction to permutation statistical methods and an overview and brief summaries of the next 10 chapters. Most of the substantive chapters utilize six examples or sections to illustrate the application of permutation statistical methods to one-sample tests, tests for two independent samples, matched-pairs tests, completely-randomized designs, randomized-blocks designs, linear correlation and regression, and a variety of types of contingency tables.

Chapter 2 provides a brief history and subsequent development of permutation statistical methods. Permutation statistical methods were introduced by R.A. Fisher in 1925, further developed by R.C. Geary in 1927, T. Eden and F. Yates in 1933, and H. Hotelling and M.R. Pabst in 1936, but it was E.J.G. Pitman who made permutation statistical methods explicit with three seminal articles published in 1937 and 1938. However, it took another 50 years before high-speed computing was developed and permutation statistical methods became practical.

References

1. Box, G.E.P., Andersen, S.L.: Permutation theory in the derivation of robust criteria and the study of departures from assumption (with discussion). J. R. Stat. Soc. B Meth. **17**, 1–34 (1955)
2. Dwass, M.: Modified randomization tests for nonparametric hypotheses. Ann. Math. Stat. **28**, 181–187 (1957)
3. Eden, T., Yates, F.: On the validity of Fisher's z test when applied to an actual example of non-normal data. J. Agric. Sci. **23**, 6–17 (1933)
4. Fisher, R.A.: The arrangement of field experiments. J. Am. Stat. Assoc. **33**, 503–513 (1926)
5. Freeman, G.H., Halton, J.H.: Note on an exact treatment of contingency, goodness of fit and other problems of significance. Biometrika **38**, 141–149 (1951)
6. Geary, R.C.: Some properties of correlation and regression in a limited universe. Metron **7**, 83–119 (1927)
7. Hotelling, H., Pabst, M.R.: Rank correlation and tests of significance involving no assumption of normality. Ann. Math. Stat. **7**, 29–43 (1936)
8. Howell, D.C.: Statistical Methods for Psychology, 8th edn. Wadsworth, Belmont (2013)
9. Kendall, M.G.: Rank Correlation Methods. Griffin, London (1948)
10. Kruskal, W.H., Wallis, W.A.: Use of ranks in one-criterion variance analysis. J. Am. Stat. Assoc. **47**, 583–621 (1952). [Erratum: J. Am. Stat. Assoc. **48**, 907–911 (1953)]
11. Mann, H.B., Whitney, D.R.: On a test of whether one of two random variables is stochastically larger than the other. Ann. Math. Stat. **18**, 50–60 (1947)
12. Mielke, P.W., Berry, K.J.: Permutation Methods: A Distance Function Approach. Springer, New York (2001)
13. Mielke, P.W., Berry, K.J.: Permutation Methods: A Distance Function Approach, 2nd edn. Springer, New York (2007)
14. Pitman, E.J.G.: Significance tests which may be applied to samples from any populations. Suppl. J. R. Stat. Soc. **4**, 119–130 (1937)
15. Pitman, E.J.G.: Significance tests which may be applied to samples from any populations: II. The correlation coefficient test. Suppl. J. R. Stat. Soc. **4**, 225–232 (1937)
16. Pitman, E.J.G.: Significance tests which may be applied to samples from any populations: III. The analysis of variance test. Biometrika **29**, 322–335 (1938)
17. Wilcoxon, F.: Individual comparisons by ranking methods. Biometrics Bull. **1**, 80–83 (1945)

Chapter 2
A Brief History of Permutation Methods

Abstract This chapter provides a brief history and overview of the early beginnings and subsequent development of permutation statistical methods, organized by decades from the 1920s to the present.

A variety of books and articles have been written on the history of statistics and statistical methods. Five of the better-known books are by Stephen Stigler titled *American Contributions to Mathematical Statistics in the Nineteenth Century, Vol. I* [92], *American Contributions to Mathematical Statistics in the Nineteenth Century, Vol. II* [93], *The History of Statistics: The Measurement of Uncertainty Before 1900* [94], *Statistics on the Table: The History of Statistical Concepts and Methods* [95], and *The Seven Pillars of Statistical Wisdom* [96].[1]

Other notable books are *Studies in the History of Probability and Statistics: I. Dicing and Gaming* and *Games, Gods, and Gambling: The Origin and History of Probability and Statistical Ideas from the Earliest Times to the Newtonian Era* by F.N. David [23, 24], *The Making of Statisticians* by J. Gani [40], *History of Probability and Statistics and Their Applications Before 1750* and *A History of Mathematical Statistics from 1750 to 1930* by A. Hald [47, 48], *Studies in the History of Statistics and Probability, Vol. II* by M.G. Kendall and R.L. Plackett [58], *Statistics in Britain, 1865–1930: The Social Construction of Scientific Knowledge* by D. MacKenzie [64], *Studies in the History of Statistics and Probability, Vol. I* by E.S. Pearson and M.G. Kendall [79], *The Rise of Statistical Thinking, 1820–1900* by T.M. Porter [84], and *The Lady Tasting Tea: How Statistics Revolutionized Science in the Twentieth Century* by D.S. Salsburg [87].[2]

This chapter provides a brief history and overview of the early beginnings and subsequent development of permutation statistical methods organized by decades. Because of the audience for whom this book is intended as well as space limitations,

---

[1] Authors' note: *Statistics on the Table* and *The Seven Pillars of Statistical Wisdom* by Stephen Stigler are comprehensible and lucid texts written for readers with limited statistical training.

[2] Authors' note: *The Rise of Statistical Thinking* by Theodore Porter and *The Lady Tasting Tea* by David Salsburg are well-written and appropriate for readers with limited statistical training.

© Springer Nature Switzerland AG 2019

K. J. Berry et al., *A Primer of Permutation Statistical Methods*,

https://doi.org/10.1007/978-3-030-20933-9_2

only a small sample of contributions and contributors to the permutation literature is presented for each 10-year period. For more comprehensive histories of the development of permutation statistical methods, see two articles in *WIREs Computational Statistics* on "Permutation methods," [9] and "Permutation methods. Part II" [13], and a book on *A Chronicle of Permutation Statistical Methods* by the authors [10]. Much of the material in this chapter has been adapted from these three sources.

2.1   The Period from 1920 to 1929

The 1920s marked the very beginnings of permutation statistical methods. Only two articles and one chapter pertaining to permutation statistical methods were published between 1920 and 1929. First was an article by J. Spława-Neyman, "On the application of probability theory to agricultural experiments," published in *Annals of Agricultural Sciences* in 1923; second was a chapter by R.A. Fisher, published in Fisher's first book titled *Statistical Methods for Research Workers* in 1925; and third was an article by R.C. Geary on "Some properties of correlation and regression in a limited universe," published in *Metron* in 1927. However, the importance of these early contributions cannot be overstated.

2.1.1   J.S. Neyman

In 1923 Jerzy Spława-Neyman introduced a completely-randomized permutation model for the analysis of field experiments conducted for the purpose of comparing a number of crop varieties [90].[3] The article was part of his doctoral thesis submitted to the University of Warsaw in 1924 and based on research that he had previously carried out at the Agricultural Institute of Bydgoszcz in Northern Poland. The article was written in Polish and was essentially lost to permutation researchers for 66 years until it was translated by D.M. Dabrowska and T.P. Speed and re-published in *Statistical Science* in 1990 [22].

2.1.2   R.A. Fisher

In 1925 Ronald Aylmer Fisher calculated an exact probability value using the binomial probability distribution in his first book titled *Statistical Methods for*

---

[3]Jerzy Spława-Neyman later shortened his name to Jerzy Neyman, emigrated to the USA, and assumed a position at the University of California, Berkeley, in 1938. Neyman founded the Department of Statistics at UC Berkeley in 1955.

Research Workers [35]. Although the use of the binomial distribution to obtain a probability value is not usually considered to be a permutation test per se, Henry Scheffé, writing in *The Annals of Mathematical Statistics*, considered it to be the first application in the literature of a permutation test [88, p. 318]. Also, the binomial distribution does yield an exact probability value and Fisher found it useful, calculating the exact expected values for experimental data. Fisher wrote that the utility of any statistic depends on the original distribution and "appropriate use of exact methods," which he noted have been worked out for only a few cases. Fisher explained that the application is greatly extended as many statistics tend to the normal distribution as the sample size increases, acknowledging that it is therefore customary to assume normality and to limit consideration of statistical variability to calculations of the standard error.

Fisher provided two examples, of which only the first is described here. The example utilized data from the evolutionary biologist Raphael Weldon who threw 12 dice 26,306 times for a total of 315,672 observations, recording the number of times a 5 or a 6 occurred, which Weldon considered to be a "success." Fisher used the binomial distribution to obtain the exact expected value for each of the possible outcomes of 0, 1, ..., 12. For example, the exact binomial probability value for six of 12 dice showing either a 5 or a 6 is

$$p(6|12) = \binom{12}{6} \left(\frac{2}{6}\right)^6 \left(\frac{4}{6}\right)^{12-6} = (924)(0.0014)(0.0878) = 0.1113 \,.$$

Multiplying $p = 0.1113$ by $N = 23{,}306$ trials yields an expectation of 2927.20. Fisher concluded the dice example by calculating a chi-squared goodness-of-fit test and a normal approximation to the discrete binomial distribution. For the chi-squared goodness-of-fit analysis Fisher reported a chi-squared value of $\chi^2 = 35.49$ and a probability value of $P = 0.0001$, and for the normal approximation analysis Fisher reported a standard score of $z = +5.20$ and a two-tail probability value of $P = 0.20 \times 10^{-6}$.

From this example it is clear that Fisher demonstrated a preference for exact solutions, eschewing the normal approximation to the discrete binomial distribution even though the sample sizes were very large. Fisher was to go on to develop other permutation methods and this early work provides a glimpse into how Fisher advanced exact solutions for statistical problems.

2.1.3   R.C. Geary

In 1927 Robert Charles Geary was the first to use an exact permutation analysis to demonstrate the utility of asymptotic approaches for data analysis in an investigation of the properties of linear correlation and regression in finite populations [41]. In his 1927 paper published in *Metron*, Geary examined the mathematical principles underlying a method for indicating the correlation between two variates, arguing that "the formal theory of correlation . . . makes too great demands upon the slender mathematical equipment of even the intelligent public" [41, p. 83].

For his data, Geary considered potato consumption and the incidence of cancer deaths in Ireland. Repeating the experiment 1000 times while holding the marginal frequency totals constant, Geary found that cell arrangements greater than those of the actual experiment occurred in just 231 of the 1000 repetitions yielding a probability value of $P = 0.2310$. Geary concluded that the relationship between potato consumption and cancer was not statistically significant.

2.2 The Period from 1930 to 1939

A number of notable threads of inquiry were established in the period from 1930 to 1939 that were destined to become important in the development of permutation statistical methods. First, there was widespread recognition of the computational difficulties inherent in constructing permutation tests. Second, there was general acceptance that permutation tests were data-dependent, relying solely on the information contained in the observed sample without any reference to the population from which the sample had been drawn. Third, it was recognized that permutation tests were distribution-free and made no assumptions about the population(s) from which the samples had been drawn, such as normality or homogeneity of variance. Fourth, it was generally recognized that it was not necessary to calculate an entire test statistic when undertaking a permutation test. Only that portion of the statistic that varied under permutation was required and the invariant portion could therefore be ignored for permutation purposes, leading to increased computational efficiency. Finally, Monte Carlo permutation methods were recognized to be an efficient alternative to exact permutation methods, in which only a random sample of all possible arrangements of the observed data values was analyzed.

The 1930s witnessed a number of important articles on permutation statistical methods. A selection of nine of the most important articles published between 1930 and 1939 illustrates the development of permutation statistical methods in the 1930s: articles by O. Tedin in 1931, by T. Eden and F. Yates in 1933, by R.A. Fisher in 1935, by H. Hotelling and M.R. Pabst in 1936, three articles by E.J.G. Pitman in 1937 and 1938, an article by M.G. Kendall in 1938, and an article by M.G. Kendall and B. Babington Smith in 1939.

2.2.1 O. Tedin

Olof Tedin was a Swedish geneticist who spent most of his professional career as a plant breeder with the Swedish Seed Association. In 1931 Tedin published a paper in the *Journal of Agricultural Science* in which he demonstrated that, when the assumptions of the classical analysis of variance test are met in practice, the classical test and the corresponding permutation test yielded essentially the same probability value [97].

2.2.2 T. Eden and F. Yates

Like R.C. Geary in 1927, Thomas Eden and Frank Yates utilized permutation statistical methods in 1933 to compare a theoretical distribution to an empirical distribution [26]. Eden and Yates examined height measurements of Yeoman II wheat shoots grown in eight blocks, each consisting of four sub-blocks of eight plots. The simulated and theoretical probability values for 1000 random arrangements of the observed data were compared using a chi-squared goodness-of-fit procedure and were found to be in close agreement, supporting the assumption of normality. Eden and Yates concluded that Fisher's variance-ratio z statistic could be applied to data of this type with confidence.[4] Most important to permutation statistical methods, Eden and Yates were able to considerably reduce the amount of computation required by observing that the block sum-of-squares and the total sum-of-squares would be constant for all 1000 samples; consequently, the value of z for each sample would be solely determined by the value of the treatment sum-of-squares.

2.2.3 R.A. Fisher

In 1935 Ronald Aylmer Fisher published a paper in *Journal of the Royal Statistical Society* in which he analyzed data on 30 criminal same-sex twins that had been previously published by Dr. Johannes Lange, Chief Physician at the Munich–Schwabing Hospital and Director of the German Experimental Station for Psychiatry [37]. The point of the twin example—that for small samples exact tests are possible, thereby eliminating the need for estimation—indicates an early understanding of the superiority of exact probability values computed from known discrete distributions over approximations based on assumed theoretical distributions. As Fisher pointed out, "The test of significance is therefore direct, and exact for small samples. No process of estimation is involved" [36, p. 50]. Today the test is known as Fisher's exact probability (FEP) test for 2×2 contingency tables and is included in most statistical computing packages.[5]

---

[4]The original symbol for the variance-ratio test statistic used by Fisher was z. In 1934 George Snedecor published tabled values in a small monograph for Fisher's z statistic and rechristened the test statistic F [89].

[5]The exact probability test for 2×2 contingency tables was independently developed by Frank Yates in 1934 [104] and Joseph Irwin in 1935 [52].

2.2.4   H. Hotelling and M.R. Pabst

In 1936 Harold Hotelling and Margaret Richards Pabst at Columbia University used permutation methods to calculate exact probability values for small samples of rank data in their research on simple bivariate correlation [51]. Noting that tests of significance are primarily based on the assumption of a normal distribution in a hypothetical population from which the observations are assumed to be a random sample, Hotelling and Pabst developed permutation methods of statistical inference without assuming any particular distribution of the variates in the population from which the sample had been drawn. Hotelling and Pabst utilized the calculation of a probability value that incorporated all possible permutations of the data, under the null hypothesis that all permutations were equally-likely. This 1936 article may well have been the first example that detailed the method of calculating a permutation test using all possible arrangements of the observed data.

2.2.5   E.J.G. Pitman

In three papers published in 1937 and 1938, Edwin James George Pitman demonstrated how researchers, using exact permutation structures, could devise valid tests of significance that made no assumptions about the distributions of the sampled populations [81–83]. While much credit must go to R.A. Fisher and R.C. Geary for their early contributions to permutation statistical methods, it was E.J.G. Pitman at the University of Tasmania who made permutation methods explicit in these three papers.

In the first of these three seminal papers published in 1937, Pitman demonstrated how researchers could devise valid tests of significance between two independent samples that made no assumptions about the distributions of the sampled populations [81]. In addition, Pitman showed how precise limits could be determined for the difference between two independent means, again without making any assumptions about the populations from which the samples had been obtained. The second paper, also published in 1937, developed permutation statistical methods for the Pearson product-moment correlation coefficient "which makes no assumptions about the population sampled" [81, p. 232].

In the third paper published in 1938, Pitman proposed a permutation test for the analysis of variance "which involved no assumptions of normality" [83, p. 335]. Pitman noted that in the form of analysis of variance test discussed in the paper (randomized-blocks) the observed values were not regarded as a sample from a larger population. This early statement is possibly the first pronouncement that permutation statistical methods do not require random sampling from a well-defined infinite population.

2.2.6 M.G. Kendall

Also in 1938 Maurice George Kendall incorporated exact probability values utilizing the "entire universe" of permutations in the construction of test statistic τ, a new measure of rank-order correlation that was based on the difference between the sums of concordant and discordant pairs of observations that he labeled S [55]. A clever recursion procedure permitted the efficient calculation of all possible arrangements of the observed data. Utilizing this powerful recursion technique, Kendall constructed a table of the distribution of test statistic S for values of n from 1 to 10, thereby providing exact probability values.

2.2.7 M.G. Kendall and B. Babington Smith

In 1939 Maurice George Kendall and Bernard Babington Smith considered the problem of m rankings [57]. They defined a coefficient of concordance as

$$W = \frac{12S}{m^2(n^3 - n)} \, ,$$

where m denotes the number of rankings, n denotes the number of rank scores in each ranking, and S denotes the observed sum-of-squares of the deviations of sums of ranks from the mean value. Since $m^2(n^3 - n)$ and the constant 12 are invariant under permutation of the observed data, Kendall and Babington Smith showed that to test whether an observed value of test statistic W is statistically significant it is only necessary to consider the distribution of S over all possible permutations of the n observed values.[6]

2.3 The Period from 1940 to 1949

Since permutation methods are by their very nature computationally intensive, permutation statistical methods developed between 1940 and 1949 were characterized by researchers expressing frustration over difficulties in computing a sufficient number of permutations of the observed data in a reasonable time. To compensate for the difficulty, many researchers turned to rank-order statistics, which were much more amenable to permutation methods. Thus this period from 1940 to 1949 was distinguished by a plethora of rank-order tests. Prominent in this period was H. Scheffé with an article in 1943, F. Wilcoxon with an article in 1945, L. Festinger with an article in 1946, H.B. Mann and D.R. Whitney with an article in 1947,

---

[6]Also see an article on this topic by E.J. Burr in 1960 [19].

M.G. Kendall with a short book in 1948, and S.S. Wilks with an article in 1948. These articles led to the publication of numerous tables of exact probability values for rank-order tests of differences.

2.3.1   H. Scheffé

In 1943 Henry Scheffé published what soon became a seminal article on non-parametric inference [88]. In an extensive review and highly mathematical summary of the non-parametric literature of the time, Scheffé provided an excellent description of permutation statistical methods, attributing the origins of permutation methods to the work of R.A. Fisher in 1925. Scheffé expressed dissatisfaction with those cases in which the author of the test provided an approximation to the discrete permutation distribution by means of some familiar continuous distribution. This 1943 paper by Scheffé provided an important impetus to the development of permutation statistical methods in the 1940s.

2.3.2   F. Wilcoxon

In 1945 Frank Wilcoxon, a chemist by training, introduced two test statistics for rank-order values in *Biometrics Bulletin* [102]. In this very brief paper of only three and a half pages, Wilcoxon considered the case of two samples of equal sizes and provided a table of exact probability values for the lesser of the two sums of ranks for both paired and unpaired experiments. In the case of unpaired samples, a table provided exact probability values for 5–10 replicates in each sample, and for paired samples, a table provided exact probability values for 7–16 paired comparisons. Ralph Bradley referred to Wilcoxon's unpaired and paired rank tests as the catalysts for the flourishing of non-parametric statistics [50] and E. Bruce Brooks described the 1945 Wilcoxon article as "a bombshell which broke new and permanent ground" and pronounced the paired and unpaired rank-sum tests as "cornerstones in the edifice of nonparametric statistics"[18].

2.3.3   L. Festinger

In 1946 psychologist Leon Festinger introduced a statistical test of differences between two independent samples by first converting raw scores to ranks, then testing the difference between the means of the ranks [34]. Festinger provided tables for tests of significance based on exact probability values for 0.05 and 0.01 confidence levels for $n = 2(1), \ldots, 15$, the smaller of the two samples, and $m = 2(1), \ldots, 38$, the larger of the two samples. Festinger's approach to the two-sample rank-sum test was developed independently of Wilcoxon's. Moreover, Festinger's tables considered both equal and unequal sample sizes, whereas Wilcoxon's method allowed for only equal sample sizes. While both approaches generated all possible permutations of outcomes, Festinger's method was much more general and simpler to implement.

2.3.4 H.B. Mann and D.R. Whitney

In 1947 mathematicians Henry Berthold Mann and Donald Ransom Whitney, acknowledging the previous work by Wilcoxon on the two-sample rank-sum test, proposed an equivalent test statistic, U, based on the relative ranks of two independent samples [65]. Using a recurrence relation, Mann and Whitney constructed tables of exact probability values up to and including $n = m = 8$, where n and m denoted the number of rank scores in each of the two samples. Finally, from the recurrence relation Mann and Whitney derived explicit expressions for the mean, variance, and various higher moments for U, showing that the limit of the distribution approached normality as $\min(n, m) \to \infty$.

2.3.5 M.G. Kendall

In 1948 Maurice George Kendall published a small volume titled *Rank Correlation Methods* [56]. The importance of Kendall's book on rank-order correlation methods cannot be overstated. The title of Kendall's book was perhaps a little misleading as the book contained much more than rank-correlation methods, including an extensive summary of permutation methods. Of particular relevance to permutation statistical methods, Kendall included descriptive summaries of articles that contained permutation statistics per se and tables of exact probability values obtained from permutation distributions. For example, Kendall summarized articles by H. Hotelling and M.R. Pabst that used permutation methods for calculating exact probability values for small samples of rank-score data [51], E.J.G. Pitman on permutation tests for two independent samples, linear correlation, and randomized-blocks designs [81–83], F. Wilcoxon on tables of exact probability values for the two-sample test for rank-order statistics [102], and H.B. Mann and D.R. Whitney on exact probability values for the two-sample rank-sum test [65].

2.3.6 S.S. Wilks

Kendall's book on *Rank Correlation Methods* was quickly followed by a substantial and sophisticated exposition of rank-order statistics by Samuel Stanley Wilks in

1948 [103]. In a highly structured organization, Wilks provided a lengthy discourse on rank-order statistics, summarizing the results on rank-order statistics, and listing all the references up to that time. Although the title of the article was "Order statistics," the article was also a rich source on permutation statistical methods. The article by Wilks on order statistics comprised some 45 pages in *Bulletin of the American Mathematical Society* and included summaries of the contributions to permutation statistical methods by R.A. Fisher, H. Hotelling and M.R. Pabst, E.J.G. Pitman, M. Friedman, H. Scheffé, and many others.

2.4   The Period from 1950 to 1959

Like the 1940s, permutation statistical methods in the 1950s were characterized by extensive analyses of rank-score data. The exact analysis of contingency tables by G.H. Freeman and J.H. Halton in 1951, exact probability values for the Wilcoxon two-sample rank-sum test by C. White in 1952, exact probability values for an analysis of variance for ranks by W.H. Kruskal and W.A. Wallis in 1952, the promotion of exact permutation methods by G.E.P. Box and S.L. Andersen in 1955, and the rigorous investigation into the precision of Monte Carlo permutation methods by M. Dwass in 1957 illustrate the development of permutation statistical methods between 1950 and 1959.

2.4.1   G.H. Freeman and J.H. Halton

In 1951 Gerald Freeman and John H. Halton published a short but influential article in *Biometrika* that addressed exact methods for analyzing two-way and three-way contingency tables, given fixed marginal frequency totals [38]. The approach adopted by Freeman and Halton for two-way contingency tables utilized the conventional hypergeometric probability distribution. This was the same approach put forward by R.A. Fisher in 1935 for 2×2 contingency tables. A three-way contingency table is more complex than a two-way table, but Freeman and Halton developed an innovative permutation method. Freeman and Halton concluded that the exact method they proposed was generally useful in cases where a chi-squared test would normally be utilized, but should not be used because the observed and expected cell values were too small. The method, they explained, was also useful when a chi-squared test was wholly unsuitable, such as when the entire population contained so few members that a chi-squared test was not appropriate.

2.4.2   C. White

Although trained as a medical doctor, Colin White nevertheless contributed to the field of permutation statistics. In 1952 White recursively generated tables of exact probability values for the Wilcoxon two-sample rank-sum test in which the sample sizes, n_1 and n_2, could be either equal or unequal [101]. White provided three tables that gave critical values of rank sums for $n_1 = 2(1), \ldots, 15$ and $n_2 = 4(1), \ldots, 28$ for critical values of $\alpha = 0.05$, $n_1 = 2(1), \ldots, 15$ and $n_2 = 5(1), \ldots, 28$ for critical values of $\alpha = 0.01$, and $n_1 = 3(1), \ldots, 15$ and $n_2 = 7(1), \ldots, 27$ for critical values of $\alpha = 0.001$.

2.4.3   W.H. Kruskal and W.A. Wallis

Also in 1952 William Henry Kruskal and Wilson Allen Wallis proposed an exact C-sample rank-sum test that they denoted as H [60]. Although H is asymptotically distributed as chi-squared with $C - 1$ degrees of freedom, Kruskal and Wallis provided tables based on exact probability values for $C = 3$ independent samples, with each sample equal to or less than $n = 5$ for $\alpha = 0.10, 0.05$, and 0.01 levels of significance. Kruskal and Wallis compared the exact probability values with three moment approximations: the first based on the chi-squared distribution, the second based on the incomplete gamma distribution, and the third based on the incomplete beta distribution. Finally, Kruskal and Wallis observed that when $C = 2$, H was equivalent to the Wilcoxon [102], Festinger [34], and Mann–Whitney [65] two-sample rank-sum tests.

2.4.4   G.E.P. Box and S.L. Andersen

In 1955 George Edward Pelham Box and Sigurd Lökken Andersen published an important and influential paper on "Permutation theory in the derivation of robust criteria and the study of departures from assumption" in *Journal of the Royal Statistical Society* [15]. This was a lengthy paper of 35 pages and included discussions by several prominent members of the Royal Statistical Society. Box and Andersen noted that in practical circumstances little is usually known of the validity of assumptions, such as the normality of the error distribution. They argued for statistical procedures that were insensitive to changes in extraneous factors not under test, but sensitive to those factors under test; that is, procedures both robust and powerful. In this context, they addressed permutation theory as a robust method and applied it to comparisons of means and variances. Box and Andersen pointed out that tests on differences between variances could be so misleading as to be valueless, unless the resulting distribution was very close to normal. They then stated that an assertion of normality would certainly not be justified. The solution, they proposed, was the use of "a remarkable new class of tests" called permutation tests [15, p. 3].

2.4.5 P.H. Leslie

Also in 1955 Patrick Holt Leslie published a short paper of only one-and-a-half folio pages on "a simple method of calculating the exact probability in 2×2 contingency tables with small marginal totals" [62]. Consider a simple example with $n_1. = 7$, $n_{.1} = 6$, $N = 16$, and $n_{11} = 5$. The essential values are the binomial coefficients for $n_1. = 7$, constituting $n_{11} = 0, \ldots, n_{.1}$, and in reverse order, the binomial coefficients for $N - n_1. = 9$, constituting $n_{11} = n_{.1}, \ldots, 0$. As Leslie showed, the required binomial coefficients could easily be obtained from the first $n + 1$ terms of the expanded binomial series; for example,

$$1 + \frac{n}{1!} + \frac{n(n-1)}{2!} + \frac{n(n-1)(n-2)}{3!} + \cdots + \frac{n!}{n!} = \sum_{i=0}^{n} \binom{n}{i} = 2^n .$$

2.4.6 M. Dwass

Meyer Dwass provided the first rigorous investigation into the precision of Monte Carlo probability approximations. In 1957 Dwass published an article on modified permutation tests for non-parametric hypotheses [25] that relied heavily on previously-published theoretical contributions by Erich Lehmann and Charles Stein [61]. Dwass noted that a practical shortcoming of exact permutation procedures was the great difficulty in enumerating all the possible arrangements of the observed data. Dwass then proposed "the most obvious procedure" of examining a random sample drawn without replacement from all possible permutations of the observed data and making the decision to accept or reject the null hypothesis on the basis of those permutations only. Dwass observed that while it is true that the size of the random sample would necessarily have to be very large, the optimum exact permutation test is usually impossible to calculate.

2.5 The Period from 1960 to 1969

Permutation statistical methods are, by their very nature, computationally intensive methods and it took the development of high-speed computing for permutation methods to achieve their potential. In the period prior to 1960, computers were large, slow, expensive, and input was usually by way of punch cards. In large part their use was restricted to military and industrial applications. In the 1960s many permutation algorithms and associated computer programs were developed for mainframe computers. Most of the programs were written in an early version of FORTRAN, which had been developed by IBM in 1956 for scientific and engineering applications. Two articles on computing exact probability values for 2×2 contingency tables illustrate this early development: one article by W.A. Robertson in 1960 and another by I.D. Hill and M.C. Pike in 1965.

In contrast, Eugene Edgington at the University of Calgary dominated the literature on permutation statistical methods in the 1960s. Edgington published four major articles with an emphasis on permutation tests for differences in 1964, nonrandom samples in 1966, statistical inference in 1967, and Monte Carlo permutation methods in 1969. Also in 1969, Edgington published a book on *Statistical Inference* that contained a substantial chapter on permutation statistical methods.

2.5.1   W.H. Robertson

A number of articles were published on the computation of exact probability values for contingency tables and goodness-of-fit tests between 1960 and 1969. In 1960 William H. Robertson published an article on programming Fisher's exact probability method of comparing two percentages [85]. In this paper Robertson described the application of a high-speed computer for determining the exact probability associated with the problem of comparing two percentages utilizing the Fisher–Yates exact probability method.[7] In programming the Fisher–Yates exact probability method, Robertson was forced to rely on stored logarithms of factorial expression, given the limited capabilities of digital computers in 1960.

2.5.2   E.S. Edgington

In terms of permutation statistical methods, the period 1960–1969 could be labeled the Edgington decade. Beginning in the early 1960s, Eugene Sinclair Edgington published a number of articles and books on permutation methods, which he called "randomization" methods, and was an influential voice in promoting the use of permutation tests and measures. In 1964 Edgington published a descriptive article

---

[7]Relatively speaking, there were no "high-speed" computers in 1960. Since Robertson worked at the Sandia National Laboratory in Albuquerque, New Mexico, he had access to a Royal McBee LGP-30. The Royal McBee Librascope General Purpose (LGP) computer was considered a desktop computer, even though it weighed 740 pounds. The LGP-30 contained a 4096-word magnetic drum, and had a clock rate of only 120 kHz.

on permutation tests in *The Journal of Psychology* [27]. In this brief but formative article, Edgington defined a permutation test as a statistical test that derives a sampling distribution of a statistic from repeated computations of the statistic for various ways of pairing, arranging, or dividing the scores. Edgington considered three types of permutation statistical tests: tests for differences between independent samples, tests for differences between paired samples, and tests for measures of correlation. Edgington noted that permutation tests could be particularly useful whenever the assumptions of parametric tests could not be met, when samples were very small, and when exact probability tables for the desired test statistic were not available.

2.5.3   I.D. Hill and M.C. Pike

In the period from 1960 to 1969 there appeared a multitude of computer algorithms and sequence generators, all essential to the computation of exact and Monte Carlo permutation methods. One interesting and representative algorithm was by I.D. Hill and M.C. Pike. In 1965 Hill and Pike designed an algorithm for computing tail-area probability values for 2×2 contingency tables that was based on an exact method for fixed marginal frequency totals [49]. It was an interesting algorithm because it provided an exact one-tailed probability value by summing the individual probability values that are equal to or less than the observed probability value, and then provided two quite different two-tailed exact probability values. One two-tailed probability value was obtained from the one-tailed probability value and a probability value calculated in similar fashion from the second tail. The second two-tailed probability value was obtained by including in the second tail all those terms that gave an inverse odds-ratio statistic at least as great as the odds-ratio statistic for the observed table.

2.5.4   E.S. Edgington

Eugene Edgington was especially critical of the use of normal-theory methods when applied to nonrandom samples. In 1966 Edgington published a controversial article in *Psychological Bulletin* that focused on statistical inference and nonrandom sampling [28]. Writing primarily for psychologists, Edgington pointed out that since experimental psychologists seldom sample randomly, it was difficult for psychologists to justify using hypothesis-testing procedures that required the assumption of random sampling of the population or populations about which inferences were to be made. Edgington stated his position unequivocally: "statistical inferences cannot be made concerning populations that have not been randomly sampled" [28, p. 485].

In 1967 Eugene Edgington published an article on making statistical inferences from a sample of $N = 1$ [29]. Edgington clarified the problem of making statistical inferences with permutation methods. He noted that while it was certainly correct that a researcher could not statistically generalize to a population from only one subject, it was also correct that a researcher could not statistically generalize to a population from which the researcher had not taken a random sample of subjects. Edgington noted that this observation precluded making inferences to populations for virtually all experiments, both those with large and small sample sizes. Finally, Edgington noted that hypothesis testing was still possible without random sampling, but that significance statements were consequently limited to the effect of the experimental treatment on the subjects actually used in the experiment.

In 1969 Eugene Edgington elaborated on approximate permutation tests; that is, Monte Carlo permutation tests [30]. Edgington defined an approximate permutation test as a test in which the significance of an obtained statistic was determined by using a distribution consisting of a random sample of test statistics drawn from the entire sampling distribution. Edgington noted that an approximate permutation test could thereby greatly reduce the amount of computation required to a practical level. At the time, in 1969, Edgington and others were recommending approximate permutation tests based on 1000 random samples. Today, 1,000,000 random samples is fairly standard and easily accomplished with modern desktop computers, workstations, and even laptops.

Also in 1969 Eugene Edgington published a book titled *Statistical Inference: The Distribution-free Approach* that contained an entire chapter on permutation tests for experiments [31]. In this lengthy chapter of 76 pages, Edgington examined inferences concerning hypotheses about experimental treatment effects with finite populations, with no assumptions about the shapes of the populations, and for nonrandom samples. He explored in great detail and with many examples, permutation tests for paired comparisons, contingency tables, correlation, interactions, differences between independent samples, and other lesser permutation tests such as differences between medians, ranges, and standard deviations. Edgington concluded the chapter with a discussion of normal-theory tests as approximations to permutation tests.

2.5.5   O. Kempthorne and T.E. Doerfler

In 1969 Oscar Kempthorne and Thomas E. Doerfler published a paper examining the behavior of selected tests of significance under experimental randomization [54]. Kempthorne and Doerfler selected three tests for a matched-pairs design and concluded that the Fisher permutation test was to be preferred over the Wilcoxon matched-pairs rank-sum test, which, not surprisingly, was to be preferred over the sign test. All comparisons were based on Monte Carlo permutation test procedures with 50 sets of randomly-generated data from eight distributions for experiments on 3–6 pairs of observations.

While the purported purpose of the paper was to compare matched-pairs designs, the paper actually contained a great deal more. First, Kempthorne and Doerfler objected to the use of specified cut-off points for the significance level, α, and to classifying the conclusion as being simply significant or not significant. They argued that the use of such a dichotomy was inappropriate in the reporting of experimental data as it resulted in a loss of information. Second, they objected to the common practice of adding very small values to measurements so as to avoid ties when converting raw scores to ranks. Third, they suggested that the term "significance level" of a test be retired from the statistical vocabulary. Finally, they dismissed the assumption of random samples in comparative populations and praised permutation tests for their ability to answer the question "What does this experiment, on its own, tell us?" [54, p. 235].

2.6   The Period from 1970 to 1979

Like the 1960s, the 1970s witnessed the development of computer algorithms for exact permutation methods. Researchers were focused on defining efficient methods for computing exact probability values. By 1979 punch cards had largely disappeared and desktop computers, although not common, were available to many researchers. In 1973 Alvan Feinstein produced one of the best introductions to permutation methods ever published and in 1976 Paul Mielke, with his collaborators at Colorado State University, published the first of what would become several hundred articles and books on exact and Monte Carlo permutation statistical methods.

2.6.1   A.W. Ghent

No account of the analysis of contingency tables would be complete without mention of the work of Arthur W. Ghent, who significantly extended the method of binomial coefficients first proposed by Patrick Leslie in 1955 [62]. In 1972 Ghent examined the literature on the alignment and multiplication of appropriate binomial coefficients for computing the Fisher–Yates exact probability test for 2×2 contingency tables with fixed marginal frequency totals [44]. In an exceptionally clear and cogent presentation, Ghent reviewed the method of binomial coefficients first proposed by Leslie in 1955 [62] and independently discovered by Sakoda and Cohen in 1957 [86].

The method of binomial coefficients was a computational procedure involving, first, the selection of the appropriate series of binomial coefficients; second, their alignment at starting points in accord with the configuration of frequencies in the observed contingency table; and finally, the multiplication of adjacent coefficients that constitute the numerators of the exact hypergeometric probability values of all 2×2 contingency tables that are equal to or more extreme than the probability of the observed contingency table, given fixed marginal frequency totals.

2.6.2   A.R. Feinstein

Trained as both a mathematician and a medical doctor, Alvan R. Feinstein published 400 original articles and six books. In 1973 Feinstein published a must-read article on permutation methods [33].[8] The importance of Feinstein's article was not that it contained new permutation methods, but that it summarized and promoted permutation methods to a new audience of clinical researchers in a cogent and lucid manner. Writing for a statistically unsophisticated readership, Feinstein distinguished between socio-political research where the purpose was usually to estimate a population parameter, and medical research where the purpose was typically to contrast a difference between two groups. Feinstein observed that a random sample is mandatory for estimating a population parameter, but "has not been regarded as equally imperative for contrasting a difference" [33, p. 899]. In a strongly worded conclusion, Feinstein argued that the ultimate value of permutation methods was that their intellectual directness, precision, and simplicity would free both the investigator and the statistician from "a deleterious pre-occupation with sampling distributions, pooled variances, and other mathematical distractions" [33, p. 914].

2.6.3   P.W. Mielke, K.J. Berry, and E.S. Johnson

In 1976 Paul W. Mielke, Kenneth J. Berry, and Earl S. Johnson published an article on "Multi-response permutation procedures for a priori classifications," which they abbreviated as MRPP for convenience [73]. Mielke, Berry, and Johnson provided an exact permutation test for analyzing multi-response data at the ordinal or higher levels. The associated test statistic, which they denoted as δ, was based on the average difference, or any specified norm, between data points within a priori disjoint subgroups of a finite population of points in an r-dimensional space, such as r measured responses from each object in a finite population of objects. In addition, alternative approximate tests based on the beta and normal distributions were provided. Two detailed examples utilizing actual social science data illustrated permutation statistical methods, including comparisons of the approximate tests. A third example described the behavior of these tests under a variety of conditions, including the inclusion of extreme values. This 1976 article by Mielke, Berry, and Johnson introduced test statistic δ, which serves as the first of the three main constructs of this book. Second, this article introduced ordinary Euclidean scaling in which absolute differences between data points were utilized instead of the more conventional squared Euclidean differences.

---

[8]Authors' note: After 40-plus years, this 1973 article by Feinstein remains as perhaps the clearest non-mathematical introduction to permutation methods ever written and should be consulted by all researchers new to the field of permutation methods.

2.6.4   B.F. Green

In 1977 Bert Green published an interactive FORTRAN program for one- and two-sample permutation tests of location [46]. Noting that Fisher's permutation tests of location had been described by Ralph Bradley as "stunningly efficient" but "dismally impractical" [17], Green proposed a practical permutation program containing two heuristics that permitted most of the permutations to be counted implicitly rather than explicitly. Both exact and Monte Carlo permutation procedures were provided in the program.

2.6.5   A. Agresti and D. Wackerly

Also in 1977, Alan Agresti and Dennis Wackerly published an article on exact conditional tests of independence for $r \times c$ contingency tables with fixed marginal frequency totals [2]. Unlike previous researchers, Agresti and Wackerly were less concerned with the exact hypergeometric probability and more concerned with the exact probability of established test statistics, such as Pearson's chi-squared statistic. Agresti and Wackerly defined the attained significance level to be the sum of the probability values of all contingency tables for which the value of the test statistic was at least as large as the value of the test statistic for the observed contingency table. This perception by Agresti and Wackerly was destined to become an important observation.

2.6.6   J.M. Boyett

In 1979 James M. Boyett published an algorithm and associated FORTRAN subroutine to generate random $r \times c$ contingency tables with given fixed row and column marginal frequency totals [16]. First, employing a uniform pseudo-random number generator and a shuffling routine, Boyett generated a random permutation of the first N integers, $x_1, x_2, \ldots, x_N$, then partitioned the permuted integers into r groups of the row variable with each group S_i containing a_i. values for $i = 1, \ldots, r$. For the column variable, the first N integers (not permuted) were partitioned into c groups with each group T_j containing $a_{.j}$ values for $j = 1, \ldots, c$. Thus,

$$S_1 = \{x_{a1.+1}, \ldots, x_{a1.+a2.}\}, \ldots, S_r = \{x_{N-a_{r.}+1}, \ldots, x_N\},$$

$$T_1 = \{1, \ldots, a_{.1}\},$$

and

$$T_2 = \{a_{.1} + 1, \ldots, a_{.1} + a_{.2}\}, \ldots, T_c = \{N - a_{.c} + 1, \ldots, N\}.$$

2.7   The Period from 1980 to 1989

Permutation statistical methods arrived at a new level of maturity in the 1980s, primarily as a result of two factors: (1) greatly improved computer clock speeds and (2) widely available desktop computers and workstations. While interest continued in the study of linear rank-order statistics, the period witnessed a dramatic shift in sources of permutation publications. Prior to 1980 nearly all published papers on permutation methods appeared in computer journals, such as *Communications of the ACM*, *Journal of Numerical Analysis*, *The Computer Journal*, and *The Computer Bulletin*. In the period between 1980 and 1989 there was a shift away from computer journals and into statistical journals, such as *Biometrika*, *Biometrics*, *Journal of Statistical Computation and Simulation*, and *Applied Statistics*.[9] An even more dramatic change occurred in this period as an increasing number of published papers on permutation statistical methods began appearing in discipline journals, such as *American Journal of Public Health*, *American Antiquity*, *Educational and Psychological Measurement*, *Journal of Applied Meteorology*, and *British Journal of Mathematical and Statistical Psychology*.

2.7.1   E.S. Edgington

In 1980 Eugene Edgington published *Randomization Tests*, the first full book devoted to permutation (randomization) statistical methods [32]. The book was intended as a practical guide for experimenters on the use of permutation tests. Edgington defined permutation tests as those in which the data are repeatedly rearranged, a test statistic is computed on each arrangement, and the proportion of the arrangements with as large a test statistic value as the value for the obtained results determines the significance of the results. Edgington argued that random assignment is the only element necessary for determining the significance of experimental results by a permutation test procedure. Therefore, assumptions regarding random sampling and assumptions regarding normality, homogeneity of variance, and other characteristics of randomly sampled populations are unnecessary. A second edition was published in 1987, a third edition was published in 1995, and a fourth edition co-authored with Patrick Onghena was published in 2007.[10]

---

[9]The journal *Applied Statistics* is also known as *Journal of the Royal Statistical Society, Series C*.

[10]Eugene Edgington, a dominating force in the promotion of permutation statistical methods for 50 years, passed away on September 2, 2013, at the age of 89.

2.7.2   K.J. Berry, K.L. Kvamme, and P.W. Mielke

Also in 1980 Kenneth J. Berry, Kenneth L. Kvamme, and Paul W. Mielke published
an article in *American Antiquity* titled "A permutation technique for the spatial
analysis of the distribution of artifacts into classes" [8]. This brief article was,
most probably, the first analysis of archaeological data using permutation methods
published in the field of anthropology. The authors argued that the identification
of localized activity areas through an analysis of artifact distribution within an
archaeological site is a complex process warranting more than visual assessment
and impressionistic interpretation and noted that quantitative approaches to date
have utilized conventional statistical tests that require indefensible assumptions to
be made about the data. Utilizing ordinary Euclidean scaling functions on data
gathered from Sde Divshon, an Upper Paleolithic site on the Divshon Palin in Israel,
the authors presented a rigorous test of the patterning of positions of end scrapers,
carinated scrapers, and burins within the archaeological site.

2.7.3   W.M. Patefield

In 1981 William M. Patefield published a subroutine for the generation of random
$r \times c$ contingency tables which was designed to be an improvement over the
previously published algorithm of Boyett [78]. As Patefield explained, under the
null hypothesis of no association between row and column categories, the joint
probability distribution of a random table is given by n_{ij}, $i = 1, \ldots, r$ and
$j = 1, \ldots, c$, conditional on the row and column totals, $n_{i.}$, $i = 1, \ldots, r$, and
$n_{.j}$, $j = 1, \ldots, c$. Patefield considered the conditional distribution of a table entry
n_{lm} given the table entries in row l; that is, n_{ij}, $i = 1, \ldots, l-1$ and $j = 1, \ldots, c$
and the previous table entries in row l; that is, n_{lj}, $j = 1, \ldots, m-1$.
    Assuming valid conditional table entries, Patefield showed that the range of the
conditional distribution is from a minimum of

$$\max \left\{ 0, n_{l.} - \sum_{j=1}^{m-1} \left[n_{lj} - \sum_{j=m+1}^{c} \left(n_{.j} - \sum_{i=1}^{l-1} n_{ij} \right) \right] \right\}$$

to a maximum of

$$\min \left[\left(n_{.m} - \sum_{i=1}^{l-1} n_{im} \right), \left(n_{l.} - \sum_{j=1}^{m-1} n_{lj} \right) \right].$$

The table entries, n_{rm}, $m = 1, \ldots, c$, in the last row of the table and n_{lc}, $l = 1, \ldots, r$, in the last column of the table, were obtained from the previous $(r -$

$1) \times (c - 1)$ table entries and the fixed row and column marginal frequency totals, $n_{i.}, i = 1, \ldots, r$, and $n_{.j}, j = 1, \ldots, c$.

2.7.4 C.R. Mehta and N.R. Patel

In 1983 Cyrus R. Mehta and Nitin R. Patel created an innovative network algorithm for the Fisher–Yates exact probability test for $r \times c$ unordered contingency tables [67]. Unlike earlier algorithms for unordered contingency tables that were based on an exhaustive enumeration of all possible tables with fixed marginal frequency totals, the Mehta–Patel network algorithm eliminated the need to completely enumerate all possible contingency tables in the permutation reference set. Today the Mehta–Patel algorithms are available in a number of platforms, the most widely distributed being StatXact.[11]

2.7.5 P.W. Mielke

In 1984 Paul W. Mielke published a chapter on "Meteorological applications of permutation techniques based on distance functions" in the *Handbook of Statistics, Vol. 4* [68]. Trained as both a meteorologist and a biostatistician, Mielke utilized meteorological applications as a vehicle for illustrating permutation statistical methods, dividing the chapter into two main sections. The first section described multi-response permutation procedures (MRPP) as a permutation generalization of completely-randomized analysis of variance designs. The second section described multivariate randomized-blocks procedures (MRBP) as a permutation generalization of randomized-blocks analysis of variance designs. This 1984 chapter contained the first formal presentation of permutation methods based on ordinary Euclidean scaling, which serves as the second of the three main constructs of this book, along with permutation test statistic δ described on p. 33.

2.7.6 K.J. Berry and P.W. Mielke

In 1985 Kenneth J. Berry and Paul W. Mielke developed non-asymptotic permutation tests for Goodman and Kruskal's τ_a and τ_b measures of nominal association [5]. The algorithm was based on the exact mean, variance, and skewness under the conditional permutation distribution, which then employed a Pearson type III

---

[11] StatXact is a statistical software package for analyzing data using exact statistics. It is marketed by Cytel Inc. [4].

probability distribution to obtain approximate probability values. Berry and Mielke found the non-asymptotic approach to be superior to the conventional asymptotic method for small samples and for unbalanced marginal frequency distributions.

2.7.7 A.K. Thakur, K.J. Berry, and P.W. Mielke

Also in 1985 Ajit K. Thakur, Kenneth J. Berry, and Paul W. Mielke published an algorithm for testing linear trend and homogeneity in proportions [98]. Trend was evaluated by the Cochran–Armitage method as well as by multiple pairwise comparisons using the Fisher–Yates exact probability method. A recursion technique with an arbitrary initial value was employed, yielding exact two-tailed probability values based on all permutations of cell frequencies with fixed marginal frequency totals.

2.7.8 K.J. Berry and P.W. Mielke

In 1988 Kenneth J. Berry and Paul W. Mielke published an article in *Educational and Psychological Measurement* in which they generalized Cohen's κ measure of agreement for categorical polytomies to ordinal and interval data and to multiple observers [6]. As originally conceived, Cohen's κ measure of agreement was appropriate only for two observers and was limited to a set of discrete unordered categories. Noting that a number of statistical problems require the measurement of agreement, rather than association or correlation, Berry and Mielke generalized Cohen's κ measure of agreement so that it would measure agreement at any level of measurement among any number of observers. The generalization required a new symbol, to distinguish it from κ. Thus this 1988 article by Berry and Mielke introduced the $\Re$ chance-corrected measure of effect size, which serves as the third of the three main constructs of this book, along with the permutation test statistic δ described on p. 33 and ordinary Euclidean scaling described on p. 37.

Also in 1988 Mielke and Berry published an article in *Biometrika* on "Cumulant methods for analyzing independence of r-way contingency tables and goodness-of-fit frequency data" [69]. Mielke and Berry showed that the cumulant methods presented in this paper for analyzing independence of r-way contingency tables and goodness-of-fit frequency data were appropriate for many cases involving sparse data, that is, small expected cell frequencies, whereas any continuous approximation would be unsatisfactory. The method was based on the exact determination of the mean, variance, and skewness of the permutation distribution.

2.7.9 M.E. Biondini, P.W. Mielke, and K.J. Berry

Also in 1988 Mario E. Biondini, Paul W. Mielke, and Kenneth J. Berry published an article on permutation methods for the analysis of ecological data [14]. Noting that while classical least squares statistics are optimal and result in maximum likelihood estimators of the unknown parameters of the model if the population is normal, or multivariate normal, with equal variances, or a variance–covariance matrix which exhibits compound symmetry, Biondini, Mielke, and Berry argued that classical least squares statistics are far from optimal when the population distribution is asymmetric or when extreme values are present. Biondini, Mielke, and Berry presented two distribution-free permutation procedures for the analysis of ecological data with ordinary Euclidean scaling as the basis of both procedures.

2.7.10 J.W. Tukey

Also in 1988 John Wilder Tukey read a paper at the Ciminera Symposium in Philadelphia, Pennsylvania. The paper was never published, but copies of this important paper continue to circulate even today [99]. Tukey began the paper by defining what he called "the three R's" as Randomization, Robustness, and Rerandomization. By "randomization" Tukey meant a controlled randomized design wherein treatments were randomly assigned to subjects in an effort to eliminate bias and to nearly balance whatever is important. By "robustness" Tukey meant to ensure high stringency, high efficiency, and high power over a wide range of probability models. By "rerandomization" Tukey meant "analysis of randomized comparative experiments by means of permutation methods to confine the probabilities to those we have ourselves made" [99, p. 17].

Tukey distinguished among three types of rerandomization. First, complete rerandomization; that is, an exact permutation analysis. Second, sampled rerandomization; that is, a Monte Carlo permutation analysis. Third, subset rerandomization; that is, a double permutation analysis. Long an advocate of permutation methods, it is in this paper that Tukey refers to rerandomization as the "platinum standard" of significance tests. After critically denouncing techniques such as the bootstrap and the jackknife, Tukey concluded the paper by arguing that when an experiment can be randomized, it should be. Then the preferred method of analysis should be based on rerandomization. In an important affirmation of permutation methods, Tukey stated that "No other class of approach provides significance information of comparable quality" [99, p. 18].

2.8 The Period from 1990 to 1999

The period from 1990 to 1999 witnessed an explosion of journal articles on permutation methods in a wide variety of disciplines and research areas; for example, animal behavior, archaeology, atmospheric science, biology, biometrics, biostatistics, chemistry, clinical trials, dental research, earth science, ecology, education, engineering, environmental health, forest research, geology, human genetics, medicine, pharmacology, physiology, psychology, toxicology, wood science, and zoology.

This period was also characterized by the publication of a number of tutorials that attempted to introduce or promote permutation methods to a variety of audiences; for example, psychologists, econometricians, teachers of mathematics, chemists, researchers in biomedicine and clinical trials, and statisticians. Earlier undertakings on the development of permutation methods, coupled with the availability of high-speed computers and efficient computing algorithms, provided a solid foundation for the development of permutation statistical methods in the 1990s.

2.8.1 R.B. May and M.A. Hunter

In 1993 Richard B. May and Michael A. Hunter published a short article on "Some advantages of permutation tests" [66]. May and Hunter laid out in an elementary and very readable fashion the rationale and advantages of permutation tests, illustrating permutation methods with the two-sample test for means. May and Hunter noted that with the normal or population model a researcher must first know something about a theoretical parent distribution and then evaluate the data in light of the model. On the other hand, the permutation model starts with the data at hand and generates a set of outcomes to which the obtained outcome is compared. The reference, or permutation, distribution is generated from all possible arrangements of the data.

2.8.2 P.W. Mielke and K.J. Berry

In 1994 Paul W. Mielke and Kenneth J. Berry presented permutation tests for common locations among g samples with unequal variances [70]. As Mielke and Berry explained, in completely-randomized experimental designs where population variances are equal under the null hypothesis, it is not uncommon to have multiplicative treatment effects that produce unequal variances under the alternative hypothesis. Mielke and Berry presented permutation procedures to test for (1) median location and scale shifts, (2) scale shifts only, and (3) mean location shifts only. In addition, corresponding multivariate extensions were provided.

2.8.3 P.E. Kennedy and B.S. Cade

In 1996 Peter E. Kennedy and Brian S. Cade published an article on permutation tests for multiple regression [59]. In this article Kennedy and Cade examined four generic methods for conducting a permutation test in the context of linear multiple regression. Using the classical linear regression model given by

$$y = \mathbf{X}\beta + \mathbf{Z}\theta + \epsilon \, ,$$

where β and θ are parameter vectors and $\mathbf{X}$ and $\mathbf{Y}$ are corresponding matrices of observations on explanatory variables, Kennedy and Cade sought to test $\theta = 0$.

The first method calculated the F statistic for testing $\theta = 0$ and compared the F test statistic with F statistics produced by shuffling the $\mathbf{Z}$ variables as a group. The second method calculated the F statistic for testing $\theta = 0$ and compared the F test statistic with F statistics produced by shuffling the y variable. The third method calculated the F statistic for testing $\theta = 0$ and compared the F test statistic with F statistics produced by shuffling the $\mathbf{Z}$ variables on a residualized y variable. First, y was residualized for $\mathbf{X}$ and, second, the residualized y was treated as the dependent variable. The fourth method calculated the F statistic for testing $\theta = 0$ and compared the F test statistic with F statistics produced by residualizing both y and $\mathbf{Z}$. Kennedy and Cade recommended the fourth method as it alone possessed desirable repeated-sample properties.

2.8.4 P.W. Mielke, K.J. Berry, and C.O. Neidt

Also in 1996 Paul W. Mielke, Kenneth J. Berry, and Charles O. Neidt published a new permutation procedure for Hotelling's multivariate matched-pairs T^2 test [74]. They explained that since Hotelling's T^2 test obtains a vector of measurements on each subject in each of two time periods, the test is applicable to two different analyses. Consider n subjects and c raters. It is possible to block on the n subjects and examine the multivariate difference among the c raters at the two time periods. Alternatively, it is also possible to block on the c raters and examine the multivariate difference among the n subjects at the two time periods.

In the first scenario, Hotelling's T^2 test statistic is distributed under the Neyman–Pearson null hypothesis as Snedecor's F distribution with c and $n - c$ degrees of freedom in the numerator and denominator, respectively. In the second scenario, Hotelling's T^2 test statistic is distributed under the Neyman–Pearson null hypothesis as Snedecor's F distribution with n and $n - c$ degrees of freedom in the numerator and denominator, respectively. Consequently, one of the two scenarios will yield degrees of freedom in the denominator that is equal to or less than zero. Moreover, when $n = c$ neither scenario is possible. Mielke, Berry, and Neidt developed a multivariate extension of a univariate permutation test for matched pairs that eliminated the problem and was shown to be more discriminating than Hotelling's matched-pairs T^2 test.

2.8.5   J. Ludbrook and H.A.F. Dudley

In 1998 John Ludbrook and Hugh Dudley published an influential article in *The American Statistician* titled "Why permutation tests are superior to t and F tests in biomedical research" [63]. In this article Ludbrook and Dudley noted that statisticians believe that biomedical researchers conduct most experiments by taking random samples and therefore recommend statistical procedures that are valid under the Neyman–Pearson population model of inference. Given that biomedical researchers typically do not employ random sampling, but instead rely on randomization of a nonrandom sample, Ludbrook and Dudley argued that the Neyman–Pearson population model did not apply to biomedical research and strongly recommended statistical procedures based on data-dependent permutations of the observations.

2.8.6   R.W. Frick

Also in 1998 Robert W. Frick published an article that challenged the standard textbook treatment of conventional statistical tests based on random sampling from an infinite population [39]. Frick termed this standard treatment the "population-based" interpretation of statistical testing and noted three problems with the population-based treatment. First, researchers rarely make any attempt to randomly sample from a defined population. Second, even if random sampling actually occurred, conventional statistical tests do not precisely describe the population. Third, researchers do not generally use statistical testing to generalize to a population. Against the population-based interpretation Frick proposed what he called a "process-based" interpretation, arguing that random sampling is a process, not the outcome of a process. To this end, Frick recommended consideration of permutation statistical methods.

2.8.7   J. Gebhard and N. Schmitz

Also in 1998 Jens Gebhard and Norbert Schmitz published two articles on permutation methods [42, 43]. In the first article Gebhard and Schmitz showed that permutation methods possess optimum properties for both continuous and discrete distributions. A variety of examples illustrated permutation tests for the continuous distributions: normal, gamma, exponential, chi-squared, and Weibull;

and for the discrete distributions: Poisson, binomial, and negative binomial. In the second article Gebhard and Schmitz formulated an efficient computer algorithm for computing the critical regions.

2.9   The Period from 2000 to 2009

If permutation methods might be said to have "arrived" in the period between 1980 and 1999, they might be said to have "erupted" in the period from 2000 to 2009. Significant advances in computing, including increased speed, enlarged memory and capacity, canned statistical packages that included permutation add-ons or modules, and the development of a new computer language, R, by Ross Ihaka and Robert Gentleman enabled a virtual explosion of new permutation methods and applications.[12] After the year 2000, permutation methods continued to be introduced into, spread to, or expanded in a number of different fields and disciplines, most notably in medicine, psychology, clinical trials, biology, ecology, environmental science, earth science, and atmospheric science.

Along with a proliferation of journal articles, a multitude of books on permutation methods appeared during this period. Having all the information collected and organized in one compact source instead of scattered among many journal in myriad disciplines made it easier for the user to learn about new and existing permutation methods. Included among these books were volumes on *Data Analysis by Resampling: Concepts and Applications* by C.E. Lunneborg in 2000; *Permutation Tests: A Practical Guide to Resampling Methods for Testing Hypotheses* and *Permutation, Parametric and Bootstrap Tests of Hypotheses* by P.I. Good in 2000; *Permutation Methods: A Distance Function Approach* by P.W. Mielke and K.J. Berry, *Resampling Methods: A Practical Guide to Data Analysis* by P.I. Good, and *Multivariate Permutation Tests: With Applications in Biostatistics* by F. Pesarin in 2001; *Resampling Methods for Dependent Data* by S.N. Lahiri in 2003; *Permutation, Parametric and Bootstrap Tests of Hypotheses* by P.I. Good in 2005; a second edition of *Resampling Methods: A Practical Guide to Data Analysis* by P.I. Good and *Exact Analysis of Discrete Data* by K.F. Hirji in 2006; *Randomization Tests* by E.S. Edgington and P. Onghena, *Randomization and Monte Carlo Methods in Biology* by B.F.J. Manly, and a second edition of *Permutation Methods: A Distance Function Approach* by P.W. Mielke and K.J. Berry in 2007.

---

[12]Technically, R was first developed in 1995, but only came into wide use in the period 2000–2009.

2.9.1   K.J. Berry and P.W. Mielke

In 2000 Kenneth J. Berry and Paul W. Mielke utilized Monte Carlo permutation methods to investigate the Fisher Z transformation of the sample product-moment correlation coefficient between variables x and y [7]. Utilizing Monte Carlo permutation methods Berry and Mielke compared combinations of sample sizes and population parameters for seven bivariate distributions. Both confidence intervals and hypothesis testing were examined for robustness and non-normality. Each Monte Carlo simulation was based on 1,000,000 bivariate random samples of sizes $n = 20$ and $n = 80$ for $\rho_{xy} = 0.00$ and $\rho_{xy} = +0.60$, and compared to nominal upper-tail probability values of $\alpha = 0.99$, 0.90, 0.75, 0.50, 0.25, 0.10, and 0.01. Based on the results of the permutation simulations, Berry and Mielke concluded that considerable caution should be exercised when using the Fisher Z transformation.

2.9.2   A. Agresti

In 2001 Alan Agresti published a lengthy article in *Statistics in Medicine* on recent advances associated with exact inference for categorical data [1]. The article was, in part, an overview article, but also one that examined and summarized some of the criticisms of exact methods. For example, the conservative nature of exact methods due to the inherent discreteness of the permutation distribution. Agresti devoted two sections of the paper to complications from discreteness, illustrating the problem with numerous examples involving samples with small sample sizes. Agresti explained that in the real world it is rarely possible to achieve an arbitrary critical value such as $\alpha = 0.05$ under permutation and noted that some researchers argued that fixing an unachievable α level is artificial and that one should merely report the probability value. Finally, Agresti offered a compromise: use adjustments of exact methods based on the mid-P value. The mid-P procedure, Agresti explained, uses one-half the probability of the observed contingency table, plus the probability values of those contingency tables that are less than that of the observed contingency table.

2.9.3   P.W. Mielke and K.J. Berry

Also in 2001 Paul W. Mielke and Kenneth J. Berry published a research monograph titled *Permutation Methods: A Distance Function Approach* [71]. The book provided exact probability values and approximate probability values based on Monte Carlo and moment techniques for univariate and multivariate data. Metric Euclidean distance functions were emphasized, in contrast to the non-metric squared Euclidean functions common to statistical tests that rely on the assumption of normality.

In 2002 Paul Mielke and Kenneth Berry published an article on a multivariate multiple regression analysis for experimental designs [72]. Mielke and Berry used permutation methods to evaluate multivariate residuals obtained from a regression algorithm. As they noted, applications included various completely randomized and randomized-blocks experimental designs such as one-way, Latin square, factorial, nested, and split-plot analysis of variance designs, both with and without covariates. Unlike parametric procedures, the only requirement was the randomization of subjects to treatments. When compared with classical parametric approaches, Mielke and Berry found permutation methods to be exceedingly robust to the presence of extreme values and, because the methods were based on permutations of the observed data, no assumptions such as normality, homogeneity, and independence were required.

2.9.4   F. Pesarin and L. Salmaso

Also in 2002 Fortunato Pesarin and Luigi Salmaso published an article in which they explored exact permutation methods in unreplicated two-level multi-factorial designs [80]. The approach of Pesarin and Salmaso preserved the exchangeability of error components by testing up to k effects in 2^k designs. Pesarin and Salmaso further discussed the advantages and limitations of exact permutation procedures and executed a simulation study utilizing the Iris data of Fisher based on a paired permutation strategy.

2.9.5   A. Janssen and T. Pauls

In 2003 Arnold Janssen and Thorsten Pauls published a lengthy, highly technical article in *The Annals of Statistics* titled "How do bootstrap and permutation tests work?" [53]. This was an ambitious paper of 40 pages that considered a comprehensive and unified approach for the conditional and unconditional analysis of linear Monte Carlo permutation methods. Under fairly mild assumptions, Janssen and Pauls proved tightness and an asymptotic series representation for weak accumulation points. The results lead Janssen and Pauls to a discussion of the asymptotic correctness of Monte Carlo permutation methods as well as applications in testing hypotheses.

2.9.6   B.S. Cade and J.D. Richards

In 2006 Brian S. Cade and Jon D. Richards published a permutation test statistic for quantile regression [20]. Cade and Richards observed that estimating the quantiles of a response variable conditioned on a set of covariances in a linear model has many applications in the biological and ecological sciences, as quantile regression models allow the entire conditional distribution of a response variable y to be related to some covariates $\mathbf{X}$, providing a richer description of functional changes that is possible by simply focusing on just the mean or other central statistics.

2.9.7   P.W. Mielke, K.J. Berry, and J.E. Johnston

In 2007 Paul W. Mielke, Kenneth J. Berry, and Janis E. Johnston presented a Monte Carlo permutation algorithm for the enumeration of a subset of all possible r-way contingency tables with fixed marginal frequency totals [75]. The algorithm provided analyses for any r-way contingency table with an integral value of $r \geq 2$. This had long been a perplexing problem. There had been published any number of algorithms for $r \times c$ contingency tables. For example, Boyett in 1979 [16] and Patefield in 1981 [78] had developed Monte Carlo permutation algorithms for $r \times c$ contingency tables with fixed marginal frequency totals. Both algorithms enumerated a subset of all possible two-way contingency tables from an observed contingency table. The algorithm by Mielke, Berry, and Johnston was not an extension of either the Boyett or Patefield algorithms, but an entirely new, highly efficient, Monte Carlo permutation approach. The algorithm was later employed in a number of applications [76].

2.9.8   R.A. Gianchristofaro, F. Pesarin et al.

Also in 2007 Rosa A. Gianchristofaro, Fortunato Pesarin, and Luigi Salmaso published an article in which they considered permutation statistical methods for testing ordered variables based on the nonparametric combination of permutation dependent tests [45]. As Gianchristofaro, Pesarin, and Salmaso noted, several solution had been proposed to cope with univariate testing problems on ordered categorical data, most of which were based on the restricted maximum likelihood-ratio test. These solutions were generally criticized because the degree of accuracy of their asymptotic null and alternative distributions was difficult to assess and to characterize. The authors offered a new exact solution based on simultaneous analysis of a finite set of sampling moments of ranks assigned to ordered classes and processed by the nonparametric permutation method.

2.9.9 P.W. Mielke, M.A. Long et al.

In 2009 Paul W. Mielke, Michael A. Long, Kenneth J. Berry, and Janis E. Johnston extended the two-treatment ridit analysis developed by I.D.J. Bross to $g \geq 2$ treatment groups [77]. Ridit is an acronym for Relative to an Identified Distribution, where the suffix "it" represents a type of data transformation similar to logit and probit. The most common application of ridit analysis compares two independent treatment groups in which ridit scores are calculated for the c ordered category frequencies of the first treatment group and applied to the c ordered categories of the second treatment group, and vice versa. Mielke, Long, Berry, and Johnston used a Monte Carlo permutation procedure to generate L sets of N random assignments selected from the c^N assignment configurations of the g treatment groups.

2.10 The Period from 2010 to 2018

Three features of permutation statistical methods were especially prominent in the period 2010–2018. The first entailed an increasing criticism of rank-order statistical procedures with their attendant loss of information due to the substitution of rank-order statistics for numerical values. In lieu of rank-order statistical procedures, many researchers advocated the use of permutation methods that utilized the original numerical values and did not depend on the assumption of normality.

The second feature was a criticism of permutation statistical methods based on squared Euclidean scaling that gave artificial weight to extreme scores and implied a geometry of the analysis space that differed from the geometry of the ordinary Euclidean data space. The alternative was to develop permutation tests and measures based on ordinary Euclidean scaling that proved to be very robust relative to outliers, extreme values, and highly skewed distributions.

The third feature in this period was a heavy reliance on Monte Carlo permutation methods instead of time-consuming exact permutation methods. Monte Carlo permutation methods with a large number of replications yielded results very close to exact results. Moreover, in many cases Monte Carlo procedures proved to be more efficient, especially in the analysis of contingency tables.

2.10.1 K.J. Berry, J.E. Johnston, and P.W. Mielke

In 2011 Kenneth J. Berry, Janis E. Johnston, and Paul W. Mielke published an overview article in *WIREs Computational Statistics* simply titled "Permutation methods" [9]. Organized by decades, the article chronicled the development of permutation statistical methods from 1920 to 2010. Special attention was paid to the differences between the Neyman–Pearson population model of statistical inference and the Fisher–Pitman permutation model, as well as to the differences between ordinary and squared Euclidean scaling functions.

2.10.2 D. Curran-Everett

In 2012 Douglas Curran-Everett published his eighth installment in a series on Explorations in Statistics [21]. The eighth article focused on permutation statistical methods. As Curran-Everett described, permutation methods operate on the observed data from an experiment or survey and answer the question: out of all the possible ways we can arrange the observed data, in what proportion of those arrangements is a specified sample statistic at least as extreme as the one observed? Curran-Everett explained that the proportion is the desired probability value.

2.10.3 J. Stelmach

In 2013 Jacek Stelmach published a paper on permutation tests to compare two populations [91]. As Stelmach explained, one of the practical problems in estimating real processes with regression models is the inevitable obsolescence of the models as a result of changes in these processes. Stelmach observed that parametric tests are usually carried out but these tests require a set of assumptions related to the knowledge of a distribution, but permutation tests do not require any knowledge of the distribution of examined populations. To this end Stelmach proposed a permutation test to test the null hypothesis of equality of two multi-dimensional populations.

2.10.4 K.J. Berry, J.E. Johnston, and P.W. Mielke

In 2014 Kenneth J. Berry, Janis E. Johnston, and Paul W. Mielke published a research monograph titled *A Chronicle of Permutation Statistical Methods: 1920–2000, and Beyond* [10]. The book traced the historical development of permutation statistical methods from the early works of R.A. Fisher, R.C. Geary, and E.J.G. Pitman in the 1920s and 1930s to 2010. Because the development of permutation statistical methods was so closely tied to the development of high-speed computing, the book traces the development of permutation methods and computing as parallel structures.

2.10.5   I.S. Amonenk and J. Robinson

In 2015 Inga S. Amonenk and John Robinson published a paper in which they introduced a new nonparametric test statistic for the permutation test in complete block designs [3]. Amonenk and Robinson determined the region in which the test statistic existed, its properties on the boundary of the region, and proved that saddlepoint approximations for tail probability values could be obtained inside the interior of the region. Finally, Amonenk and Robinson provided numerical examples showing that both the accuracy and the power of the new statistic improved on the properties of the classical F-ratio test statistic under some non-Gaussian models and equaled the properties for the Gaussian case.

2.10.6   K.J. Berry, J.E. Johnston, and P.W. Mielke

In 2016 Kenneth J. Berry, Janis E. Johnston, and Paul W. Mielke published a research monograph titled *Permutation Statistical Methods: An Integrated Approach* [11]. The book provided a synthesis of a number of statistical tests and measures which, at first consideration, appear disjoint and unrelated. Numerous comparisons of permutation and classical statistical methods were presented, and the two methods were compared via probability values and, where appropriate, measures of effect size. The Neyman–Pearson population model was introduced and compared with the Fisher–Pitman permutation model of statistical inference. Permutation tests and measures were described for a variety of completely-randomized designs with interval-, ordinal-, and nominal-level data, and for randomized-blocks designs with interval-, ordinal-, and nominal-level data.

2.10.7   M. Umlauft, F. Konietschke, and M. Pauly

In 2017 Maria Umlauft, Frank Konietschke, and Marcus Pauly published an article on inference methods for null hypotheses formulated in terms of distribution functions in general nonparametric factorial designs [100]. Umlauft, Konietschke, and Pauly proposed a permutation approach which they described as a flexible generalization of the Kruskal–Wallis g-sample rank-sum test to all types of factorial designs with independent observations. The authors showed that the permutation principle is asymptotically correct while keeping its finite exactness property when the data are exchangeable.

2.10.8   I.K. Yeo

Also in 2017 In-Kwan Yeo proposed an efficient computer algorithm for computing the exact distribution of the Wilcoxon signed-rank test [105]. Even at this late date computer algorithms were still being proposed that were either faster, more efficient, or more elegant than previous algorithms. Yeo noted that the proposed algorithm was straightforward and easy to program even if ranks scores were tied. Yeo performed a simulation study to compare the exact distribution and the normal approximation and also compared computing times of the proposed algorithm with those of other algorithms. Finally, Yeo presented the R computer program in which the algorithm was coded.

2.10.9   K.J. Berry, J.E. Johnston, and P.W. Mielke

In 2018 Kenneth J. Berry, Janis E. Johnston, and Paul W. Mielke published a research monograph titled *The Measurement of Association: A Permutation Statistical Approach* [12]. The book utilized exact and Monte Carlo permutation statistical methods to generate probability values and measures of effect size for a variety of measures of association. Association was broadly defined to include measures of correlation for two interval-level variables, measures of association for two nominal-level variables or two ordinal-level variables, and measures of agreement for two nominal-level or two ordinal-level variables. Additionally, measures of association for mixtures of the three levels of measurement were considered: nominal–ordinal, nominal–interval, and ordinal–interval measures. Numerous comparisons of permutation and classical statistical methods were presented.

Also in 2018 Kenneth Berry, Janis Johnston, and Paul Mielke published an overview article in *WIREs Computational Statistics* titled "Permutation methods. Part II" [13]. The article was an extension of the authors' previous article published in 2011 in the same journal. The earlier article chronicled the development of permutation statistical methods from its beginnings in the 1920s to 2010. This article concentrated on computation efficiencies for permutation methods. Four calculation efficiencies were highlighted. First, the advent and availability of high-speed computing. Second, the reliance on all combinations of values of the observed data instead of all permutations. Third, the use of mathematical recursion to eliminate many of the calculations. Fourth, the use of only the variable components of the selected test statistic and the elimination of those components that are invariant under permutation.

2.11 Summary

This chapter provided a brief history and overview of the early beginnings and subsequent development of permutation statistical methods, roughly organized by decades. Because of space limitations, only a small sample of contributions and contributors to the permutation literature was presented for each 10-year period. The early contributors to permutation statistical methods did not possess the computing power to make permutation methods feasible. Throughout the early decades this was a constant theme: there simply was no practical way to calculate the probability values needed for an exact permutation analysis. Eventually modern computing made permutation methods both feasible and practical. Thus the histories of computing and permutation methods go hand-in-hand. Presently there is sufficient computing power in any desktop, workstation, or laptop computer to generate the many thousands of arrangements of the observed data needed for a permutation statistical analysis.

Chapter 3 presents two models of statistical inference: the Neyman–Pearson population model and the Fisher–Pitman permutation model. The population model is the standard model taught in all introductory classes and will be familiar to most readers. The permutation model will be unfamiliar to many readers and is the main reason this book is being written. As noted in this chapter, permutation methods can be computationally intensive. Thus Chap. 3 presents five computational efficiencies for permutation statistical methods.

References

1. Agresti, A.: Exact inference for categorical data: recent advances and continuing controversies. Stat. Med. **20**, 2709–2722 (2001)
2. Agresti, A., Wackerly, D.: Some exact conditional tests of independence for $R \times C$ cross-classification tables. Psychometrika **42**, 111–125 (1977)
3. Amonenk, I.S., Robinson, J.: A new permutation test statistic for complete block designs. Ann. Stat. **43**, 90–101 (2015)
4. Author: StatXact for Windows. Cytel Software, Cambridge (2000)
5. Berry, K.J., Mielke, P.W.: Goodman and Kruskal's tau-b statistic: a nonasymptotic test of significance. Sociol. Method. Res. **13**, 543–550 (1985)
6. Berry, K.J., Mielke, P.W.: A generalization of Cohen's kappa agreement measure to interval measurement and multiple raters. Educ. Psychol. Meas. **48**, 921–933 (1988)
7. Berry, K.J., Mielke, P.W.: A Monte Carlo investigation of the Fisher Z transformation for normal and nonnormal distributions. Psychol. Rep. **87**, 1101–1114 (2000)
8. Berry, K.J., Kvamme, K.L., Mielke, P.W.: A permutation technique for the spatial analysis of artifacts into classes. Am. Antiquity **45**, 55–59 (1980)
9. Berry, K.J., Johnston, J.E., Mielke, P.W.: Permutation methods. Comput. Stat. **3**, 527–542 (2011)
10. Berry, K.J., Johnston, J.E., Mielke, P.W.: A Chronicle of Permutation Statistical Methods: 1920–2000 and Beyond. Springer, Cham (2014)
11. Berry, K.J., Mielke, P.W., Johnston, J.E.: Permutation Statistical Methods: An Integrated Approach. Springer, Cham (2016)

12. Berry, K.J., Johnston, J.E., Mielke, P.W.: The Measurement of Association: A Permutation Statistical Approach. Springer, Cham (2018)
13. Berry, K.J., Johnston, J.E., Mielke, P.W., Johnston, L.A.: Permutation methods. Part II. Comput. Stat. **10**, 1–31 (2018)
14. Biondini, M.E., Mielke, P.W., Berry, K.J.: Data-dependent permutation techniques for the analysis of ecological data. Vegetatio **75**, 161–168 (1988). [The name of the journal was changed to *Plant Ecology* in 1997]
15. Box, G.E.P., Andersen, S.L.: Permutation theory in the derivation of robust criteria and the study of departures from assumption (with discussion). J. R. Stat. Soc. B Methodol. **17**, 1–34 (1955)
16. Boyett, J.M.: Algorithm 144: $R \times C$ tables with given row and column totals. J. R. Stat. Soc. C Appl. **28**, 329–332 (1979)
17. Bradley, J.V.: Distribution-free Statistical Tests. Prentice–Hall, Englewood Cliffs (1968)
18. Brooks, E.B.: Frank Wilcoxon, 2 Sept 1892 – 18 Nov 1965. Tales of Statisticians. http://www.umass.edu/wsp/statistics/tales/wilcoxon.html. Accessed 1 Apr 2012
19. Burr, E.J.: The distribution of Kendall's score S for a pair of tied rankings. Biometrika **47**, 151–171 (1960)
20. Cade, B.S., Richards, J.D.: A permutation test for quantile regression. J. Agric. Biol. Environ. Stat. **11**, 106–126 (2006)
21. Curran-Everett, D.: Explorations in statistics: permutation methods. Adv. Physiol. Educ. **36**, 181–187 (2012)
22. Dabrowska, D.M., Speed, T.P.: On the application of probability theory to agricultural experiments. Essay on principles. Section 9. Stat. Sci. **5**, 465–480 (1990). [This is a translation by Dabrowska and Speed of an article originally published in Polish in *Annals of Agricultural Sciences* by Jerzy Spława–Neyman in 1923]
23. David, F.N.: Studies in the history of probability and statistics: I. Dicing and gaming. Biometrika **42**, 1–15 (1955)
24. David, F.N.: Games, Gods, and Gambling: The Origin and History of Probability and Statistical Ideas from the Earliest Times to the Newtonian Era. Hafner, New York (1962)
25. Dwass, M.: Modified randomization tests for nonparametric hypotheses. Ann. Math. Stat. **28**, 181–187 (1957)
26. Eden, T., Yates, F.: On the validity of Fisher's z test when applied to an actual example of non-normal data. J. Agric. Sci. **23**, 6–17 (1933)
27. Edgington, E.S.: Randomization tests. J. Psychol. **57**, 445–449 (1964)
28. Edgington, E.S.: Statistical inference and nonrandom samples. Psychol. Bull. **66**, 485–487 (1966)
29. Edgington, E.S.: Statistical inference from $N = 1$ experiments. J. Psychol. **65**, 195–199 (1967)
30. Edgington, E.S.: Approximate randomization tests. J. Psychol. **72**, 143–149 (1969)
31. Edgington, E.S.: Statistical Inference: The Distribution-free Approach. McGraw–Hill, New York (1969)
32. Edgington, E.S.: Randomization Tests. Marcel Dekker, New York (1980)
33. Feinstein, A.R.: Clinical Biostatistics XXIII: The role of randomization in sampling, testing, allocation, and credulous idolatry (Part 2). Clin. Pharmacol. Ther. **14**, 898–915 (1973)
34. Festinger, L.: The significance of differences between means without reference to the frequency distribution function. Psychometrika **11**, 97–105 (1946)
35. Fisher, R.A.: Statistical Methods for Research Workers. Oliver and Boyd, Edinburgh (1925)
36. Fisher, R.A.: The Design of Experiments. Oliver and Boyd, Edinburgh (1935)
37. Fisher, R.A.: The logic of inductive inference (with discussion). J. R. Stat. Soc. **98**, 39–82 (1935)
38. Freeman, G.H., Halton, J.H.: Note on an exact treatment of contingency, goodness of fit and other problems of significance. Biometrika **38**, 141–149 (1951)
39. Frick, R.W.: Interpreting statistical testing: process and propensity, not population and random sampling. Behav. Res. Methods Instrum. Comput. **30**, 527–535 (1998)

40. Gani, J. (ed.): The Making of Statisticians. Springer, New York (1982)
41. Geary, R.C.: Some properties of correlation and regression in a limited universe. Metron **7**, 83–119 (1927)
42. Gebhard, J., Schmitz, N.: Permutation tests — a revival?! I. Optimum properties. Stat. Pap. **39**, 75–85 (1998)
43. Gebhard, J., Schmitz, N.: Permutation tests — a revival?! II. An efficient algorithm for computing the critical region. Stat. Pap. **39**, 87–96 (1998)
44. Ghent, A.W.: A method for exact testing of 2×2, 2×3, 3×3, and other contingency tables, employing binomial coefficients. Am. Midl. Nat. **88**, 15–27 (1972)
45. Gianchristofaro, R.A., Pesarin, F., Salmaso, L.: Permutation Anderson–Darling type and moment-based test statistics for univariate ordered categorical data. Commun. Stat. Simul. Comput. **36**, 139–150 (2007)
46. Green, B.F.: A practical interactive program for randomization tests of location. Am. Stat. **31**, 37–39 (1977)
47. Hald, A.: History of Probability and Statistics and Their Applications Before 1750. Wiley, New York (1990)
48. Hald, A.: A History of Mathematical Statistics from 1750 to 1930. Wiley, New York (1998)
49. Hill, I.D., Pike, M.C.: Algorithm 4: TWOBYTWO. Comput. Bull. **9**, 56–63 (1965). [Reprinted in Comput J **22**, 87–88 (1979). Addenda in Comput. J. **9**, 212 (1966) and **9**, 416 (1967)]
50. Hollander, M.: A conversation with Ralph A. Bradley. Stat. Sci. **16**, 75–100 (2000)
51. Hotelling, H., Pabst, M.R.: Rank correlation and tests of significance involving no assumption of normality. Ann. Math. Stat. **7**, 29–43 (1936)
52. Irwin, J.O.: Tests of significance for differences between percentages based on small numbers. Metron **12**, 83–94 (1935)
53. Janssen, A., Pauls, T.: How do bootstrap and permutation tests work? Ann. Stat. **31**, 768–806 (2003)
54. Kempthorne, O., Doerfler, T.E.: The behaviour of some significance tests under experimental randomization. Biometrika **56**, 231–248 (1969)
55. Kendall, M.G.: A new measure of rank correlation. Biometrika **30**, 81–93 (1938)
56. Kendall, M.G.: Rank Correlation Methods. Griffin, London (1948)
57. Kendall, M.G., Babington Smith, B.: The problem of m rankings. Ann. Math. Stat. **10**, 275–287 (1939)
58. Kendall, M.G., Plackett, R.L. (eds.): Studies in the History of Statistics and Probability, vol. II. Griffin, London (1977)
59. Kennedy, P.E., Cade, B.S.: Randomization tests for multiple regression. Commun. Stat. Simul. Comput. **25**, 923–936 (1996)
60. Kruskal, W.H., Wallis, W.A.: Use of ranks in one-criterion variance analysis. J. Am. Stat. Assoc. **47**, 583–621 (1952). [Erratum: J. Am. Stat. Assoc. **48**, 907–911 (1953)]
61. Lehmann, E.L., Stein, C.M.: On the theory of some non-parametric hypotheses. Ann. Math. Stat. **20**, 28–45 (1949)
62. Leslie, P.H.: A simple method of calculating the exact probability in 2×2 contingency tables with small marginal totals. Biometrika **42**, 522–523 (1955)
63. Ludbrook, J., Dudley, H.A.F.: Why permutation tests are superior to t and F tests in biomedical research. Am. Stat. **52**, 127–132 (1998)
64. MacKenzie, D.: Statistics in Britain, 1865–1930: The Social Construction of Scientific Knowledge. Edinburgh University Press, Edinburgh (1981)
65. Mann, H.B., Whitney, D.R.: On a test of whether one of two random variables is stochastically larger than the other. Ann. Math. Stat. **18**, 50–60 (1947)
66. May, R.B., Hunter, M.A.: Some advantages of permutation tests. Can. Psychol. **34**, 401–407 (1993)
67. Mehta, C.R., Patel, N.R.: A network algorithm for performing Fisher's exact test in $r \times c$ contingency tables. J. Am. Stat. Assoc. **78**, 427–434 (1983)

68. Mielke, P.W.: Meteorological applications of permutation techniques based on distance functions. In: Krishnaiah, P.R., Sen, P.K. (eds.) Handbook of Statistics, vol. IV, pp. 813–830. North-Holland, Amsterdam (1984)
69. Mielke, P.W., Berry, K.J.: Cumulant methods for analyzing independence of r-way contingency tables and goodness-of-fit frequency data. Biometrika **75**, 790–793 (1988)
70. Mielke, P.W., Berry, K.J.: Permutation tests for common locations among samples with unequal variances. J. Educ. Behav. Stat. **19**, 217–236 (1994)
71. Mielke, P.W., Berry, K.J.: Permutation Methods: A Distance Function Approach. Springer, New York (2001)
72. Mielke, P.W., Berry, K.J.: Multivariate multiple regression analyses: a permutation method for linear models. Psychol. Rep. **91**, 3–9 (2002)
73. Mielke, P.W., Berry, K.J., Johnson, E.S.: Multi-response permutation procedures for a priori classifications. Commun. Stat. Theor. Methods **5**, 1409–1424 (1976)
74. Mielke, P.W., Berry, K.J., Neidt, C.O.: A permutation test for multivariate matched-pairs analyses: comparisons with Hotelling's multivariate matched-pairs T^2 test. Psychol. Rep. **78**, 1003–1008 (1996)
75. Mielke, P.W., Berry, K.J., Johnston, J.E.: Resampling programs for multiway contingency tables with fixed marginal frequency totals. Psychol. Rep. **101**, 18–24 (2007)
76. Mielke, P.W., Berry, K.J., Johnston, J.E.: Resampling probability values for weighted kappa with multiple raters. Psychol. Rep. **102**, 606–613 (2008)
77. Mielke, P.W., Long, M.A., Berry, K.J., Johnston, J.E.: g-treatment ridit analysis: resampling permutation methods. Stat. Methodol. **6**, 223–229 (2009)
78. Patefield, W.M.: Algorithm 159: an efficient method of generating random $r \times c$ tables with given row and column totals. J. R. Stat. Soc. C Appl. **30**, 91–97 (1981)
79. Pearson, E.S., Kendall, M.G. (eds.): Studies in the History of Statistics and Probability, vol. I. Griffin, London (1970)
80. Pesarin, F., Salmaso, L.: Exact permutation tests for unreplicated factorials. Appl. Stoch. Model. Bus. **18**, 287–299 (2002)
81. Pitman, E.J.G.: Significance tests which may be applied to samples from any populations. Suppl. J. R. Stat. Soc. **4**, 119–130 (1937)
82. Pitman, E.J.G.: Significance tests which may be applied to samples from any populations: II. The correlation coefficient test. Suppl. J. R. Stat. Soc. **4**, 225–232 (1937)
83. Pitman, E.J.G.: Significance tests which may be applied to samples from any populations: III. The analysis of variance test. Biometrika **29**, 322–335 (1938)
84. Porter, T.M.: The Rise of Statistical Thinking, 1820–1900. Princeton University Press, Princeton (1986)
85. Robertson, W.H.: Programming Fisher's exact method of comparing two percentages. Technometrics **2**, 103–107 (1960)
86. Sakoda, J.M., Cohen, B.H.: Exact probabilities for contingency tables using binomial coefficients. Psychometrika **22**, 83–86 (1957)
87. Salsburg, D.S.: The Lady Tasting Tea: How Statistics Revolutionized Science in the Twentieth Century. Holt, New York (2001)
88. Scheffé, H.: Statistical inference in the non-parametric case. Ann. Math. Stat. **14**, 305–332 (1943)
89. Snedecor, G.W.: Calculation and Interpretation of Analysis of Variance and Covariance. Collegiate Press, Ames (1934)
90. Spława–Neyman, J.: Próba uzasadnienia zastosowań rachunku prawdopodobieństwa do doświadczeń polowych (On the application of probability theory to agricultural experiments. Essay on principles. Section 9). Rocz Nauk Rolnicz (Ann. Agric. Sci.) **10**, 1–51 (1923). [Translated from the original Polish by D. M. Dabrowska and T. P. Speed and published in Statist. Sci. **5**, 465–472 (1990)]
91. Stelmach, J.: On permutation tests with several test statistics to compare two populations. In: Vojackova, H. (ed.) Mathematical Methods in Economics 2013, pp. 850–855. Coll Polytechnics Jihlava, Jihlava (2013)

92. Stigler, S.M.: American Contributions to Mathematical Statistics in the Nineteenth Century, vol. I. Arno Press, New York (1980)

93. Stigler, S.M.: American Contributions to Mathematical Statistics in the Nineteenth Century, vol. II. Arno Press, New York (1980)

94. Stigler, S.M.: The History of Statistics: The Measurement of Uncertainty Before 1900. Harvard University Press, Cambridge (1986)

95. Stigler, S.M.: Statistics on the Table: The History of Statistical Concepts and Methods. Harvard University Press, Cambridge (1999)

96. Stigler, S.M.: The Seven Pillars of Statistical Wisdom. Harvard University Press, Cambridge (2016)

97. Tedin, O.: The influence of systematic plot arrangements upon the estimate of error in field experiments. J. Agric. Sci. **21**, 191–208 (1931)

98. Thakur, A.K., Berry, K.J., Mielke, P.W.: A FORTRAN program for testing trend and homogeneity in proportions. Comput. Prog. Biomed. **19**, 229–233 (1985)

99. Tukey, J.W.: Randomization and re-randomization: the wave of the past in the future. In: Statistics in the Pharmaceutical Industry: Past, Present and Future. Philadelphia Chapter of the American Statistical Association (1988). [Presented at a Symposium in Honor of Joseph L. Ciminera held in June 1988 at Philadelphia, Pennsylvania]

100. Umlauft, M., Konietschke, F., Pauly, M.: Rank-based permutation approaches for non-parametric factorial designs. Brit. J. Math. Stat. Psychol. **70**, 368–390 (2017)

101. White, C.: The use of ranks in a test of significance for comparing two treatments. Biometrics **8**, 33–41 (1952)

102. Wilcoxon, F.: Individual comparisons by ranking methods. Biometrics Bull. **1**, 80–83 (1945)

103. Wilks, S.S.: Order statistics. Bull. Am. Math. Soc. **54**, 6–50 (1948)

104. Yates, F.: Contingency tables involving small numbers and the χ^2 test. Suppl. J. R. Stat. Soc. **1**, 217–235 (1934)

105. Yeo, I.K.: An algorithm for computing the exact distribution of the Wilcoxon signed-rank statistic. J. Korean Stat. Soc. **46**, 328–338 (2017)

Chapter 3
Permutation Statistical Methods

Abstract This chapter presents two models of statistical inference: the conventional Neyman–Pearson population model that is taught in every introductory course and the Fisher–Pitman permutation model with which the reader is assumed to unfamiliar. The Fisher–Pitman model consists of three different permutation methods: exact permutation methods, Monte Carlo permutation methods, and moment-approximation permutation methods. The three methods are described and illustrated with example analyses.

This chapter presents two competing models of statistical inference: the population (normal) model and the permutation model. The Neyman–Pearson population model is the standard model taught in all introductory classes and is familiar to most readers.[1] The Neyman–Pearson population model was specifically designed to make inferences about population parameters, provide approximate probability values, and is characterized by the assumptions of random sampling, a normally-distributed population, and homogeneity of variance when appropriate. The Fisher–Pitman permutation model of statistical inference is less well known and includes three different permutation methodologies, each of which is described and illustrated in this chapter: exact permutation methods, Monte Carlo permutation methods, and moment-approximation permutation methods.[2] In contrast to conventional statistical tests based on the Neyman–Pearson population model, tests based on the Fisher–Pitman permutation model are distribution-free, entirely data-dependent, appropriate for nonrandom samples, provide exact probability values, and are ideal for small sets of data.

---

[1]The Neyman–Pearson population model of statistical inference is named for Jerzy Neyman (1894–1981) and Egon Pearson (1895–1980).

[2]The Fisher–Pitman permutation model of statistical inference is named for R.A. Fisher (1890–1962) and E.J.G. Pitman (1897–1993).

© Springer Nature Switzerland AG 2019   57
K. J. Berry et al., *A Primer of Permutation Statistical Methods*,
https://doi.org/10.1007/978-3-030-20933-9_3

On the other hand, permutation tests can be computationally intensive, often requiring many millions of calculations. Five computational efficiencies for permutation statistical tests are described in this chapter. First, the development of high-speed computing has made permutation methods feasible. Second, the examination of all combinations of the observed data instead of all permutations of the data greatly reduces the amount of calculation required. Third, the use of mathematical recursion simplifies calculations of both test statistics and probability values. Fourth, calculation of only the variable portion of the selected test statistic minimizes the calculations required. Fifth, holding one array of the observed data constant reduces the number of arrangements required for exact permutation analyses.

As documented in Chap. 2, the permutation model of statistical inference had its beginnings in the 1920s and 1930s with the works of Fisher [12], Geary [14], Eden and Yates [9], Hotelling and Pabst [18], and Pitman [36–38]. Constrained by the difficulty of computing tens of thousands of statistical values on tens of thousands of arrangements of the observed data, permutation methods languished for many years until the advent of high-speed computing. Presently, statistical methods under the Fisher–Pitman permutation model is a rapidly developing field of statistical methodology and finds increasing utility in a large number of academic fields and disciplines.

3.1   The Neyman–Pearson Population Model

In contemporary research two competing models of statistical inference coexist: the population model and the permutation model.[3] The population model of statistical inference, formally proposed by Jerzy Neyman and Egon Pearson in a seminal two-part article on statistical inference published in 1928, is the model taught almost exclusively in introductory courses, although in most textbooks the presentation of the population model espoused by Neyman and Pearson is often conflated with an approach espoused by Fisher [19].

The Neyman–Pearson population model of statistical inference assumes random sampling with replacement from one or more specified populations [34, 35]. Under the Neyman–Pearson population model the level of statistical significance that results from applying a statistical test to the results of an experiment or survey corresponds to the frequency with which the null hypothesis would be rejected in repeated random samplings from the same specified population(s). Because repeated sampling of the specified population(s) is usually prohibitive, it is assumed that an approximating theoretical distribution such as a z, t, F, or χ^2 distribution conforms

---

[3]There are, of course, other models of statistical inference. A third model, the Bayesian inference model, is also very popular, especially in the decision-making sciences.

to the discrete sampling distribution of the test statistics generated under repeated random sampling.

Under the Neyman–Pearson population model two hypotheses concerning a population parameter or parameters are advanced: the null hypothesis symbolized by H_0 and a mutually-exclusive, exhaustive alternative hypothesis symbolized by H_1.[4] The probability of rejecting a true H_0 is determined by the researcher and specified as type I or α error, a region of rejection in the tail or tails of the theoretical distribution is delimited corresponding to α; for example, $\alpha = 0.05$ or $\alpha = 0.01$, and H_0 is rejected if the observed test statistic value falls into the region(s) of rejection with probability of type I error equal to or less than α.

Technically, under the Neyman–Pearson population model of statistical inference the null hypothesis is rejected if the computed test statistic value falls into the region of rejection defined by α. For example, if $\alpha = 0.05$ with a two-tail test and the critical values defining the region of rejection are ± 1.96, then a test statistic value more extreme than ± 1.96 in either direction implies rejection of the null hypothesis with a probability of type I error usually expressed as $p < 0.05$. In this research monograph asymptotic probability values under the Neyman–Pearson population model are given to four decimal places for comparison with exact probability values under the Fisher–Pitman permutation model of statistical inference.

3.2   The Fisher–Pitman Permutation Model

While the Neyman–Pearson population model of statistical inference is familiar to most researchers, the Fisher–Pitman permutation model of inference may be less familiar. Permutation statistical methods were introduced by R.A. Fisher in 1925 [12], further developed by Geary in 1927 [14], Eden and Yates in 1933 [9], Hotelling and Pabst in 1936 [18], and made explicit by Pitman in 1937 and 1938 [36–38]. For the interested reader, a number of excellent presentations of the two models are available. See especially, discussions by Curran-Everett [8], Feinstein [11], Hubbard [19], Kempthorne [23], Kennedy [24], Lachin [25], Ludbrook [26, 27], and May and Hunter [30].

For a permutation statistical test in its most basic form, a test statistic is computed on the observed data—often the same test statistic as in the Neyman–Pearson population model. The observations are then permuted over all possible arrangements of the observed data and the specified statistic is computed for each possible, equally-likely arrangement of the observed data. The proportion of arrangements in the reference set of all possible arrangements possessing test statistic values that are equal to or more extreme than the observed test statistic value constitutes the probability of the observed test statistic value.

---

[4]Some introductory textbooks denote the alternative hypothesis by H_A.

Figure 3.1 presents a flowchart detailing the calculation of an exact permutation probability value under the Fisher–Pitman model. The first step is to initialize two counters; in this case, Counter A and Counter B. Counter A provides a count of all test statistic values that are equal to or greater than the observed test statistic value. Counter B provides a count of all possible arrangements of the observed data. Second, the desired test statistic is calculated on the observed set of data. Third, a new arrangement of the observed data is generated, while preserving the sample size(s) and Counter B is increased by 1. Fourth, the desired test statistic is calculated on the new arrangement of the observed data and compared with the original test statistic value calculated on the observed set of data. If the value of the new test statistic is equal to or greater than the value of the observed test statistic, Counter A is increased by 1. If not, a check is made to see if this arrangement is the last in the reference set of all possible arrangements. If it is, then Counter A divided by Counter B yields the exact probability value; that is, the proportion of all possible test statistic values that are equal to or greater than the observed test statistic value. Otherwise, a new arrangement of the observed data is generated and the process is repeated.

Statistical tests and measures based on the Fisher–Pitman permutation model possess several advantages over statistical tests and measures based on the Neyman–Pearson population model. First, tests based on the permutation model are much less complex than tests based on the population model. Therefore, the results are much easier to communicate to unsophisticated or statistically naïve audiences. Second, permutation tests provide exact probability values based on the discrete permutation distribution of equally-likely test statistic values. Tests based on the Neyman–Pearson population model only provide vague results such as $P < 0.05$.[5] Third, permutation tests are entirely data-dependent in that all the information required for analysis is contained within the observed data—also called "the data at hand method" [16]. There is no reliance on factors external to the observed data, such as population parameters, assumptions about theoretical approximating distributions, and alternative hypotheses. Fourth, permutation tests are appropriate for nonrandom samples, such as are common in many fields of research. Fifth, permutation tests are distribution-free in that they do not depend on the assumptions associated with conventional tests under the population model, such as normality and homogeneity of variance. Sixth, permutation tests are ideal for small data sets, where conventional tests often are problematic when attempting to fit a continuous theoretical distribution to only a few discrete values.

Because permutation statistical methods are inherently computationally-intensive, it took the development of high-speed computing for permutation methods to achieve their potential. Today, a small laptop computer outperforms even the largest mainframe computers of previous decades. Three types of permutation tests are common in the literature: exact, Monte Carlo, and moment-approximation permutation tests.

---

[5]In this book, an upper-case letter P indicates a cumulative probability value and a lower-case letter p indicates a point probability value.

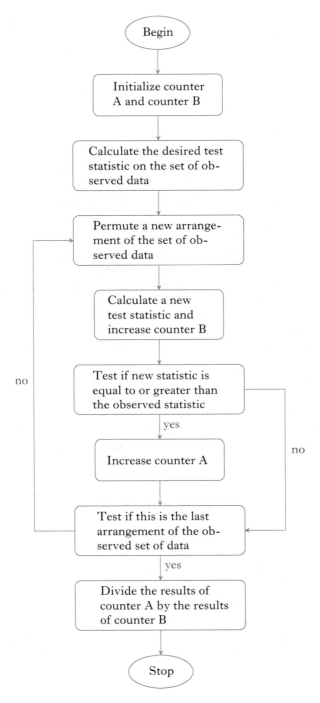

Fig. 3.1 Flowchart for the calculation of an exact permutation probability value

Table 3.1
Cross-classification of
variables A and B

Variable A	Variable B		Total
	b	$\bar{b}$	
a	9	9	18
$\bar{a}$	0	12	12
Total	9	21	30

3.2.1 Exact Permutation Tests

The first step in an exact permutation test is to calculate a test statistic value for the observed data. Second, a reference set of all possible, equally-likely arrangements of the observed data is systematically generated. Third, the desired test statistic is calculated for each arrangement in the reference set. Fourth, the probability of obtaining the observed value of the test statistic, or one more extreme, is the proportion of the test statistics in the reference set with values that are equal to or more extreme than the value of the observed test statistic.

To be perfectly clear, in practice a different order is followed. First, a test statistic value for the observed data is calculated. Second, the first of a reference set of all possible, equally-likely arrangements of the observed data is generated. Third, a test statistic value for the new arrangement of the observed data is calculated and compared with the original test statistic value. Fourth, if the new value is equal to or exceeds the original test statistic value, a counter is increased by one. The process is repeated until all possible arrangements of the observed data have been generated and evaluated. Finally, the probability of obtaining the observed value of the test statistic, or one more extreme, is the proportion of the test statistics in the reference set with values that are equal to or more extreme than the value of the observed test statistic. In this manner it is not necessary to store the reference set of all possible arrangements of the observed data, which is often quite large.

An Exact Permutation Example

To illustrate an exact permutation test, consider the small set of data given in Table 3.1. Fisher's exact probability test is the iconic permutation test.[6] Fisher's exact test calculates the hypergeometric point probability value for the reference set of all possible arrangements of cell frequencies, given the observed marginal frequency totals. The two-tail probability value of the observed arrangement of cell frequencies is the sum of the observed probability value and all probability values that are equal to or less than the observed probability value. Because Fisher's exact test simply yields a probability value, there is no test statistic defined in the

---

[6]Fisher's exact test was independently developed by R.A. Fisher, Joseph Irwin, and Frank Yates in the early 1930s [13, 21, 40].

Table 3.2 Conventional notation for a 2×2 contingency table

		Variable B	
Variable A	b	$\bar{b}$	Total
a	n_{11}	n_{12}	$n_{1.}$
$\bar{a}$	n_{21}	n_{22}	$n_{2.}$
Total	$n_{.1}$	$n_{.2}$	N

usual sense. Thus the first step is to determine the reference set of all possible arrangements of the four cell frequencies, given the observed marginal frequency totals. For a 2×2 contingency table, it is relatively easy to determine the total number of possible tables in the reference set.

Consider the 2×2 contingency table in Table 3.2. Denote by a dot ($\cdot$) the partial sum of all rows or all columns, depending on the position of the ($\cdot$) in the subscript list. If the ($\cdot$) is in the first subscript position, the sum is over all rows and if the ($\cdot$) is in the second subscript position, the sum is over all columns. Thus $n_{i.}$ denotes the marginal frequency total of the ith row, $i = 1, \ldots, r$, summed over all columns, and $n_{.j}$ denotes the marginal frequency total of the jth column, $j = 1, \ldots, c$, summed over all rows. Thus $n_{1.}$ and $n_{2.}$ denote the marginal frequency totals for rows 1 and 2, $n_{.1}$ and $n_{.2}$ denote the marginal frequency totals for columns 1 and 2, n_{ij} denotes the cell frequencies for $i, j = 1, 2$, and $N = n_{11} + n_{12} + n_{21} + n_{22}$. The total number of possible values for any cell frequency, say n_{11}, is given by

$$M = \min(n_{1.}, n_{.1}) - \max(0, n_{11} - n_{22}) + 1 .$$

Thus, for the frequency data given in Table 3.1 there are

$$M = \min(18, 9) - \max(0, 8 - 11) + 1 = 9 - 0 + 1 = 10$$

possible arrangements of cell frequencies in the reference set, given the observed row and column marginal frequency distributions, {18, 12} and {9, 21}, respectively.

The reference set of the $M = 10$ arrangements of cell frequencies and the associated hypergeometric point probability values are listed in Table 3.3. For any 2×2 contingency table, such as depicted in Table 3.2, the hypergeometric point probability of any specified cell, say cell (1,1), is given by

$$p(n_{11}|n_{1.}, n_{.1}, N) = \binom{n_{.1}}{n_{11}}\binom{n_{.2}}{n_{12}}\binom{N}{n_{1.}}^{-1} = \frac{n_{1.}!\, n_{2.}!\, n_{.1}!\, n_{.2}!}{N!\, n_{11}!\, n_{12}!\, n_{21}!\, n_{22}!} .$$

For the frequency data given in Table 3.1, the two-tail probability value is the sum of the probability value of the observed contingency table and all probability values that are equal to or less than the probability value of the observed table. Thus Table 10 in Table 3.3 (the observed table) has a hypergeometric point probability value of $p_{10} = 0.3398 \times 10^{-2}$ and only Tables 3.1 and 3.2 possess point probability values that are less than $p = 0.3398 \times 10^{-2}$; that is, $p_1 = 0.1538 \times 10^{-4}$ and

Table 3.3 Listing of the $M = 10$ possible 2×2 contingency tables in the reference set from the frequency data given in Table 3.1 with associated exact hypergeometric point probability values

Table 1		Probability	Table 2		Probability
0	18	0.1538×10^{-4}	1	17	0.6228×10^{-3}
9	3		8	4	
Table 3		Probability	Table 4		Probability
2	16	0.8470×10^{-2}	3	15	0.5270×10^{-1}
7	5		6	6	
Table 5		Probability	Table 6		Probability
4	14	0.1694×10^{-1}	5	13	0.2964
5	7		7	8	
Table 7		Probability	Table 8		Probability
6	12	0.2855	7	11	0.1468
3	9		5	10	
Table 9		Probability	Table 10		Probability
8	10	0.3670×10^{-1}	9	9	0.3398×10^{-2}
1	11		0	12	

Table 3.4 Listing of the 3×5 cell frequencies with rows (R_1, R_2, R_3) and columns $(C_1, C_2, C_3, C_4, C_5)$ for an exact probability example

	B_1	B_2	B_3	B_4	B_5	Total
A_1	4	7	2	9	0	22
A_2	1	5	2	7	6	21
A_3	4	5	10	18	0	37
Total	9	17	14	34	6	80

$p_2 = 0.6228 \times 10^{-3}$, respectively. The cumulative probability value of the three tables is

$$P = p\{9|18, 9, 30\} + p\{0|18, 9, 30\} + p\{1|18, 9, 30\}$$

$$= \frac{18! \, 12! \, 9! \, 21!}{30! \, 9! \, 9! \, 0! \, 12!} + \frac{18! \, 12! \, 9! \, 21!}{30! \, 0! \, 18! \, 9! \, 3!} + \frac{18! \, 12! \, 9! \, 21!}{30! \, 1! \, 17! \, 8! \, 4!}$$

$$= 0.3398 \times 10^{-2} + 0.1538 \times 10^{-4} + 0.6228 \times 10^{-3}$$

$$= 0.4036 \times 10^{-2} \, .$$

A Second Exact Permutation Test Example

For a second example of an exact permutation analysis, consider the 3×5 contingency table with $N = 80$ cell frequencies given in Table 3.4. Pearson's chi-squared test statistic for an $r \times c$ contingency table is taught in every introductory course and is given by

$$\chi^2 = N \left(\sum_{i=1}^{r} \sum_{j=1}^{c} \frac{n_{ij}^2}{n_{i.}n_{.j}} - 1 \right),$$

where $n_{i.}$ denotes a row marginal frequency total for $i = 1, \ldots, r$, $n_{.j}$ denotes a column marginal frequency total for $j = 1, \ldots, c$, n_{ij} denotes an observed cell frequency for $i = 1, \ldots, r$ and $j = 1, \ldots, c$, and N is the total of the cell frequencies; in this case, $N = 80$. For the frequency data given in Table 3.4 with row marginal frequency totals $\{22, 21, 37\}$ and column marginal frequency totals $\{9, 17, 14, 34, 6\}$, the observed value of Pearson's chi-squared test statistic is

$$\chi^2 = N \left(\sum_{i=1}^{r} \sum_{j=1}^{c} \frac{n_{ij}^2}{n_{i.}n_{.j}} - 1 \right)$$

$$= 80 \left(\frac{4^2}{(22)(9)} + \frac{7^2}{(22)(17)} + \cdots + \frac{0^2}{(37)(6)} - 1 \right) = 25.1809.$$

The exact probability value of $\chi^2 = 25.1809$ under the Fisher–Pitman permutation model is the sum of the hypergeometric point probability values associated with the chi-squared values calculated on the reference set of all M possible arrangements of the cell frequencies, given the observed marginal frequency totals. For the frequency data given in Table 3.4, there are $M = 21{,}671{,}722$ possible, equally-likely arrangements of the cell frequencies given the observed marginal frequency totals, of which $16{,}498{,}422$ chi-squared values are equal to or greater than the observed chi-squared value of $\chi^2 = 25.1809$, yielding an exact hypergeometric probability value of $P = 0.1009 \times 10^{-2}$.

For comparison, the chi-squared test statistic is asymptotically distributed as Pearson's χ^2 with $(r - 1)(c - 1)$ degrees of freedom under the Neyman–Pearson null hypothesis. With $(r - 1)(c - 1) = (3 - 1)(5 - 1) = 8$ degrees of freedom, the asymptotic probability value of $\chi^2 = 25.1809$ is $P = 0.1449 \times 10^{-2}$.

Comparison with Fisher's Exact Probability Test

Although Fisher's exact probability test is typically limited to 2×2 contingency tables, it is possible to compute Fisher's exact test on larger tables, such as the 3×5 contingency table given in Table 3.4 [32]. It is important to note that Fisher's exact probability test and an exact chi-squared test of independence are constructed quite differently, although both tests will occasionally yield identical probability values.

Fisher's exact test generates a reference set of all M possible arrangements of cell frequencies given the observed marginal frequency totals, computes the hypergeometric point probability value for each arrangement of the observede data, and sums the probability values that are equal to or less than the probability value obtained from the observed arrangement of cell frequencies. On the other hand, an exact chi-squared test generates a reference set of all M possible arrangements of cell frequencies given th observed marginal frequency totals, calculates the chi-squared value for each arrangement of cell frequencies, computes the hypergeometric point probability value for each arrangement, and sums the probability values associated with those chi-squared values that are equal to or greater than the chi-squared value obtained from the observed arrangement of cell frequencies.

For the frequency data given in Table 3.4, the point probability value for the observed arrangement of cell frequencies is $p = 0.5164 \times 10^{-8}$. There are $M = 21{,}671{,}722$ possible, equally-likely arrangements of the cell frequencies in Table 3.4, of which $18{,}683{,}509$ hypergeometric point probability values are equal to or greater than $p = 0.5164 \times 10^{-8}$, yielding an exact probability value of $P = 0.5174 \times 10^{-2}$.

3.2.2 Monte Carlo Permutation Tests

As sample sizes increase, the size of the reference set of all possible arrangements of the observed data can become quite large and exact permutation methods are quickly rendered impractical. For example, permuting two samples of sizes $n_1 = n_2 = 35$ generates

$$M = \frac{(n_1 + n_2)!}{n_1!\, n_2!} = \frac{(35 + 35)!}{35!\, 35!} = 112{,}186{,}277{,}816{,}662{,}845{,}432$$

equally-likely arrangements of the observed data; or in words, 112 billion billion different arrangements of the observed data—too many statistical values to compute in a reasonable amount of time.

When exact permutation procedures become intractable, a random subset of all possible arrangements of the observed data can be substituted, providing approximate, but highly accurate, probability values. Monte Carlo permutation methods generate and examine a random subset of all possible, equally-likely arrangements of the observed data. For each randomly-selected arrangement of the observed data, the desired test statistic is calculated. The probability of obtaining the observed value of the test statistic, or one more extreme, is the proportion of the randomly-selected test statistics with probability values that are equal to or more extreme than the probability value of the observed test statistic. With a sufficient number of randomly-selected samples, a probability value can be computed to any reasonable accuracy. Provided the probability value is not too small, the current recommended practice is to use $L = 1{,}000{,}000$ randomly-selected arrangements of the observed data to ensure a probability value with three decimal places of accuracy. To ensure four decimal places of accuracy, the number of randomly-selected arrangements must be increased by two magnitudes of order; that is, $L = 100{,}000{,}000$ [22].

A Monte Carlo Permutation Example

Consider once again the frequency data given in Table 3.4 on p. 64 with $N = 80$ observations. In many cases the exact analysis of $M = 21,671,722$ arrangements of cell frequencies would be considered impractical. In such cases a random sample of cell arrangements can yield an approximate probability value with considerable accuracy. Based on $L = 1,000,000$ randomly-selected cell arrangements given the observed marginal frequency totals, the Monte Carlo probability value of $\chi^2 = 25.1809$ is $P = 0.1055 \times 10^{-2}$, which compares favorably with the exact probability value of $P = 0.1009 \times 10^{-2}$.

3.2.3 Moment-Approximation Permutation Tests

Monte Carlo permutation methods can be inefficient when desired probability values are very small; for example, probability values on the order of 10^{-6}, as the Monte Carlo permutation method requires a large number of randomly-selected test statistics to approximate such a small probability value. Prior to the development of high-speed computing that made exact and Monte Carlo permutation methods possible, researchers relied on moment-approximation procedures to provide approximate probability values. The moment-approximation of a test statistic requires calculation of the exact moments of the test statistic, assuming equally-likely arrangements of the observed data. The exact moments are then used to fit a specified distribution that approximates the underlying discrete permutation distribution and provide an approximate, but often highly accurate, probability value.

For many years the beta distribution was used for the approximating distribution. Presently, the approximating distribution of choice is the Pearson type III probability distribution, which depends on the exact mean, variance, and skewness of the test statistic under consideration, say δ, given by

$$\mu_\delta = \frac{1}{M} \sum_{i=1}^{M} \delta_i \, ,$$

$$\sigma_\delta^2 = \frac{1}{M} \sum_{i=1}^{M} \left(\delta_i - \mu_\delta \right)^2 \, ,$$

and

$$\gamma_\delta = \frac{1}{\sigma_\delta^3} \left[\frac{1}{M} \sum_{i=1}^{M} \left(\delta_i - \mu_\delta \right)^3 \right] \, ,$$

respectively, where M denotes the total number of possible, equally-likely arrangements of the observed data. The standardized statistic given by

$$T = \frac{\delta_0 - \mu_\delta}{\sigma_\delta}$$

follows the Pearson type III distribution, where δ_0 denotes the observed value of test statistic δ. It should be noted that while the moments are exact, the resultant Pearson type III probability value is always approximate.

A Moment-Approximation Permutation Example

For the frequency data given in Table 3.4 on p. 64, the observed value of the permutation test statistic is $\delta_0 = 24.8661$, the expected value of test statistic δ is $\mu_\delta = 8.00$, the variance of test statistic δ is $\sigma_\delta^2 = 14.5148$, the standardized test statistic is

$$T = \frac{\delta_0 - \mu_\delta}{\sigma_\delta} = \frac{24.8661 - 8.00}{\sqrt{14.5148}} = +4.4270 \,,$$

and the moment-approximation probability value based on the Pearson type III probability distribution is $P = 0.9763 \times 10^{-3}$.

A Comparison of the Three Approaches

The three approaches to determining permutation probability values (exact, Monte Carlo, and moment-approximation) often yield similar probability values. The difference between the moment-approximation probability value ($P = 0.9763 \times 10^{-3}$) and the exact probability value based on all $M = 21,671,722$ arrangements of the observed data in Table 3.4 ($P = 0.1009 \times 10^{-4}$) is only

$$\Delta_P = 0.9763 \times 10^{-3} - 0.1009 \times 10^{-4} = 0.9662 \times 10^{-3} \,,$$

the difference between the moment-approximation probability value ($P = 0.9763 \times 10^{-3}$) and the Monte Carlo probability value based on a sample of $L = 1,000,000$ random arrangements of the observed data in Table 3.4 ($P = 0.1055 \times 10^{-2}$) is only

$$\Delta_P = 0.1055 \times 10^{-2} - 0.9763 \times 10^{-3} = 0.7870 \times 10^{-4} \,,$$

and the difference between the Monte Carlo probability value based on a sample of $L = 1,000,000$ random arrangements of the observed data in Table 3.4 ($P = 0.1055 \times 10^{-2}$) and the exact probability value based on all $M = 21,671,722$ arrangements of the observed data in Table 3.4 ($P = 0.1009 \times 10^{-2}$) is only

$$\Delta_P = 0.1055 \times 10^{-2} - 0.1009 \times 10^{-2} = 0.4600 \times 10^{-4} \,.$$

3.3 Permutation and Parametric Statistical Tests

Permutation statistical tests, based on the Fisher–Pitman permutation model, differ from traditional parametric tests, based on the Neyman–Pearson population model, in several ways. First, permutation tests are entirely data-dependent in that all the information required for analysis is contained within the observed data set [4, 33]. Second, permutation tests are appropriate for nonrandom samples, such as are common in many fields of research [38]. Third, permutation tests are distribution-free in that they do not depend on the assumptions associated with traditional parametric tests, such as normality and homogeneity of variance [5]. Fourth, permutation tests provide exact probability values based on the discrete permutation distribution of equally-likely test statistic values, rather than approximate probability values based on a theoretical approximating distribution, such as a z, χ^2, t, or F distribution [11]. Fifth, permutation tests are ideal for small data sets, whereas distribution functions often provide poor fits to the underlying discrete sampling distribution. Of these five differences, the requirements of random sampling and normality greatly limit the application of statistical tests and measures based on the Neyman–Pearson population model.

3.3.1 The Assumption of Random Sampling

It is important to note that the mathematical theorems that justify most statistical procedures under the Neyman–Pearson population model of statistical inference apply only to random samples drawn with replacement from a completely-specified sampling frame. However, if the sample is not a random sample from a well-defined population, then the validity of the hypothesis test is questionable [38]. There are, admittedly, some applications in statistical analysis in which random sampling from a specified population is neither attempted nor considered important. The fact that medical researchers seldom use random samples often comes as a surprise to investigators who work in other domains [11].

Research psychologists have been especially concerned with problems of random sampling. Writing in *Psychological Bulletin* in 1966, psychologist Eugene Edgington stated his position unequivocally: "statistical inferences cannot be made concerning populations that have not been randomly sampled" [10, p. 485]. Writing in *Canadian Psychology* in 1993, psychologists Michael Hunter and Richard May noted that random sampling is of particular relevance to psychologists, "who rarely use random sampling or any other sort of probability sampling" [20, p. 385]. In 1988 psychologist William Hays wrote:

> The point is that *some* probability structure must be known or assumed to underlie the occurrence of samples if statistical inference is to proceed. This point is belabored only because it is so often overlooked, and statistical inferences are so often made with only the most casual attention to the process by which the sample was generated. The assumption

of some probability structure underlying the sampling is a little "price tag" attached to a statistical inference. It is a sad fact that if one knows nothing about the probability of occurrence for particular samples of units for observation, very little of the machinery we are describing here applies. This is why our assumption of random sampling is not to be taken lightly.... Unless this assumption is at least reasonable, the probability results of inferential methods mean very little, and these methods might as well be omitted [17, p. 212].[7]

In summary, conventional sampling distributions require random sampling whereas permutation distributions do not [20, p. 387].

3.3.2   The Assumption of Normality

The assumption of normality is so basic to classical statistics that it deserves special attention. Two points should be emphasized. First, permutation tests make no distributional assumptions and, therefore, do not depend on the assumption of normality. Second, the assumption of normality by conventional tests is always unrealistic and never justified in practice [5, 29].

In 1927 R.C. Geary famously proclaimed: "Normality is a myth; there never has, and never will be, a normal distribution" [15, p. 241] and in 1938 Joseph Berkson wrote: "we may assume that it is practically certain that any series of real observations does not actually follow a normal curve *with absolute exactitude in all respects*" [2, p. 526] (see footnote 7). Robert Matthews once described the normal distribution as "beautiful, beguiling and thoroughly dangerous" [29, p. 193] and in 1954 I.D.J. Bross pointed out that statistical methods "are based on certain assumptions—assumptions which not only can be wrong, but in many situations *are* wrong" [6, p. 815] (see footnote 7). Others have empirically demonstrated the prevalence of highly-skewed and heavy-tailed distributions in a variety of academic disciplines, the best-known of which is Theodore Micceri's widely quoted 1989 article on "The unicorn, the normal curve, and other improbable creatures" [31].

3.4   Advantages of Permutation Methods

Alvan Feinstein was a strong advocate for permutation methods. Trained as both a mathematician and a medical doctor, Feinstein is widely regarded as the founder of clinical epidemiology and patient-oriented medicine and the originator of clinimetrics: the application of mathematics to the field of medicine [3, p. 246]. In 1973 Feinstein published a formative article titled "The role of randomization in sampling, testing, allocation, and credulous idolatry" [11]. As Feinstein's focus

---

[7]Emphasis in the original.

was on medical investigations, he detailed the major violations of the assumptions underlying tests of two groups:

1. The groups studied in modern clinical or epidemiologic research are seldom selected as random samples.
2. For the many clinical and epidemiology research projects that are performed as surveys, the subjects are not randomly assigned.
3. The distribution of the target variable is usually unknown in the parent population.
4. It is usually known that the target variable does not have a Gaussian distribution, and often departs from it dramatically.
5. It is usually known that the variances of the two samples are not remotely similar.

Feinstein then put forth some advantages of tests under the Fisher–Pitman permutation model that were insightful for the time and foreshadowed later research:

1. The result of a permutation test is a direct, exact probability value for the random likelihood of the observed difference.
2. Permutation tests do not require any unwarranted inferential estimations of means, variances, pooled variances, or other parameters of an unobserved, hypothetical parent population. The tests are based solely on the evidence that was actually obtained.
3. The investigator is not forced into making any erroneous assumptions either that the contrasted groups were chosen as random samples from a parent population or that treatments under study were randomly allocated to the two groups.
4. The investigator is not forced into making any erroneous or unconfirmable assumptions about a Gaussian (or any other) distribution for the parent population, or about equal variances in the contrasted groups.
5. A permutation test can be applied to groups of any size, no matter how large or small. There are no degrees of freedom to be considered. In the case of a contingency table, there is no need to worry about the magnitude of the expected value, no need to calculate expectations based on fractions of people, and no need to worry about applying, or not applying, Yates' correction for continuity.

To summarize, permutation statistical methods yield exact probability values, are completely data-dependent, do not require random sampling, make no assumptions about distributions, and can be applied to very small samples. The one drawback to permutation tests, as noted by Feinstein in 1973, is that permutation tests are notoriously difficult to calculate. While this statement was certainly true in 1973, in the age of high-speed computing the statement is most certainly no longer accurate.

3.5   Calculation Efficiency

Although permutation statistical methods do not require random sampling, normality, homogeneity, or large sample sizes, a potential drawback is the sheer
amount of computation required, with exact permutation tests being unrealistic for
many statistical analyses. Even Monte Carlo permutation methods often require the
enumeration of millions of random arrangements of the observed data in order to
provide a desired accuracy.

Five innovations mitigate the computation problem. First, high-speed computing
makes possible exact permutation statistical methods in which all possible arrangements of the observed data are generated and examined. Second, the examination
of all combinations of the observed data instead of all permutations of the observed
data provides the same probability value with considerable savings in computing
time. Third, mathematical recursion greatly simplifies difficult calculations. Fourth,
calculation of only the variable components of the selected test statistic reduces
the amount of calculation required for each of the enumerated arrangements. Fifth,
holding one array of the observed data constant in any type of block design can
substantially lessen the number of arrangements required for an exact permutation
analysis.

3.5.1   High-Speed Computing

One has only to observe the hordes of the digitally distracted trying to navigate
a crowded sidewalk with their various smart-phones, pads, pods, ear-buds, and
tablets to realize that computing power, speed, and accessibility have finally arrived.
Permutation methods are, by their very nature, computationally intensive and
required the development of high-speed computing to achieve their potential. Prior
to 1960, computers were large, slow, and expensive. In large part their use was
restricted to military and industrial applications. In the 1960s, mainframe computers
became widely available to academicians at major research universities. By 1980
desktop computers and workstations, although not common, were available to many
researchers. In addition, the speed of computing increased greatly between 1960 and
1980. All this paved the way for the rapid development of permutation statistical
methods.

While not widely available to researchers, by 2010 mainframe computers were
measuring computing speeds in teraflops. To emphasize the progress of computing,
in 1951 the Remington Rand Corporation introduced the UNIVAC computer
running at 1905 flops, which with ten mercury delay line memory tanks could store
20,000 bytes of information; in 2008 the IBM Corporation supercomputer, code-

named Roadrunner, reached a sustained performance of one petaflops[8]; in 2010 the Cray Jaguar was named the world's fastest computer performing at a sustained speed of 1.75 petaflops with 360 terabytes of memory; and in November of 2010 China exceeded the computing speed of the Cray Jaguar by 57% with the introduction of China's Tianhe-1A supercomputer performing at 2.67 petaflops [28].

In October of 2011, China broke the petaflops barrier again with the introduction of the Sunway Bluelight MPP [1]. In late 2011 the IBM Yellowstone supercomputer was installed at the National Center for Atmospheric Research (NCAR) Wyoming Supercomputer Center in Cheyenne, Wyoming. After months of testing, the Wyoming Supercomputer Center officially opened on Monday, 15 October 2012. Yellowstone was a 1.6 petaflops machine with 149.2 terabytes of memory and 74,592 processor cores and replaced an IBM Bluefire supercomputer installed in 2008 that had a peak speed of 76 teraflops. Also in late 2011, IBM unveiled the Blue Gene\P and \Q supercomputing processing systems that can achieve 20 petaflops. At the same time, IBM filed a patent for a massive supercomputing system capable of 107 petaflops. In June of 2018 IBM unveiled the Summit supercomputer at Oak Ridge National Laboratory in Tennessee that achieved sustained computing speeds of 200 petaflops.

On the near horizon are so-called quantum computers. The basic element of a quantum computer is the qubit. Unlike a standard bit (binary digit), which can take on a value of either 0 or 1, a qubit (quantum bit) can be either 0, 1, or a combination of the two. Because qubits can represent 0 and 1 simultaneously, they can encode a wealth of information. As Thomas Siegfried explained it, five bits represent *one* out of $2^5 = 32$ possible permutations, but five qubits represent *all* of $2^5 = 32$ possible permutations [39]. Teams from academia and industry are working on versions of quantum computers with 50–100 qubits, enough to perform calculations that the most powerful supercomputers of today cannot accomplish in a reasonable time [7]. Google, which has already developed a nine qubit computer, has aggressive plans to scale up to 49 qubits, and IBM, which has developed a 16 qubit prototype, announced in early 2017 that it would build a 50 qubit quantum computer in the next few years [7].

Finally, high-speed computers have dramatically changed the field of computational statistics. The future of high-speed computing appears very promising for exact and Monte Carlo permutation statistical methods. Combined with other efficiencies, it can safely be said that permutation methods have the potential to provide exact or Monte Carlo probability values in an efficient manner for a wide variety of statistical applications.

---

[8]One petaflops indicates a quadrillion operations per second, or a 1 with 15 zeroes following it.

3.5.2   Analysis with Combinations

Although permutation statistical methods are known by the attribution "permutation," they are generally not based on all possible permutations of the observed data. Instead, exact permutation methods are based on all possible *combinations* of arrangements of the observed data. Since, in general, there are fewer combinations than permutations, analysis of combinations of the observed data greatly reduces the amount of calculation required.

To illustrate the efficiency achieved by analyzing all combinations of the observed data instead of all permutations, consider $N = 10$ observations that are to be randomized into two groups, A and B, where $n_A = n_B = 5$ observations. Suppose that the purpose is to compare differences between the two groups, such as a mean difference. Let the $n_A = 5$ observations be designated as a through e and the $n_B = 5$ observations be designated as f through j. For Group A, the first observation can be chosen in 10 different ways, the second observation in nine ways, the third observation in eight ways, the fourth observation in seven ways, and the fifth observation in six ways. Once the five observations of Group A have been chosen, the remaining five observations are assigned to Group B.

Of the $10 \times 9 \times 8 \times 7 \times 6 = 30{,}240$ ways in which the five observations can be arranged for Group A, each individual quintet of observations will appear in a series of permutations. Thus, the quintet $\{a, b, c, d, e\}$ can be permuted as $\{a, b, c, e, d\}$, $\{a, b, d, e, c\}$, $\{a, b, d, c, e\}$, and so on. Each permutation of the five observations will yield the same mean value. The number of different permutations for a group of five observations is $5! = 120$. Thus, each distinctive quintet will appear in 120 ways among the 30,240 possible arrangements. Therefore, 30,240 divided by 120 yields 252 distinctive quintets of observations that can be formed by dividing $N = 10$ observations into two groups of five observations each. The number of quintets can conveniently be expressed as

$$\frac{(n_A + n_B)!}{n_A! \, n_B!} = \frac{(5+5)!}{5! \, 5!} = 252 \ .$$

However, half of these arrangements are similar, but opposite. Thus, a quintet such as $\{a, b, c, d, e\}$ might be assigned to Group A and the quintet $\{f, g, h, i, j\}$ might be assigned to Group B, or vice versa, yielding the same absolute mean difference. Consequently, there are only $252/2 = 126$ distinctly different pairs of quintets to be considered. A substantial amount of calculation can be eliminated by considering all possible combinations of arrangements of the observed data in place of all possible permutations with no loss of accuracy. Even in this small example, a reduction from 30,240 equally-likely arrangements of the observed data to 126 arrangements constitutes a substantial increase in efficiency.

3.5.3 *Mathematical Recursion*

Mathematical recursion is a process by which an initial probability value of a test statistic is calculated, then successive probability values are generated from the initial value by a recursive process. The initial value need not be an actual probability value, but can be a completely arbitrary positive value by which the resultant relative probability values are adjusted for the initializing value at the conclusion of the recursion process.

A Recursion Example

Consider a 2×2 contingency table using the notation in Table 3.5. Denote by a dot ($\cdot$) the partial sum of all rows or all columns, depending on the position of the ($\cdot$) in the subscript list. If the ($\cdot$) is in the first subscript position, the sum is over all rows and if the ($\cdot$) is in the second subscript position, the sum is over all columns. Thus, $n_{i\cdot}$ denotes the marginal frequency total of the ith row, $i = 1, \ldots, r$, summed over all columns, $n_{\cdot j}$ denotes the marginal frequency total of the jth column, $j = 1, \ldots, c$, summed over all rows, and $N = n_{11} + n_{12} + n_{21} + n_{22}$ denotes the table frequency total. The probability value corresponding to any set of cell frequencies in a 2×2 contingency table, n_{11}, n_{12}, n_{21}, n_{22}, is the hypergeometric point probability value given by

$$p = \binom{n_{\cdot 1}}{n_{11}} \binom{n_{\cdot 2}}{n_{12}} \binom{N}{n_{1\cdot}}^{-1} = \frac{n_{1\cdot}!\, n_{2\cdot}!\, n_{\cdot 1}!\, n_{\cdot 2}!}{N!\, n_{11}!\, n_{12}!\, n_{21}!\, n_{22}!} \,.$$

Since the exact probability value of a 2×2 contingency table with fixed marginal frequency totals and one degree of freedom is equivalent to the probability value of any one cell, determining the probability value of the cell containing n_{11} observations is sufficient.

If

$$p\{n_{11} + 1 | n_{1\cdot}, n_{\cdot 1}, N\} = p\{n_{11} | n_{1\cdot}, n_{\cdot 1}, N\} \times f(n_{11}) \,,$$

Table 3.5 Conventional notation for a 2×2 contingency table

		Category		
Category		1	2	Total
1		n_{11}	n_{12}	$n_{1\cdot}$
2		n_{21}	n_{22}	$n_{2\cdot}$
Total		$n_{\cdot 1}$	$n_{\cdot 2}$	N

then solving for $f(n_{11})$ produces

$$f(n_{11}) = \frac{p\{n_{11} + 1 | n_1., n_{.1}, N\}}{p\{n_{11} | n_1., n_{.1}, N\}}$$

$$= \frac{n_{11}! \, n_{12}! \, n_{21}! \, n_{22}!}{(n_{11} + 1)! \, (n_{12} - 1)! \, (n_{21} - 1)! \, (n_{22} + 1)!}$$

and, after cancelling, yields

$$f(n_{11}) = \frac{n_{12} \, n_{21}}{(n_{11} + 1)(n_{22} + 1)} . \tag{3.1}$$

To illustrate mathematical recursion with an arbitrary initial value, consider the 2×2 contingency table given in Table 3.6 with $N = 24$ observations. For the cell containing $n_{11} = 6$ observations there are

$$M = \min(n_1., n_{.1}) - \max(0, n_{11} - n_{22}) + 1$$

$$= \min(10, 8) - \max(0, 6 - 12) + 1 = 8 - 0 + 1 = 9$$

possible arrangements of cell frequencies, given the observed marginal frequency totals. Table 3.7 lists the reference set of the $M = 9$ cell arrangements along with the associated hypergeometric point probability values to six decimal places.

To illustrate the use of an arbitrary origin in a recursion procedure, consider Table 3.1 in Table 3.7 and set relative probability value $H\{n_{11} = 0 | 10, 8, 24\}$ to a small arbitrarily-chosen positive value, say 1.00. Thus, $H\{n_{11} = 0 | 10, 8, 24\} = 1.00$. Then, following Eq. (3.1), a recursion procedure produces

$$H\{n_{11} = 1 | 10, 8, 24\} = 1.000000 \times \frac{(10)(8)}{(0 + 1)(6 + 1)} = 11.428571 ,$$

$$H\{n_{11} = 2 | 10, 8, 24\} = 11.428571 \times \frac{(9)(7)}{(1 + 1)(7 + 1)} = 45.000000 ,$$

$$H\{n_{11} = 3 | 10, 8, 24\} = 45.000000 \times \frac{(8)(6)}{(2 + 1)(8 + 1)} = 80.000000 ,$$

$$H\{n_{11} = 4 | 10, 8, 24\} = 80.000000 \times \frac{(7)(5)}{(3 + 1)(9 + 1)} = 70.000000 ,$$

Table 3.6 Example data for a recursion process with an arbitrary initial value

	Variable B		
Variable A	b	$\bar{b}$	Total
a	6	4	10
$\bar{a}$	2	12	14
Total	8	16	24

Table 3.7 Listing of the
$M = 9$ possible $2{\times}2$
contingency tables from
Table 3.6 in the reference set
with associated exact
hypergeometric probability
values to six decimal places

Table 1		Probability	Table 2		Probability
0	10	0.004083	1	9	0.046664
8	6		7	7	
Table 3		Probability	Table 4		Probability
2	8	0.183739	3	7	0.326648
6	8		5	9	
Table 5		Probability	Table 6		Probability
4	6	0.285817	5	5	0.124720
4	10		3	11	
Table 7		Probability	Table 8		Probability
6	4	0.025983	7	3	0.002284
2	12		1	13	
Table 9		Probability			
8	2	0.000061			
0	14				

$$H\{n_{11} = 5|10, 8, 24\} = 70.000000 \times \frac{(6)(4)}{(4+1)(10+1)} = 30.545455 \,,$$

$$H\{n_{11} = 6|10, 8, 24\} = 30.545455 \times \frac{(5)(3)}{(5+1)(11+1)} = 6.363636 \,,$$

$$H\{n_{11} = 7|10, 8, 24\} = 6.363636 \times \frac{(4)(2)}{(6+1)(12+1)} = 0.559441 \,,$$

and

$$H\{n_{11} = 8|10, 8, 24\} = 0.559441 \times \frac{(3)(1)}{(7+1)(13+1)} = 0.014985 \,,$$

for a total of

$$T = \sum_{i=0}^{8} H\{n_{11} = i|10, 8, 24\}$$

$$= 1.000000 + 11.428571 + \cdots + 0.014985 = 244.912088 \,.$$

The desired exact point probability values are then obtained by dividing each relative probability value, $H\{n_{11}|n_{1.}, n_{.1}, N\}$, by the recursively-obtained total, T.

For example,

$$p\{n_{11} = \ 0|10, 8, 24\} = \frac{H_1}{T} = \frac{1.000000}{244.912088} = 0.004083 \,,$$

$$p\{n_{11} = \ 1|10, 8, 24\} = \frac{H_2}{T} = \frac{11.428571}{244.912088} = 0.046664 \,,$$

$$p\{n_{11} = \ 2|10, 8, 24\} = \frac{H_3}{T} = \frac{45.000000}{244.912088} = 0.183739 \,,$$

$$p\{n_{11} = \ 3|10, 8, 24\} = \frac{H_4}{T} = \frac{80.000000}{244.912088} = 0.326648 \,,$$

$$p\{n_{11} = \ 4|10, 8, 24\} = \frac{H_5}{T} = \frac{70.000000}{244.912088} = 0.285817 \,,$$

$$p\{n_{11} = \ 5|10, 8, 24\} = \frac{H_6}{T} = \frac{30.545455}{244.912088} = 0.124720 \,,$$

$$p\{n_{11} = \ 6|10, 8, 24\} = \frac{H_7}{T} = \frac{6.363636}{244.912088} = 0.025983 \,,$$

$$p\{n_{11} = \ 7|10, 8, 24\} = \frac{H_8}{T} = \frac{0.559441}{244.912088} = 0.002284 \,,$$

and

$$p\{n_{11} = \ 8|10, 8, 24\} = \frac{H_9}{T} = \frac{0.014985}{244.912088} = 0.000061 \,.$$

In this manner, the entire analysis is conducted utilizing an arbitrary initial value and a recursion procedure, thereby eliminating all factorial expressions. When the number of potential contingency tables given by $\max(n_{11}) - \min(n_{11}) + 1$ is large, the computational savings can be substantial.

3.5.4   Variable Components of a Test Statistic

Under permutation, only the variable components of the specified test statistic need to be calculated for each arrangement of the observed data. As this component is often a very small piece of the desired test statistic, calculations can often be reduced by several factors. To illustrate, consider the raw-score expression for a conventional Pearson product-moment correlation coefficient between variables x and y given by

$$r_{xy} = \frac{\sum\limits_{i=1}^{N} x_i y_i - \left(\sum\limits_{i=1}^{N} x_i \sum\limits_{i=1}^{N} y_i\right)\Big/N}{\sqrt{\left[\sum\limits_{i=1}^{N} x_i^2 - \left(\sum\limits_{i=1}^{N} x_i\right)^2\Big/N\right]\left[\sum\limits_{i=1}^{N} y_i^2 - \left(\sum\limits_{i=1}^{N} y_i\right)^2\Big/N\right]}}, \tag{3.2}$$

where N is the number of bivariate measurements. For Pearson's correlation coefficient given in Eq. (3.2)

$$N, \quad \sum_{i=1}^{N} x_i, \quad \sum_{i=1}^{N} x_i^2, \quad \sum_{i=1}^{N} y_i, \quad \text{and} \quad \sum_{i=1}^{N} y_i^2$$

are invariant under permutation. Thus, it is sufficient to calculate only $\sum_{i=1}^{N} x_i y_i$ for each permutation of the observed data, eliminating a great deal of calculation. In addition, it is only necessary to permute either variable x or variable y, leaving the other variable fixed.

3.5.5 Holding an Array Constant

In the special case of block designs, such as matched-pairs and randomized-blocks analysis of variance, it is possible to reduce the number of arrangements to be examined by holding one of the arrays (treatment values) constant, while permuting the other arrays. For example, given $g = 3$ treatments and $b = 10$ subjects (blocks) in each treatment, there are

$$M = (g!)^b = (3!)^{10} = 60{,}466{,}176$$

arrangements of the observed data to be considered. Holding one of the b sets of blocks constant, relative to the other $b - 1$ sets of blocks, there are

$$M = (g!)^{b-1} = (3!)^{10-1} = 10{,}077{,}696$$

arrangements of the observed data to be considered, a reduction of 50,388,480 arrangements, or 83%.

These five features, high-speed computing, mathematical recursion with an arbitrary initial value, computation of only the variable components of the test statistic under permutation, holding an array of the observed data constant, and utilizing combinations instead of permutations, produce a highly efficient permutation statistical approach that makes permutation statistical methods both feasible and practical for many research applications.

3.6 Summary

This chapter opened with a description of two models of statistical inference: the population model first put forward by Jerzy Neyman and Egon Pearson in 1928 and the permutation model developed by R.A. Fisher, R.C. Geary, T. Eden, F. Yates, H. Hotelling, M.R. Pabst, and E.J.G. Pitman in the 1920s and 1930s. Three types of permutation statistical methods were described and illustrated: exact, Monte Carlo, and moment-approximation permutation methods.

Permutation statistical methods were shown to differ from traditional parametric methods in five ways. First, unlike conventional parametric methods, permutation statistical methods are data-dependent methods in that all the information required for analysis is contained within the observed data. Second, permutation methods neither assume nor require random sampling from a defined population, which is essential for parametric methods. Third, permutation methods are distribution-free and do not depend on the usual assumptions associated with conventional parametric methods, such as normality and homogeneity of variance. Fourth, permutation methods provide exact probability values based on the discrete permutation probability distribution, in contrast to parametric methods that provide approximate probability values based on a theoretical approximating distribution. Finally, permutation methods are suitable for small samples, whereas parametric distribution functions often provide very poor fits to the underlying discrete distribution when sample sizes are small.

On the other hand, permutation methods are computationally intensive, oftentimes requiring millions of calculations. A number of calculation efficiencies mitigate the calculation problem, including the recent development of high-speed computing, analyses based on all combinations of the observed data in place of all permutations of the data, the use of mathematical recursion, calculations based on only the variable components of a specified test statistic, and holding constant one treatment array in block designs.

Chapter 4 describes measures of central tendency and variability with which the reader is assumed to be familiar. Emphasized in Chap. 4 is the property of the arithmetic mean as the point about which the sum-of-squared deviations is minimized and the property of the median as the point about which the sum of absolute deviations is minimized. An alternative approach to the mean and median based on paired-squared and paired-absolute differences is introduced.

References

1. Barboza, D., Markoff, J.: Power in numbers: China aims for high-tech primacy. N.Y. Times **161**, D2–D3 (2011)
2. Berkson, J.: Some difficulties of interpretation encountered in the application of the chi-square test. J. Am. Stat. Assoc. **33**, 526–536 (1938)
3. Berry, K.J., Johnston, J.E., Mielke, P.W.: A Chronicle of Permutation Statistical Methods: 1920–2000 and Beyond. Springer, Cham (2014)
4. Biondini, M.E., Mielke, P.W., Berry, K.J.: Data-dependent permutation techniques for the analysis of ecological data. Vegetatio **75**, 161–168 (1988) [The name of the journal was changed to *Plant Ecology* in 1997]
5. Box, G.E.P., Andersen, S.L.: Permutation theory in the derivation of robust criteria and the study of departures from assumption (with discussion). J. R. Stat. Soc. B Methodol. **17**, 1–34 (1955)
6. Bross, I.D.J.: Is there an increased risk? Fed. Proc. **13**, 815–819 (1954)
7. Conover, E.: Quantum computers get real. Sci. News Mag. **191**, 28–33 (2017)
8. Curran-Everett, D.: Explorations in statistics: standard deviations and standard errors. Adv. Physiol. Educ. **32**, 203–208 (2008)
9. Eden, T., Yates, F.: On the validity of Fisher's z test when applied to an actual example of non-normal data. J. Agric. Sci. **23**, 6–17 (1933)
10. Edgington, E.S.: Statistical inference and nonrandom samples. Psychol. Bull. **66**, 485–487 (1966)
11. Feinstein, A.R.: Clinical Biostatistics XXIII: the role of randomization in sampling, testing, allocation, and credulous idolatry (Part 2). Clin. Pharmacol. Ther. **14**, 898–915 (1973)
12. Fisher, R.A.: Statistical Methods for Research Workers. Oliver and Boyd, Edinburgh (1925)
13. Fisher, R.A.: The logic of inductive inference (with discussion). J. R. Stat. Soc. **98**, 39–82 (1935)
14. Geary, R.C.: Some properties of correlation and regression in a limited universe. Metron **7**, 83–119 (1927)
15. Geary, R.C.: Testing for normality. Biometrika **34**, 209–242 (1947)
16. Haber, M.: Comments on "The test of homogeneity for 2×2 contingency tables: a review of and some personal opinions on the controversy" by G. Camilli. Psychol. Bull. **108**, 146–149 (1990)
17. Hays, W.L.: Statistics. Holt, Rinehart and Winston, New York (1988)
18. Hotelling, H., Pabst, M.R.: Rank correlation and tests of significance involving no assumption of normality. Ann. Math. Stat. **7**, 29–43 (1936)
19. Hubbard, R.: Alphabet soup: blurring the distinctions between p's and α's in psychological research. Theor. Psychol. **14**, 295–327 (2004)
20. Hunter, M.A., May, R.B.: Some myths concerning parametric and nonparametric tests. Can. Psychol. **34**, 384–389 (1993)
21. Irwin, J.O.: Tests of significance for differences between percentages based on small numbers. Metron **12**, 83–94 (1935)
22. Johnston, J.E., Berry, K.J., Mielke, P.W.: Permutation tests: precision in estimating probability values. Percept. Motor Skill. **105**, 915–920 (2007)
23. Kempthorne, O.: Why randomize? J. Stat. Plan. Infer. **1**, 1–25 (1977)
24. Kennedy, P.E.: Randomization tests in econometrics. J. Bus. Econ. Stat. **13**, 85–94 (1995)
25. Lachin, J.M.: Statistical properties of randomization in clinical trials. Control. Clin. Trials **9**, 289–311 (1988)
26. Ludbrook, J.: Advantages of permutation (randomization) tests in clinical and experimental pharmacology and physiology. Clin. Exp. Pharmacol. Physiol. **21**, 673–686 (1994)
27. Ludbrook, J.: Issues in biomedical statistics: comparing means by computer-intensive tests. Aust. NZ J. Surg. **65**, 812–819 (1995)
28. Lyons, D.: In race for fastest computer, China outpaces U.S. Newsweek **158**, 57–59 (2011)

29. Matthews, R.: Beautiful, but dangerous. Significance **13**, 30–31 (2016)
30. May, R.B., Hunter, M.A.: Some advantages of permutation tests. Can. Psychol. **34**, 401–407 (1993)
31. Micceri, T.: The unicorn, the normal curve, and other improbable creatures. Psychol. Bull. **105**, 156–166 (1989)
32. Mielke, P.W., Berry, K.J.: Fisher's exact probability test for cross-classification tables. Educ. Psychol. Meas. **52**, 97–101 (1992)
33. Mielke, P.W., Berry, K.J.: Data-dependent analyses in psychological research. Psychol. Rep. **91**, 1225–1234 (2002)
34. Neyman, J., Pearson, E.S.: On the use and interpretation of certain test criteria for purposes of statistical inference: part I. Biometrika **20A**, 175–240 (1928)
35. Neyman, J., Pearson, E.S.: On the use and interpretation of certain test criteria for purposes of statistical inference: part II. Biometrika **20A**, 263–294 (1928)
36. Pitman, E.J.G.: Significance tests which may be applied to samples from any populations. Suppl. J. R. Stat. Soc. **4**, 119–130 (1937)
37. Pitman, E.J.G.: Significance tests which may be applied to samples from any populations: II. The correlation coefficient test. Suppl. J. R. Stat. Soc. **4**, 225–232 (1937)
38. Pitman, E.J.G.: Significance tests which may be applied to samples from any populations: III. The analysis of variance test. Biometrika **29**, 322–335 (1938)
39. Siegfried, T.: Birth of the qubit. Sci. News Mag. **191**, 34–37 (2017)
40. Yates, F.: Contingency tables involving small numbers and the χ^2 test. Suppl. J. R. Stat. Soc. **1**, 217–235 (1934)

Chapter 4
Central Tendency and Variability

Abstract This chapter provides an overview of the concepts of central tendency and variability. For measures of central tendency, the sample mode, median, and mean are described and illustrated. For measures of variability, the sample standard deviation, sample variance, and mean absolute deviation are described and illustrated. An alternative to the mean and median based on paired squared and absolute differences between values is introduced.

The two most central concepts in statistical analysis involve the measurement of central tendency and variability. This chapter presents three test statistics that represent the "center" of a distribution of values. In general, these statistics are referred to as measures of central tendency or measures of location. Later in this chapter, two test statistics are presented that deal with how values are dispersed around a measure of central tendency. In general, these statistics are referred to as measures of variability or measures of scale. The three major measures of central tendency are the mode, the median, and the arithmetic mean.[1] For permutation statistical methods, only the arithmetic mean and the median are important. The two major measures of variability are the sample standard deviation for dispersion around the mean and the mean absolute deviation for dispersion around the median. No measure of variability exists for dispersion around the mode.

---

[1]Two other measures of central tendency that are often found in the research literature are the geometric mean and the harmonic mean.

© Springer Nature Switzerland AG 2019

K. J. Berry et al., *A Primer of Permutation Statistical Methods*,

https://doi.org/10.1007/978-3-030-20933-9_4

4.1   The Sample Mode

The sample mode is defined simply as the most common score in a distribution of N scores. More precisely, the mode is the sample score or category with the largest frequency. For example, for the following $N = 13$ scores,

$$\overbrace{}^{\text{mode}}$$
$$12,\ 12,\ 11,\ 9,\ 9,\ \ 8,\ 8,\ 8,\ 8,\ 7,\ 5,\ 5,\ 3\ ,$$

the mode is 8, as there are four 8s, more than any other score. For the frequency distribution given in Table 4.1, the sample mode is 72 as it has the largest frequency ($f = 23$). And for the frequency distribution in Table 4.2, the modal luxury automobile in a country club parking lot is BMW as it has the largest frequency ($f = 17$). There is no formula in the usual sense for the sample mode and no generally agreed-upon symbol.

Table 4.1 Example frequency data for the sample mode with scores

Score	f
90	2
88	4
85	7
80	11
76	15
72 (mode)	23
69	19
65	14
64	10
60	8
55	4
53	1

Table 4.2 Example frequency data for the sample mode with categories

Automobile	f
Acura	5
Alpha Romeo	1
Audi	8
BMW (mode)	17
Cadillac	10
Genesis	1
Infiniti	4
Jaguar	2
Lexus	7
Lincoln	8
Mercedes-Benz	11
Volvo	14

Oftentimes the sample mode is reported in newspapers and magazines without being labeled as such. For any ordered list of popularity items, the first item listed is usually the mode. For example, the Social Security Administration might report that the most popular female baby name last year was "Emma," a magazine article might state that the most popular name for a pet cat or dog in the USA is "Max," or it may be revealed that the most popular computer password is "password."[2] In such cases, Emma, Max, and password have the largest frequency of usage. Despite its widespread use, the mode finds little to no use in permutation statistical methods. The sample mode is very unstable in that a change in one value can oftentimes greatly alter the mode; many distributions have no mode, such as the uniform distribution; and some distributions have two modes (bimodal) or even many modes (multimodal). Thus the mode is not a very useful measure of central tendency in permutation statistical analyses where the emphasis is on exactness.

4.2 The Sample Mean

The arithmetic mean is the second most basic process in all of statistics. The first is the simple act of counting. For a sample of N values, the arithmetic mean is given by

$$\bar{x} = \frac{1}{N} \sum_{i=1}^{N} x_i \; ,$$

where N is the total sample size and x_i for $i = 1, \ldots, N$ denote the sample values.[3] To illustrate, consider a set of $N = 6$ values where $x_1 = 3$, $x_2 = 7$, $x_3 = 11$, $x_4 = 15$, $x_5 = 20$, and $x_6 = 28$. Then the sample mean is

$$\bar{x} = \frac{1}{N} \sum_{i=1}^{N} x_i = \frac{3 + 7 + 11 + 15 + 20 + 28}{6} = \frac{84}{6} = 14 \; .$$

There are two important properties of the sample mean. First, the sum of deviations about the mean can be shown to be zero. Let $x_1, x_2, \ldots, x_N$ denote an unordered set of N sample values and define the sum of deviations about any point, say θ, as

$$D_\theta = \sum_{i=1}^{N} \left(x_i - \theta \right) \; .$$

---

[2] Actually, the most common password used to be "password," but it has been replaced by "123456."

[3] For a brief history of the arithmetic mean, see a 2018 article by Simon Raper in *Significance* [6].

Theorem *For any finite set of N values of x in* $\mathbb{R}$, *the sum of deviations about a point* θ *is zero when* $\theta = \bar{x}$.

Proof

$$\sum_{i=1}^{N} (x_i - \theta)$$

$$= \sum_{i=1}^{N} x_i - \sum_{i=1}^{N} \theta$$

$$= \sum_{i=1}^{N} x_i - N\theta .$$

Then,

$$\theta = \frac{1}{N} \sum_{i=1}^{N} x_i = \bar{x} .$$

However, the most important statistical property of the sample mean is that the sum-of-squared deviations about the mean can be shown to be a minimum. Let $x_1, x_2, \ldots, x_N$ denote an unordered set of N sample values and define the sum of the squared deviations about any point, say θ, as

$$D_\theta = \sum_{i=1}^{N} (x_i - \theta)^2 .$$

Theorem *For any finite set of N values of x in* $\mathbb{R}$, *the sum-of-squared deviations about a point* θ *is minimized when* $\theta = \bar{x}$.

Proof

$$\sum_{i=1}^{N} (x_i - \theta)^2$$

$$= \sum_{i=1}^{N} (x_i^2 - 2x_i\theta + \theta^2)$$

$$= \sum_{i=1}^{N} x_i^2 - 2\theta \sum_{i=1}^{N} x_i + N\theta^2 .$$

Table 4.3 Sums of deviations and squared deviations about the arithmetic mean ($\bar{x} = 14$)

Object	x	$x - \bar{x}$	$(x - \bar{x})^2$
1	28	+14	196
2	20	+6	36
3	15	+1	1
4	11	−3	9
5	7	−7	49
6	3	−11	121
Sum		0	412

Table 4.4 Sums of deviations and squared deviations about a value less than the arithmetic mean ($\theta = 12$)

Object	x	$x - 12$	$(x - 12)^2$
1	28	+16	256
2	20	+8	64
3	15	+3	9
4	11	−1	1
5	7	−5	25
6	3	−9	81
Sum		+12	436

Taking the derivative with respect to θ yields

$$\frac{d\left(\sum_{i=1}^{N} x_i^2 - 2\theta \sum_{i=1}^{N} x_i + N\theta^2\right)}{d\theta} = -2\sum_{i=1}^{N} x_i + 2N\theta \ ,$$

and solving for θ yields

$$\theta = \frac{1}{N} \sum_{i=1}^{N} x_i = \bar{x} \ .$$

To illustrate both proofs, consider the small set of example data listed in Table 4.3 where $\bar{x} = 14$. For the example data listed in Table 4.3,

$$\sum_{i=1}^{N} \left(x_i - \bar{x}\right) = 0$$

and

$$\sum_{i=1}^{N} (x_i - \bar{x})^2 = 412 \ ,$$

which is a minimum. Now consider a constant somewhat smaller than $\bar{x} = 14$, say $\theta = 12$, as shown in Table 4.4. For the example data listed in Table 4.4,

$$\sum_{i=1}^{N} \left(x_i - 12\right) = +12 \ ,$$

Table 4.5 Sums of
deviations and squared
deviations about a value
greater than the arithmetic
mean ($\theta = 15$)

Object	x	$x - 15$	$(x - 15)^2$
1	28	+13	169
2	20	+5	25
3	15	0	0
4	11	−4	16
5	7	−8	64
6	3	−12	144
Sum		−6	418

which is greater than zero, and

$$\sum_{i=1}^{N}(x_i - 12)^2 = 436 \, ,$$

which is greater than 412 and is, therefore, not a minimum. Finally, consider a constant greater than $\bar{x} = 14$, say $\theta = 15$, as shown in Table 4.5. For the example data listed in Table 4.5,

$$\sum_{i=1}^{N}\left(x_i - 15\right) = -6 \, ,$$

which is less than zero, and

$$\sum_{i=1}^{N}(x_i - 15)^2 = 418 \, ,$$

which is greater than 412 and is, therefore, not a minimum.

4.2.1   The Sample Standard Deviation

The conventional measure of variability about the sample mean is the sample standard deviation given by[4]

$$s_x = \left[\frac{1}{N-1} \sum_{i=1}^{N} \left(x_i - \bar{x}\right)^2 \right]^{1/2} \, ,$$

---

[4] Technically, the estimated population standard deviation.

where $N - 1$ is the degrees of freedom (df). Thus for the x_i values, $i = 1, \ldots, N$, listed in Table 4.3 for which the sample mean is $\bar{x} = 14$,

$$s_x = \left\{ \frac{1}{6-1} \left[(28-14)^2 + (20-14)^2 + \cdots + (3-14)^2 \right] \right\}^{1/2}$$

$$= \left(\frac{412}{5} \right)^{1/2} = 9.0774 \ .$$

Both the sample mean and the sample standard deviation are expressed in the units of measurement of the original data.

Also in wide use is the sample variance given by[5]

$$s_x^2 = \frac{1}{N-1} \sum_{i=1}^{N} (x_i - \bar{x})^2 \ .$$

For the x_i values, $i = 1, \ldots, N$, listed in Table 4.3 the sample variance is

$$s_x^2 = \frac{1}{6-1} \left[(28-14)^2 + (20-14)^2 + \cdots + (3-14)^2 \right] = 82.3992 \ .$$

Because degrees of freedom are not relevant to permutation methods under the Fisher–Pitman model, the sample standard deviation and sample variance under permutation are often defined as

$$S_x = \left[\frac{1}{N} \sum_{i=1}^{N} (x_i - \bar{x})^2 \right]^{1/2}$$

and

$$S_x^2 = \frac{1}{N} \sum_{i=1}^{N} (x_i - \bar{x})^2 \ ,$$

respectively, and denoted by the upper-case letter S to distinguish the sample standard (S_x) and variance (S_x^2) from the estimated population standard deviation (s_x) and variance (s_x^2).

---

[5]Technically, the estimated population variance.

For the example data listed in Table 4.3, the sample standard deviation is

$$S_x = \left\{ \frac{1}{6} \left[(28 - 14)^2 + (20 - 14)^2 + \cdots + (3 - 14)^2 \right] \right\}^{1/2}$$

$$= \left(\frac{412}{6} \right)^{1/2} = 8.2865$$

and the sample variance is

$$S_x^2 = \frac{1}{6} \left[(28 - 14)^2 + (20 - 14)^2 + \cdots + (3 - 14)^2 \right] = \frac{412}{6} = 68.6667 \ .$$

The reader may have noticed that only sample statistics have thus far been defined; for example, the sample mean, standard deviation, and variance. Permutation statistical methods are data-dependent methods and do not utilize population parameters. All the information for a permutation statistical analysis is contained in the sample. Therefore, the population mean (μ_x), the population standard deviation (σ_x), and the population variance (σ_x^2) are not defined in this chapter, as they would be in a conventional introductory book in statistics.

4.3 The Sample Median

The sample median is typically defined as the point below which half the values fall or the 50th percentile, where the scores are assumed to be ordered. Despite its long history in statistical methods, no agreed-upon symbol for the median has been defined—here, $\tilde{x}$ designates the sample median.[6]

Calculation of the sample median depends on whether N is odd or even. If N is odd, the sample median is given by $\tilde{x} = x_{(N+1)/2}$. To illustrate, consider $N = 5$ ordered values with $x_1 = 3$, $x_2 = 7$, $x_3 = 11$, $x_4 = 15$, and $x_5 = 20$. Then,

$$\tilde{x} = x_{(N+1)/2} = x_{(5+1)/2} = x_3 = 11 \ .$$

If N is even, the sample median is given by

$$\tilde{x} = \frac{x_{N/2} + x_{N/2+1}}{2} \ .$$

---

[6]Francis Galton first used the term "median" in 1882 [2, p. 245], although it had a long history in other languages prior to 1882 [1, p. 125].

To illustrate, consider $N = 6$ ordered values with $x_1 = 3$, $x_2 = 7$, $x_3 = 11$, $x_4 = 15$, $x_5 = 20$, and $x_6 = 28$. Then,

$$\tilde{x} = \frac{x_{N/2} + x_{N/2+1}}{2} = \frac{x_{6/2} + x_{6/2+1}}{2} = \frac{x_3 + x_4}{2} = \frac{11 + 15}{2} = \frac{26}{2} = 13 .$$

When N is even, the median value is not unique. While $\tilde{x} = 13$ would be the most commonly reported value for the median, any value between and including $x_3 = 11$ and $x_4 = 15$ is technically the median of the $N = 6$ values: 3, 7, 11, 15, 20, and 28.

The most important property of the sample median is that the sum of the absolute deviations about the median can be shown to be a minimum. The usual proof is by induction, but the proof by induction can be difficult to follow. The following non-mathematical proof based on set theory is adapted from Schwertman et al. [8].

Let $x_1 \leq x_2 \leq \cdots \leq x_N$ denote an ordered set of N values and define the sum of the absolute deviations about any point, say θ, as

$$D_\theta = \sum_{i=1}^{N} |x_i - \theta| .$$

Theorem *For any finite set of N values of x in $\mathbb{R}$, the sum of absolute deviations about a point θ is minimized when $\theta = \tilde{x}$.*

Proof Recall that the median of $x_1, \ldots, x_N$ is $x_{(N+1)/2}$ if N is odd and if N is even the median is not unique and any number m for $x_{N/2} \leq m \leq x_{N/2+1}$ is a median. When $N = 1$, then N is odd and $x_{(N+1)/2} = x$ and the result is trivial; that is, $\tilde{x} = x_1$.

Now consider any $N = 2$ x values, $x_2 > x_1$. For any point θ such that θ is included in the set $\{x_1, x_x\}$; that is, $\theta \in \{x_1, x_2\}$, the sum of the absolute deviations about θ is

$$\theta - x_1 + x_2 - \theta = x_2 - x_1 .$$

Thus, for example, if $x_1 = 3$ and $x_2 = 7$, the sum of the absolute deviations is $x_2 - x_1 = 7 - 3 = 4$. To illustrate, if $x_1 = 3$, $x_2 = 7$, and $\theta = 3$,

$$\theta - x_1 + x_2 - \theta = 3 - 3 + 7 - 3 = 0 + 4 = 4 ;$$

if $x_1 = 3$, $x_2 = 7$, and $\theta = 4$,

$$\theta - x_1 + x_2 - \theta = 4 - 3 + 7 - 4 = 1 + 3 = 4 ;$$

if $x_1 = 3$, $x_2 = 7$, and $\theta = 5.6$,

$$\theta - x_1 + x_2 - \theta = 5.6 - 3 + 7 - 5.6 = 2.6 + 1.4 = 4 ;$$

and if $x_1 = 3$, $x_2 = 7$, and $\theta = 7$,

$$\theta - x_1 + x_2 - \theta = 7 - 3 + 7 - 7 = 4 + 0 = 4 .$$

However, for $\theta \notin \{x_1, x_2\}$ and $\theta < x_1$, the sum of the absolute deviations is

$$x_1 - \theta + x_2 - \theta = x_1 + x_2 - 2\theta ,$$

which is greater than $x_2 - x_1$. Thus if $x_1 = 3$ and $x_2 = 7$, $x_2 = x_1 = 7 - 3 = 4$. To illustrate, consider $x_1 = 3$, $x_2 = 7$, and $\theta = 2$, then

$$x_1 + x_2 - 2\theta = 3 + 7 - (2)(2) = 1 - 4 = 6 .$$

For $\theta \notin \{x_1, x_2\}$ and $\theta > x_2$, the sum of absolute deviations is

$$\theta - x_1 + \theta - x_2 = 2\theta - x_1 - x_2 ,$$

which is greater than $x_2 - x_1$. Thus if $x_1 = 3$ and $x_2 = 7$, $x_2 - x_1 = 7 - 3 = 4$. To illustrate, consider $x_1 = 3$, $x_2 = 7$, and $\theta = 8$, then

$$2\theta - x_1 - x_2 = (2)(8) - 3 - 7 = 16 - 10 = 6 .$$

Therefore, for any two x values, the sum of the absolute deviations about point θ is minimized when $\theta \in \{x_1, x_2\}$ and, as shown, the sum of absolute deviations is equal to $x_2 - x_1$.

Now consider the successively nested intervals,

$$\{x_1, x_N\}, \{x_2, x_{N-1}\}, \{x_3, x_{N-2}\}, \ldots, \{x_i, x_{N+1-i}\} ,$$

where $x_1 \le x_2 \le \cdots \le x_N$, $i = 1, 2, \ldots, c$, $c = N/2$ if N is even, and $c = (N + 1)/2$ if N is odd. Note that when N is even, the innermost interval is $\{x_{N/2}, x_{N/2+1}\}$ and when N is odd, the innermost interval is $\{x_{(N+1)/2}, x_{(N+1)/2}\}$.

Example of the Median with N Even
For example, consider N even where $x_1 = 3$, $x_2 = 7$, $x_3 = 11$, $x_4 = 15$, $x_5 = 20$, and $x_6 = 28$ and the median is

$$\tilde{x} = \frac{x_{N/2} + x_{N/2+1}}{2} = \frac{x_{6/2} + x_{6/2+1}}{2} = \frac{x_3 + x_4}{2} = \frac{11 + 15}{2} = 13 .$$

The outermost interval is $\{x_1, x_N\} = \{x_1, x_6\} = \{3, 28\}$ and the median of $\{3, 7, 11, 15, 20, 28\}$ is $\tilde{x} = 13$.

The first nested interval is $\{x_2, x_{N-1}\} = \{x_2, x_{6-1}\} = \{x_2, x_5\} = \{7, 20\}$ and the median of $\{7, 11, 15, 20\}$ is $\tilde{x} = 13$. The innermost nested interval is $\{x_3, x_{N-2}\} = \{x_3, x_{6-2}\} = \{x_3, x_4\} = \{11, 15\}$ and the median of $\{11, 15\}$ is

$\tilde{x} = 13$, which corresponds to

$$\{x_{N/2}, x_{N/2+1}\} = \{x_{6/2}, x_{6/2+1}\} = \{x_3, x_4\} \, .$$

Thus when N is even, θ is contained in each interval, the sum within each set of nested intervals is minimized and, therefore, the total sum of absolute deviations, D_θ, is also minimized.

Example of the Median with N Odd

Next consider N odd where, for example, $x_1 = 3$, $x_2 = 7$, $x_3 = 11$, $x_4 = 15$, and $x_5 = 20$ and the median is

$$\tilde{x} = x_{(N+1)/2} = x_{(5+1)/2} = x_3 = 11 \, .$$

The outermost interval is $\{x_1, x_N\} = \{x_1, x_5\} = \{3, 20\}$ and the median of $\{3, 7, 11, 15, 20\}$ is $\tilde{x} = 11$.

The first nested interval is $\{x_2, x_{N-1}\} = \{x_2, x_{5-1}\} = \{x_2, x_4\} = \{7, 15\}$ and the median of $\{7, 11, 15\}$ is $\tilde{x} = 11$. The innermost nested interval is $\{x_3, x_{N-2}\} = \{x_3, x_{5-2}\} = x_3, x_3 = \{11, 11\} = 11$ and the median of $\{11, 11\}$ is $\tilde{x} = 11$, which corresponds to

$$\{x_{(N+1)/2}, x_{(N+1)/2}\} = \{x_{(5+1)/2}, x_{(5+1)/2}\} = \{x_3, x_3\} \, .$$

Thus when N is odd the innermost interval is equal to the median. Since θ is contained in each interval, the sum within each set of nested intervals is minimized and, therefore, the total sum of absolute deviations, D_θ, is also minimized.

4.3.1   The Sample Mean Absolute Deviation

The conventional measure of variability about the sample median is the mean absolute deviation given by

$$\text{MAD} = \frac{1}{N} \sum_{i=1}^{N} |x_i - \tilde{x}| \, .$$

Thus for the sample data given in Table 4.6 the sample median is

$$\tilde{x} = \frac{x_{N/2} + x_{N/2+1}}{2} = \frac{x_{6/2} + x_{6/2+1}}{2} = \frac{x_3 + x_4}{2} = \frac{11 + 15}{2} = \frac{26}{2} = 13$$

and the mean absolute deviation is

$$\text{MAD} = \frac{|28 - 13| + |20 - 13| + \cdots + |3 - 13|}{6} = \frac{42}{6} = 7.00 \, .$$

Table 4.6 Example
calculations for the mean
absolute deviation

Object	x	$x - \tilde{x}$	$|x - \tilde{x}|$
1	28	+15	15
2	20	+7	7
3	15	+2	2
4	11	-2	2
5	7	-6	6
6	3	-10	10
Sum			42

Table 4.7 Example
frequency data for an
open-ended distribution

Income	f
More than 99,999	12
80,000–99,999	31
60,000–79,999	54
40,000–59,999	45
20,000–39,999	26
0–19,999	17

4.4   Comparisons Among the Three Measures

For symmetrical, unimodal distributions, the arithmetic mean, the median, and the mode yield approximately the same value. For asymmetrical, skewed, unimodal distributions, the mean, the median, and the mode usually diverge yielding somewhat different values, depending on the degree and direction of skewness. For negatively skewed distributions, the mean is usually the lowest of the three values, the median is usually the middle of the three values, and mode is usually the highest of the three values. As a handy mnemonic, the three values appear as they do in a dictionary, starting from the left tail: mean, median, and mode. For positively skewed unimodal distributions, the order is mean, median, and mode, starting from the right tail.

The sample mode is the only measure of central tendency appropriate for categorical data and that is its primary role in contemporary statistics. The sample median is usually the measure of choice for skewed distributions, as it is largely unaffected by a few extreme values, and open-ended distributions where the upper limit of the top category is undetermined, as illustrated in Table 4.7. As one humorist put it long ago, the arithmetic mean is the mode in statistical analysis, meaning it is the most frequently used measure of central tendency. The sample mean possesses mathematical properties that become very important under the Neyman–Pearson population model of inference. A principal disadvantage of the arithmetic mean is that it can be greatly affected by even a few extreme values.

4.4.1   The Effects of Extreme Values

Extreme values, or outliers, are the bugbear of applied research and occur commonly. Sometimes extreme values are due to coding errors, but more often than not extreme values occur because the variable of interest is skewed. In the social sciences, the skew is most often positive, leading to extreme values in the right-hand tail. Examples of positively skewed distributions are family income, prices of houses, age at first marriage, length of engagement or marriage, birth weight of infants, and body weight of adults. Micceri provided a number of examples of skewed distributions in psychology, finding that fewer than 7% of large sample data sets displayed tail weights and symmetry similar to a normal distribution [4]. Newman, in discussing power-law distributions, provides other examples of positively skewed distributions: sales of book titles, populations of cities, frequencies of words in human languages, the number of "hits" on web pages, the number of citations of academic papers, the financial net worth of individuals, the magnitudes of earthquakes and solar flares, and the sizes of craters on the moon [5].

In 2017 David Salsburg recounted an experience he once had at Pfizer Pharmaceutical Corporation (PPC) when analyzing the weights of rats in a toxicological experiment [7, pp. 85–86]. The strain of rats used in the study usually weighed between 200 and 300 g, with females weighing slightly less than males. He was surprised to discover in the data a single female rat weighing 2000 g and even more surprised to discover that it was not a coding error and was a bona fide rat from the same species. Salsburg noted:

> Just because a value is an outlier, it doesn't mean it should not be used. Throwing out data that appear to be wild shots can lead to erroneous conclusions [7, p. 91].

Salsburg concluded:

> [I]f I had used the median in my analysis of weights of rats, then the 2000 g female rat would not have pulled my estimate of the mean in its direction [7, p. 91].

4.5   An Alternative Approach

More succinctly, consider an alternate, more general, approach to the mean and median based on paired differences given by

$$\sum_{i=1}^{N-1} \sum_{j=i+1}^{N} \left| x_i - x_j \right|^v$$

where $x_1, \ldots, x_N$ are univariate response measurements. Let $x_{1,N} \leq \cdots \leq x_{N,N}$ denote the order statistics associated with $x_1, \ldots, x_N$. If $v = 1$, then the inequality given by

$$\sum_{i=1}^{N-1} \sum_{j=i+1}^{N} |x_i - x_j| \leq \sum_{i=1}^{N} |N - 2i + 1| |x_{i,N} - \theta| \tag{4.1}$$

holds for all θ and equality holds if θ is the median ($\tilde{x}$) of $x_1, \ldots, x_N$. If $v = 2$, then the inequality given by

$$\sum_{i=1}^{N-1} \sum_{j=i+1}^{N} (x_i - x_j)^2 \leq N \sum_{i=1}^{N} (x_i - \theta)^2 \tag{4.2}$$

holds for all θ and equality holds if θ is the mean ($\bar{x}$) of $x_1, \ldots, x_N$.

To illustrate Eq. (4.2), consider the small set of data with the values for $N = 6$ objects listed in Table 4.8 where the arithmetic mean is

$$\bar{x} = \frac{1}{N} \sum_{i=1}^{N} x_i = \frac{9 + 8 + 8 + 8 + 8 + 7}{6} = \frac{48}{6} = 8$$

and

$$N \sum_{i=1}^{N} (x_i - \bar{x})^2 = 6(2) = 12 \ .$$

Table 4.9 lists the pairwise differences and squared pairwise differences for the data listed in Table 4.8. Tables 4.8 and 4.9 illustrate that when θ is equal to the mean,

$$\sum_{i=1}^{N-1} \sum_{j=i+1}^{N} (x_i - x_j)^2 = N \sum_{i=1}^{N} (x_i - \bar{x})^2 \ ;$$

Table 4.8 Illustration of the sum-of-squared deviations about the mean

Object	x	$x - \bar{x}$	$(x - \bar{x})^2$
1	9	1	1
2	8	0	0
3	8	0	0
4	8	0	0
5	8	0	0
6	7	1	1
Sum	48		2

Table 4.9 Illustration of the sum-of-squared pairwise differences

Objects	Pairs	$x_i - x_j$	$(x_i - x_j)^2$
1–2	9–8	1	1
1–3	9–8	1	1
1–4	9–8	1	1
1–5	9–8	1	1
1–6	9–7	2	4
2–3	8–8	0	0
2–4	8–8	0	0
2–5	8–8	0	0
2–6	8–7	1	1
3–4	8–8	0	0
3–5	8–8	0	0
3–6	8–7	1	1
4–5	8–8	0	0
4–6	8–7	1	1
5–6	8–7	1	1
Sum			12

that is, $12 = 12$. It follows that the sample standard deviation can be defined in terms of all possible pairs; that is,

$$
s_x = \left[\frac{1}{N-1} \sum_{i=1}^{N} (x_i - \bar{x})^2 \right]^{1/2}
$$

$$
= \left[\frac{1}{N(N-1)} \sum_{i=1}^{N-1} \sum_{j=i+1}^{N} (x_i - x_j)^2 \right]^{1/2} . \qquad (4.3)
$$

The Italian statistician Corrado Gini was most probably the first to note that the sum-of-squares of deviations from the mean for N quantitative measurements can be expressed solely as a function of the squares of the pairwise differences for all $\binom{N}{2}$ pairs [3].

To illustrate the equivalence of the two equations for the sample standard deviation, consider the small set of data listed in Table 4.8 with $N = 6$ objects. For the conventional expression on the left side of Eq. (4.3),

$$
s_x = \left[\frac{(9-8)^2 + (8-8)^2 + \cdots + (7-8)^2}{6-1} \right]^{1/2} = \left(\frac{2}{5} \right)^{1/2} = 0.6325
$$

and for the pairwise expression on the right side of Eq. (4.3),

$$s_x = \left[\frac{(9-8)^2 + (9-8)^2 + (9-8)^2 + \cdots + (8-7)^2 + (8-7)^2}{6(6-1)} \right]^{1/2}$$

$$= \left(\frac{12}{30} \right)^{1/2} = 0.6325 \ .$$

To illustrate Eq. (4.1) on p. 96, consider once again the example data listed in Table 4.8 where the median is

$$\tilde{x} = \frac{x_{N/2} + x_{N/2+1}}{2} = \frac{x_{6/2} + x_{6/2+1}}{2} = \frac{x_3 + x_4}{2} = \frac{8+8}{2} = \frac{16}{2} = 8.00 \ .$$

Table 4.10 lists the pairwise absolute differences about the median for the data listed in Table 4.8. Table 4.11 illustrates the relationship between the sum of the adjusted absolute differences and the median. Tables 4.10 and 4.11 illustrate that when θ is equal to the median,

$$\sum_{i=1}^{N-1} \sum_{j=i+1}^{N} |x_i - x_j| = \sum_{i=1}^{N} |N - 2i + 1| |x_{i,N} - \tilde{x}| \ ;$$

that is, $10 = 10$.

Table 4.10 Illustration of the sum of absolute pairwise differences

Objects	Pairs	$x_i - x_j$	$|x_i - x_j|$
1–2	9–8	1	1
1–3	9–8	1	1
1–4	9–8	1	1
1–5	9–8	1	1
1–6	9–7	2	2
2–3	8–8	0	0
2–4	8–8	0	0
2–5	8–8	0	0
2–6	8–7	1	1
3–4	8–8	0	0
3–5	8–8	0	0
3–6	8–7	1	1
4–5	8–8	0	0
4–6	8–7	1	1
5–6	8–7	1	1
Sum			10

Table 4.11 Illustration of the sum of adjusted absolute differences about the median

i	$x_{i,N}$	$|N - 2i + 1|$	$|x_{i,N} - \tilde{x}|$	$|N - 2i + 1||x_{i,N} - \tilde{x}|$
1	9	$|6 - 2(1) + 1| = 5$	$|9 - 8| = 1$	5
2	8	$|6 - 2(2) + 1| = 3$	$|8 - 8| = 0$	0
3	8	$|6 - 2(3) + 1| = 1$	$|8 - 8| = 0$	0
4	8	$|6 - 2(4) + 1| = 1$	$|8 - 8| = 0$	0
5	8	$|6 - 2(5) + 1| = 3$	$|8 - 8| = 0$	0
6	7	$|6 - 2(6) + 1| = 5$	$|7 - 8| = 1$	5
Sum				10

4.6 Summary

This chapter provided an overview of the conventional measures of central tendency and variability—the two most basic and essential concepts underlying statistical methodology. For measures of central tendency, the sample mode, sample median, and sample mean were defined and illustrated. Special attention was paid to the sample mean as a minimizing function for the sum-of-squared deviations and the sample median as a minimizing function for the sum of absolute deviations. For measures of variability, the sample standard deviation and the mean absolute deviation were described and illustrated. Finally, an alternative approach to the mean and median based on paired squared and paired absolute differences between values was introduced. A recurring theme in the following chapters is the comparison between mean-based and median-based test statistics and the treatment of extreme values.

Chapter 5 considers one-sample tests of differences. The conventional one-sample t test is presented and compared to a permutation alternative based on all paired differences between values. Six examples illustrate permutation statistical methods applied to one-sample tests. The first example is deliberately kept small to illustrate the computations required for a one-sample permutation test. The second example develops a chance-corrected alternative to conventional measures of effect size for one-sample tests. The third example compares permutation statistical methods based on ordinary and squared Euclidean scaling functions. The fourth example compares exact and Monte Carlo permutation methods for one-sample tests. The fifth example illustrates the application of permutation statistical methods to univariate rank-score data. And the sixth example illustrates the application of permutation statistical methods to multivariate data.

References

1. David, H.A.: First (?) occurrence of common terms in mathematical statistics. Am. Stat. **49**, 121–133 (1995)
2. Galton, F.: Report of the anthropometric committee. Report of the 51st Meeting of the British Association for the Advancement of Science, pp. 245–260 (1882)
3. Gini, C.W.: Variabilità e Mutuabilità. Contributo allo Studio delle Distribuzioni e delle Relazioni Statistiche. C. Cuppini, Bologna (1912)
4. Micceri, T.: The unicorn, the normal curve, and other improbable creatures. Psychol. Bull. **105**, 156–166 (1989)
5. Newman, M.: Power-law distribution. Significance **14**, 10–11 (2017)
6. Raper, S.: The shock of the mean. Significance **14**, 12–16 (2017)
7. Salsburg, D.S.: Errors, Blunders, and Lies: How to Tell the Difference. CRC Press, Boca Raton (2017)
8. Schwertman, N.C., Gilks, A.J., Cameron, J.: A simple noncalculus proof that the median minimizes the sum of the absolute deviations. Am. Stat. **44**, 38–39 (1990)

Chapter 5
One-Sample Tests

Abstract This chapter introduces permutation methods for one-sample tests. Included in this chapter are six example analyses illustrating computation of exact permutation probability values for one-sample tests, calculation of measures of effect size for one-sample tests, the effect of extreme values on conventional and permutation one-sample tests, exact and Monte Carlo permutation procedures for one-sample tests, application of permutation methods to one-sample rank-score data, and analysis of one-sample multivariate data. Included in this chapter are permutation versions of Student's one-sample t test, Wilcoxon's signed-ranks test, the sign test, and a permutation-based alternative for the two conventional measures of effect size for one-sample tests: Cohen's $\hat{d}$ and Pearson's r^2.

This chapter presents exact and Monte Carlo permutation statistical methods for one-sample tests. Also presented is a permutation-based measure of effect size for one-sample tests. One-sample tests are the simplest of a large family of statistical tests and provide an introduction to the two-sample and multi-sample tests presented in later chapters.

In this chapter, permutation statistical methods for analyzing one-sample tests are illustrated with six example analyses. The first example utilizes a small set of data to illustrate the computation of exact permutation methods for a single sample, wherein the permutation test statistic, δ, is developed and compared with Student's conventional one-sample t test statistic. The second example develops a permutation-based measure of effect size as a chance-corrected alternative to the two conventional measures of effect size for one-sample tests: Cohen's $\hat{d}$ and Pearson's r^2. The third example compares permutation statistical methods based on ordinary and squared Euclidean scaling functions, with an emphasis on the analysis of data sets containing extreme values. The fourth example utilizes a larger data set for providing comparisons of exact and Monte Carlo permutation methods, demonstrating the efficiency and accuracy of Monte Carlo statistical methods for one-sample tests. The fifth example illustrates the application of permutation statistical methods to univariate rank-score data, comparing permutation statistical methods with Wilcoxon's conventional signed-ranks test and the sign test. The sixth

© Springer Nature Switzerland AG 2019

K. J. Berry et al., *A Primer of Permutation Statistical Methods*,
https://doi.org/10.1007/978-3-030-20933-9_5

example illustrates the application of permutation statistical methods to multivariate one-sample tests.

5.1 Introduction

The most popular univariate one-sample test is Student's t test wherein the null hypothesis (H_0) under the Neyman–Pearson population model posits a value for a population parameter, such as a population mean, from which a random sample is presumed to have been drawn; that is, H_0: $\mu_x = \theta$, where θ is a specified value. For example, the null hypothesis might stipulate that the average IQ score in the population from which a sample has been drawn is H_0: $\mu_x = 100$. The test does not determine whether or not the null hypothesis is true, but only provides the probability that, if the null hypothesis is true, the sample has been drawn from a population with the specified value.

Consider Student's conventional one-sample t test. Under the Neyman–Pearson population model of statistical inference the null hypothesis is given by H_0: $\mu_x = \theta$ and the two-tail alternative hypothesis is given by H_1: $\mu_x \neq \theta$, where θ is a hypothesized value for the population mean. The permissible probability of a type I error is denoted by α and if the observed value of t is more extreme than the critical values of $\pm t$ that define α, the null hypothesis is rejected with a probability of type I error equal to or less than α.

For a one-sample t test with N cases, Student's one-sample t test statistic is given by

$$ t = \frac{\bar{x} - \theta}{s_{\bar{x}}} \, , $$

where $\bar{x}$ denotes the arithmetic mean of the observed sample values given by

$$ \bar{x} = \frac{1}{N} \sum_{i=1}^{N} x_i \, , $$

x_i denotes the ith observed sample value for $i = 1, \ldots, N$, $s_{\bar{x}}$ denotes the sample-estimated standard error of $\bar{x}$ given by

$$ s_{\bar{x}} = \frac{s_x}{\sqrt{N}} \, , $$

and s_x denotes the sample-estimated population standard deviation of variable x given by

$$ s_x = \left[\frac{1}{N-1} \sum_{i=1}^{N} (x_i - \bar{x})^2 \right]^{1/2} . $$

Technically, $\bar{x}$ is the unbiased estimator of the population mean, μ_x; $s_{\bar{x}}^2$ is the unbiased estimator of the population variance, σ_x^2; s_x is the estimated population standard deviation, σ_x; and $s_{\bar{x}}$ is the estimated population standard error, $\sigma_{\bar{x}}$. For simplification, in this book $\bar{x}$ is designated the sample mean; s_x^2, the sample variance; s_x, the sample standard deviation; and $s_{\bar{x}}$, the standard error of $\bar{x}$. The null hypothesis is rejected when the observed t test statistic exceeds the critical $\pm t$ values defined by α for Student's t distribution with $N - 1$ degrees of freedom, under the assumption of normality.[1]

The assumptions underlying Student's one-sample t test are (1) the observations are independent, (2) the data are a random sample from a well-defined population, and (3) target variable x is normally distributed in the population.

5.1.1 A Permutation Approach

Consider a one-sample test under the Fisher–Pitman permutation model of statistical inference. As discussed in Chap. 3, the Fisher–Pitman permutation model differs greatly from the Neyman–Pearson population model. Under the Fisher–Pitman permutation model there is no null hypothesis specifying a population parameter. Instead, the null hypothesis simply states that all possible arrangements of the observed data occur with equal chance [17]. Also, there is no alternative hypothesis under the Fisher–Pitman permutation model, no degrees of freedom, and no specified α level. Moreover, there is no requirement of random sampling and no assumption of normality. Finally, the Fisher–Pitman permutation statistical model provides exact probability values.

A permutation alternative to a conventional one-sample t test based on paired differences between sample values is easily defined [2]. Let x_i denote the observed sample values for $i = 1, \ldots, N$. The permutation test statistic is given by

$$\delta = \binom{N}{2}^{-1} \sum_{i=1}^{N-1} \sum_{j=i+1}^{N} |x_i - x_j|^v , \tag{5.1}$$

where for correspondence with Student's one-sample t test, $v = 2$.

Under the Fisher–Pitman null hypothesis the exact probability of an observed δ is the proportion of δ test statistic values calculated on all possible arrangements of the observed data that are equal to or less than the observed value of δ; that is,

$$P(\delta \leq \delta_0 | H_0) = \frac{\text{number of } \delta \text{ values} \leq \delta_0}{M} ,$$

---

[1] The symbol α indicates the probability of type I error: rejection of a true null hypothesis. For much of the history of statistics $\alpha = 0.05$ has been almost sacred [32]. However, more stringent values of α have recently been advanced, some as small as $\alpha = 0.005$ [1, 10].

where δ_o denotes the observed value of test statistic δ and M is the number of possible, equally-likely arrangements of the observed data.

5.1.2   The Relationship Between Statistics t and δ

Whenever a one-sample t test posits a value for the population mean other than zero, comparing Student's t statistic to other test statistics requires an adjustment to compensate for the hypothesized mean value. Consider Student's one-sample t test given by

$$t = \frac{\bar{x} - \theta}{s_{\bar{x}}} \, ,$$

where θ represents a hypothesized value for the population mean. Then

$$t^2 = \frac{(\bar{x} - \theta)^2}{s_{\bar{x}}^2}$$

$$= \frac{\bar{x}^2 - 2\bar{x}\theta + \theta^2}{s_{\bar{x}}^2}$$

$$= \frac{\bar{x}^2}{s_{\bar{x}}^2} - \frac{\theta(2\bar{x} - \theta)}{s_{\bar{x}}^2} \, .$$

Let C represent the adjustment factor given by

$$C = \frac{\theta(2\bar{x} - \theta)}{s_{\bar{x}}^2} \, .$$

Then under the Neyman–Pearson null hypothesis, H_0: $\mu_x = \theta$, with $\theta \neq 0$ and $v = 2$, the relationships between δ and Student's one-sample t statistic are given by

$$\delta = \frac{2 \sum\limits_{i=1}^{N} x_i^2}{t^2 + N - 1 + C} \tag{5.2}$$

and

$$t = \left(\frac{2}{\delta} \sum\limits_{i=1}^{N} x_i^2 - N + 1 - C \right)^{1/2} . \tag{5.3}$$

5.2   Example 1: Test Statistics t and δ

An example will serve to illustrate the relationship between test statistics t and δ for a one-sample test. For simplicity, consider a small set of data with $N = 4$, $x_1 = 9$, $x_2 = 7$, $x_3 = 5$, $x_4 = 2$, and let the null hypothesis be H_0: $\mu_x = 3$. For these example data under the Neyman–Pearson population model of statistical inference the sample mean is $\bar{x} = 5.75$, the sample standard deviation is $s_x = 2.9861$, the standard error of $\bar{x}$ is

$$s_{\bar{x}} = \frac{s_x}{\sqrt{N}} = \frac{2.9861}{\sqrt{4}} = 1.4930 \, ,$$

Student's t test statistic is

$$t = \frac{\bar{x} - \mu_x}{s_{\bar{x}}} = \frac{5.75 - 3}{1.4930} = +1.8419 \, ,$$

and the adjustment factor is

$$C = \frac{\mu_x(2\bar{x} - \mu_x)}{s_{\bar{x}}^2} = \frac{3[2(5.75) - 3]}{(1.4930)^2} = 11.4393 \, .$$

Under the Neyman–Pearson null hypothesis, H_0: $\mu_x = 3$, test statistic t is asymptotically distributed as Student's t with $N - 1$ degrees of freedom. With $N - 1 = 4 - 1 = 3$ degrees of freedom, the asymptotic two-tail probability value of $t = +1.8419$ is $P = 0.1627$, under the assumption of normality.

For the same data under the Fisher–Pitman permutation model with $v = 2$, the sum of the squared differences between all pairs of observations is

$$\sum_{i=1}^{N-1} \sum_{j=i+1}^{N} |x_i - x_j|^2$$

$$= |9 - 7|^2 + |9 - 5|^2 + |9 - 2|^2 + |7 - 5|^2 + |7 - 2|^2 + |5 - 2|^2 = 107$$

and following Eq. (5.1) with $v = 2$, the observed value of test statistic δ is

$$\delta = \binom{N}{2}^{-1} \sum_{i=1}^{N-1} \sum_{j=i+1}^{N} |x_i - x_j|^2 = \binom{4}{2}^{-1} (107) = \frac{2(107)}{4(4 - 1)} = 17.8333 \, .$$

Following the expressions given in Eqs. (5.2) and (5.3) for the relationships between test statistics δ and t, the observed value of test statistic δ with respect to the observed value of test statistic t is

$$\delta = \frac{2\sum\limits_{i=1}^{N} x_i^2}{t^2 + N - 1 + C} = \frac{2(9^2 + 7^2 + 5^2 + 2^2)}{(1.8419)^2 + 4 - 1 + 11.4393} = 17.8333$$

and the observed value of test statistic t with respect to the observed value of test statistic δ is

$$t = \left(\frac{2}{\delta} \sum_{i=1}^{N} x_i^2 - N + 1 - C \right)^{1/2}$$

$$= \left[\frac{2(9^2 + 7^2 + 5^2 + 2^2)}{17.8333} - 4 + 1 - 11.4393 \right]^{1/2} = \pm 1.8419 .$$

Because of the relationship between test statistics δ and t, the probability values given by

$$P(\delta \le \delta_o) = \frac{\text{number of } \delta \text{ values } \le \delta_o}{M}$$

and

$$P(|t| \ge |t_o|) = \frac{\text{number of } |t| \text{ values } \ge |t_o|}{M}$$

are equivalent under the Fisher–Pitman null hypothesis, where δ_o and t_o denote the observed values of test statistics δ and t, respectively, and M is the number of possible, equally-likely arrangements of the observed data.

To establish the exact probability of $\delta = 17.8333$ (or $t = \pm 1.8419$) under the Fisher–Pitman permutation model, it is necessary to enumerate completely all possible arrangements of the observed data, of which there are only

$$M = 2^N = 2^4 = 16$$

possible, equally-likely arrangements in the reference set of all permutations of the observed data. It is imperative that the M possible arrangements be generated systematically while preserving N values for each arrangement. Only a systematic procedure guarantees M equally-likely arrangements. Simply shuffling values does not ensure the M possible, equally-likely arrangements mandated by the permutation null hypothesis: all possible arrangements of the observed data occur with equal chance [17].

Let $y_i = x_i z_i$ denote the transformed x_i values for $i = 1, \ldots, N$, where z_i is either plus or minus one. Table 5.1 lists the $M = 16$ z, y, δ, and $|t|$ values. For test statistic δ there are only two δ test statistic values that are equal to or less than

Table 5.1 Calculation of δ and $|t|$ values for $x_1 = 9$, $x_2 = 7$, $x_3 = 5$, and $x_4 = 2$

Number	z	y	δ	$|t|$
1*	$+1 \ +1 \ +1 \ +1$	$+9 \ +7 \ +5 \ +2$	17.8333	1.8419
2	$+1 \ +1 \ +1 \ -1$	$+9 \ +7 \ +5 \ -2$	45.8333	0.7311
3	$+1 \ +1 \ -1 \ +1$	$+9 \ +7 \ -5 \ +2$	77.8333	0.0801
4	$+1 \ -1 \ +1 \ +1$	$+9 \ -7 \ +5 \ +2$	92.5000	0.2206
5	$-1 \ +1 \ +1 \ +1$	$-9 \ +7 \ +5 \ +2$	101.8333	0.4905
6	$-1 \ -1 \ +1 \ +1$	$-9 \ -7 \ +5 \ +2$	92.5000	0.2206
7	$+1 \ +1 \ -1 \ -1$	$+9 \ +7 \ -5 \ -2$	92.5000	0.2206
8	$+1 \ -1 \ +1 \ -1$	$+9 \ -7 \ +5 \ -2$	101.8333	0.4905
9	$-1 \ +1 \ -1 \ +1$	$-9 \ +7 \ -5 \ +2$	101.8333	0.4905
10	$+1 \ -1 \ -1 \ +1$	$+9 \ -7 \ -5 \ +2$	105.8333	0.7561
11	$-1 \ +1 \ +1 \ -1$	$-9 \ +7 \ +5 \ -2$	105.8333	0.7561
12	$-1 \ -1 \ -1 \ +1$	$-9 \ -7 \ -5 \ +2$	45.8333	0.7311
13	$-1 \ -1 \ +1 \ -1$	$-9 \ -7 \ +5 \ -2$	77.8333	0.0801
14	$-1 \ +1 \ -1 \ -1$	$-9 \ +7 \ -5 \ -2$	92.5000	0.2206
15	$+1 \ -1 \ -1 \ -1$	$+9 \ -7 \ -5 \ -2$	101.8333	0.4905
16*	$-1 \ -1 \ -1 \ -1$	$-9 \ -7 \ -5 \ -2$	17.8333	1.8419
Sum			1272.0000	

the observed value of $\delta = 17.8333$ (numbers 1 and 16 indicated with asterisks) in Table 5.1. Then if all M arrangements of the $N = 4$ observations occur with equal chance under the Fisher–Pitman null hypothesis, the exact probability value of $\delta = 17.8333$ is

$$P(\delta \le \delta_0) = \frac{\text{number of } \delta \text{ values } \le \delta_0}{M} = \frac{2}{16} = 0.1250 \, ,$$

where δ_0 denotes the observed value of test statistic δ and M is the number of possible, equally-likely arrangements of the observed data.

Alternatively, for test statistic t there are only two $|t|$ values that are equal to or greater than the observed value of $|t| = 1.8419$ (numbers 1 and 16 indicated with asterisks) in Table 5.1. Then if all M arrangements of the $N = 4$ observations occur with equal chance, the exact probability value under the Fisher–Pitman null hypothesis is

$$P(|t| \ge |t_0|) = \frac{\text{number of } |t| \text{ values } \ge |t_0|}{M} = \frac{2}{16} = 0.1250 \, ,$$

where t_0 denotes the observed value of test statistic t.

It is readily apparent from Table 5.1 that the δ and $|t|$ values possess duplicate values, for example, $\delta_1 = \delta_{16} = 17.8333$, $\delta_2 = \delta_{12} = 45.8333$, $\delta_3 = \delta_{13} = 77.8333$, and so on. Therefore, it is only necessary to generate

$$M = 2^{N-1} = 2^{4-1} = 8 \quad \text{instead of} \quad M = 2^N = 2^4 = 16$$

Table 5.2 Calculation of δ and $|t|$ values for $x_1 = 9$, $x_2 = 7$, $x_3 = 5$, and $x_4 = 2$

Number	z	y	δ	$|t|$
1	$+1 +1 +1 +1$	$+9 +7 +5 +2$	17.8333	1.8419
2	$+1 +1 +1 -1$	$+9 +7 +5 -2$	45.8333	0.7311
3	$+1 +1 -1 +1$	$+9 +7 -5 +2$	77.8333	0.0801
4	$+1 -1 +1 +1$	$+9 -7 +5 +2$	92.5000	0.2206
5	$-1 -1 +1 +1$	$-9 -7 +5 +2$	92.5000	0.2206
6	$-1 +1 +1 +1$	$-9 +7 +5 +2$	101.8333	0.4905
7	$+1 -1 +1 -1$	$+9 -7 +5 -2$	101.8333	0.4905
8	$+1 -1 -1 +1$	$+9 -7 -5 +2$	105.8333	0.7561

equally-likely arrangements of the observed data, holding one of the four values constant. Table 5.2 lists the $M = 8$ non-duplicated values ordered by the δ values from low ($\delta_1 = 17.8333$) to high ($\delta_8 = 105.8333$).

5.2.1   The Choice Between Test Statistics t and δ

An obvious question arises at this juncture: Why introduce test statistic δ when the same exact probability value can be obtained with the more familiar t test statistic? There are two answers to this question. First, test statistic δ is a powerful substitute for Student's t test statistic as it is easily generalizable to more complex research designs. In the general form given in Eq. (5.1) on p. 103 and with small modifications, δ can replace the conventional test statistics in one-sample tests, matched-pairs tests, tests for two independent samples, the full range of completely-randomized and randomized-blocks analysis of variance designs, and a large number of parametric and nonparametric tests of differences and measures of association and correlation [3, 4].

Second, while conventional tests such as Student's t test are limited to squared Euclidean differences between values, test statistic δ has no such limitation. Test statistic δ can utilize a wide range of scaling functions, but ordinary Euclidean scaling appears to be the most useful. It is essentially true that permutation tests can be designed for any conventional test statistic.[2] Then it is simply a matter of completely enumerating all possible values of the specified test statistic and determining the exact probability of the observed value. On the other hand, test statistic δ is a general test statistic with a universe of applications, which can not

---

[2]There exists a small class of statistical tests for which a permutation approach is inappropriate. Tests such as Wald's likelihood-ratio tests for goodness-of-fit and independence rely on natural logarithms and it is inevitable that under permutation some cell arrangements will contain one or more zero values. Since $\ln(0) = -\infty$, a permutation test will fail under these conditions, unless further adjustments are made to the permuted arrangements.

only replace many conventional statistics, but also define and create new statistical tests of differences and measures of association [3, 4].

5.3 The Measurement of Effect Size

The fact that a statistical test produces low probability values indicates only that there are differences among the variables that (possibly) cannot be attributed to error. The obtained probability value does not indicate whether or not these differences are of any practical value. Measures of effect size express the practical or clinical significance of a difference between the sample mean and the hypothesized population mean, as contrasted with the statistical significance of the difference. As Roger Kirk noted many years ago, a test statistic and its associated probability value therefore provide no information as to the size of treatment effects, only whether or not the effects are statistically significant [20, p. 135]. Measures of effect size have become increasingly important in recent years as they index the magnitude of a treatment effect and indicate the practical significance of the research.

It was American psychologists who spearheaded the reporting of effect sizes in academic journals. For many years, statisticians and psychometricians who were Fellows of the American Psychological Association (APA), Division 5, urged the editors of APA journals to mandate the reporting of effect sizes. The fourth edition of the *Publication Manual of the American Psychological Association* strongly encouraged reporting measures of effect size in conjunction with tests of significance. In 1999 the APA Task Force on Statistical Inference under the leadership of Leland Wilkinson noted that "reporting and interpreting effect sizes in the context of previously reported effects is essential to good research" [34, p. 599]. Consequently, a number of editors of academic journals, both APA and others, began requiring measures of effect size as a condition of publication. In recent years, there has been increased emphasis on reporting measures of effect size in addition to tests of significance in a number of academic disciplines, recognizing that determination of a significant treatment effect does not necessarily translate into a clinical effect. As a result, numerous journals now require the reporting of measures of effect size as part of their editorial policies [8, 9].

Statisticians and quantitative methodologists have raised a number of issues and concerns with null hypothesis statistical testing (NHST). A brief overview is provided by Cowles:

> The main criticisms [of NHST], endlessly repeated, are easily listed. NHST does not offer any way of testing the alternative or research hypothesis; the null hypothesis is usually false and when differences or relationships are trivial, large samples will lead to its rejection; the method discourages replication and encourages one-shot research; the inferential model depends on assumptions about hypothetical populations and data that cannot be verified ... [14, p. 83].

In addition, there are literally hundreds of articles, chapters, editorials, and blogs dealing with the problems of NHST, far too many to be summarized here. However, a brief overview of the limitations of null hypothesis statistical testing will suffice for these purposes.

First, the null hypothesis is almost never literally true, so rejection of the null hypothesis is relatively uninformative [14]. Second, tests of significance are highly dependent on sample sizes. When sample sizes are small, important effects can be non-significant, and when sample sizes are large, even trivial effects can produce very small probability values. Third, the requirement of obtaining a random sample from a well-defined population is seldom met in practice. Fourth, the assumption of normality is never satisfied in real-data situations.

As Roger Kirk explained in 1996 [21, p. 747], the one individual most responsible for bringing the shortcomings of hypothesis testing to the attention of researchers was the psychologist Jacob Cohen with two articles in the *American Psychologist* titled "Things I have learned (so far)" in 1990 [12] and "The earth is round $(p < .05)$" in 1994 [13]. As a result of the identified challenges with null hypothesis statistical testing and the reporting of probability values, various measures of effect size have been designed to reflect the substantive importance and practical significance of differences among variables. Simply put, for a one-sample test effect size refers to the magnitude of the impact of an independent variable on a dependent variable [22, p. 97].

Three types of measures of effect size have been advanced to represent the magnitude of treatment effects [28]. One type, designated the d family, is based on one or more measures of the differences among the treatment groups or among levels of an independent variable. Representative of the d family is Cohen's $\hat{d}$, which measures the effect size by the number of standard deviations separating the sample mean from the hypothesized population mean for a one-sample test, or the sample means of the treatment groups for a two-sample test.

The second type of measure of effect size, designated the r family, represents some sort of relationship among variables. Measures of effect size in the r family are typically measures of correlation or association, the most prominent being Pearson's squared product-moment correlation coefficient; that is, Pearson's r^2 coefficient of determination.

The third type of measure of effect size, designated the $\mathfrak{R}$ family, represents chance-corrected measures of effect size, sometimes termed "improvement-over-chance" measures of effect size [16]. Chance-corrected measures have much to commend them as they provide interpretations that are easily understood by the average reader. Positive values indicate an effect size greater than expected by chance with a value of $+1$ indicating a perfect relationship among variables, negative values indicate an effect size less than expected by chance, and a value of zero indicates a chance effect size.

The usual expressions for measures of effect size for a one-sample test are Cohen's $\hat{d}$ given by

$$\hat{d} = \frac{|\bar{x} - \mu_x|}{s_x},$$

Pearson's r^2 given by

$$r^2 = \frac{t^2}{t^2 + N - 1} , \tag{5.4}$$

and Mielke and Berry's $\mathfrak{R}$ given by

$$\mathfrak{R} = 1 - \frac{\delta}{\mu_\delta} , \tag{5.5}$$

where δ is defined in Eq. (5.1) on p. 103 and μ_δ is the exact expected value of test statistic δ under the Fisher–Pitman null hypothesis given by

$$\mu_\delta = \frac{1}{M} \sum_{i=1}^{M} \delta_i , \tag{5.6}$$

where, for a one-sample test, $M = 2^N$. For calculation purposes, the exact expected value of test statistic δ under the Fisher–Pitman null hypothesis is given by

$$\mu_\delta = \frac{1}{N(N-1)} \sum_{i=1}^{N-1} \sum_{j=i+1}^{N} \left(|x_i - x_j|^2 + |x_i + x_j|^2 \right) . \tag{5.7}$$

5.4 Detailed Calculations for Statistics δ and μ_δ

In this section a detailed example illustrates the calculation of test statistics δ and μ_δ, both necessary for determining the permutation-based measure of effect size,

$$\mathfrak{R} = 1 - \frac{\delta}{\mu_\delta} .$$

Consider the one-sample data listed in Table 5.3 with observations on $N = 9$ subjects.

Table 5.3 Example data for a one-sample permutation test with $N = 9$ subjects

Subject	1	2	3	4	5	6	7	8	9
Score (x)	+2	+1	+4	−1	+2	+5	+1	−2	+4

Table 5.4 Example calculations for δ with $N = 9$ subjects

Difference	$|x_i - x_j|^2$	Difference	$|x_i - x_j|^2$
1	$|+2-(+1)|^2 = 1$	19	$|+4-(+1)|^2 = 9$
2	$|+2-(+4)|^2 = 4$	20	$|+4-(-2)|^2 = 36$
3	$|+2-(-1)|^2 = 9$	21	$|+4-(+4)|^2 = 0$
4	$|+2-(+2)|^2 = 0$	22	$|-1-(+2)|^2 = 9$
5	$|+2-(+5)|^2 = 9$	23	$|-1-(+5)|^2 = 36$
6	$|+2-(+1)|^2 = 1$	24	$|-1-(-1)|^2 = 4$
7	$|+2-(-2)|^2 = 16$	25	$|-1-(-2)|^2 = 1$
8	$|+2-(+4)|^2 = 4$	26	$|-1-(+4)|^2 = 25$
9	$|+1-(+4)|^2 = 9$	27	$|+2-(+5)|^2 = 9$
10	$|+1-(-1)|^2 = 4$	28	$|+2-(+1)|^2 = 1$
11	$|+1-(+2)|^2 = 1$	29	$|+2-(-2)|^2 = 16$
12	$|+1-(+5)|^2 = 16$	30	$|+2-(+4)|^2 = 4$
13	$|+1-(+1)|^2 = 0$	31	$|+5-(+1)|^2 = 16$
14	$|+1-(-2)|^2 = 9$	32	$|+5-(-2)|^2 = 49$
15	$|+1-(+4)|^2 = 9$	33	$|+5-(+4)|^2 = 1$
16	$|+4-(-1)|^2 = 25$	34	$|+1-(-2)|^2 = 9$
17	$|+4-(+2)|^2 = 4$	35	$|+1-(+4)|^2 = 9$
18	$|+4-(+5)|^2 = 1$	36	$|-2-(+4)|^2 = 36$
Sum			392

First, determine all

$$\binom{N}{2} = \binom{9}{2} = \frac{9(9-1)}{2} = 36$$

possible squared pairwise differences between the score (x) values and calculate the sum of the squared differences as illustrated in Table 5.4. Then the observed value of test statistic δ is

$$\delta = \binom{N}{2}^{-1} \sum_{i=1}^{N-1} \sum_{j=i+1}^{N} |x_i - x_j|^2 = \binom{9}{2}^{-1} (392) = \frac{2(392)}{9(9-1)} = 10.8889 \ .$$

Alternatively, in terms of an analysis of variance model the permutation test statistic is

$$\delta = \frac{2SS_{\text{Total}}}{N-1} = \frac{2(43.5556)}{9-1} = 10.8889 \ ,$$

where the sum of the $N = 9$ values is

$$\sum_{i=1}^{N} x_i = 2 + 1 + 4 - 1 + 2 + 5 + 1 - 2 + 4 = 16.00 \ ,$$

the sum of the $N = 9$ squared values is

$$\sum_{i=1}^{N} x_i^2 = (+2)^2 + (+1)^2 + (+4)^2 + (-1)^2 + (+2)^2 + (+5)^2$$

$$+ (+1)^2 + (-2)^2 + (+4)^2 = 72.00 ,$$

and the total sum-of-squares is

$$SS_{\text{Total}} = \sum_{i=1}^{N} x_i^2 - \left(\sum_{i=1}^{N} x_i \right)^2 \Big/ N = 72.00 - (16.00)^2 / 9 = 43.5556 .$$

To find a value for μ_δ, the exact expected value of test statistic δ, two sets of paired values are required, $|x_i - x_j|^2$ and $|x_i + x_j|^2$, and their sums, as given in Table 5.5. Then the exact expected value of test statistic δ under the Fisher–Pitman null hypothesis is

$$\mu_\delta = \frac{1}{N(N - 1)} \sum_{i=1}^{N-1} \sum_{j=i+1}^{N} \left(|x_i - x_j|^2 + |x_i + x_j|^2 \right)$$

$$= \frac{1}{9(9 - 1)} \sum_{i=1}^{9-1} \sum_{j=i+1}^{9} \left(|x_i - x_j|^2 + |x_i + x_j|^2 \right) = \frac{1152}{72} = 16.00 .$$

Finally, the observed chance-corrected measure of effect size is

$$\Re = 1 - \frac{\delta}{\mu_\delta} = 1 - \frac{10.8889}{16.00} = +0.3194 ,$$

indicating approximately 32% agreement among the $N = 9$ scores above what is expected by chance.

5.5   Example 2: Measures of Effect Size

For the example data listed on p. 105 with $N = 4$, $x_1 = 9$, $x_2 = 7$, $x_3 = 5$, $x_4 = 2$, and null hypothesis H_0: $\mu_x = 3$, Cohen's $\hat{d}$ measure of effect size is

$$\hat{d} = \frac{|\bar{x} - \mu_x|}{s_x} = \frac{|5.75 - 3|}{2.9861} = 0.9209 ,$$

Table 5.5 Example calculations for μ_δ with $N = 9$ subjects

Difference	$|x_i - x_j|^2$	$|x_i + x_j|^2$	Sum
1	$|+2 - (+1)|^2 = 1$	$|+2 + (+1)|^2 = 9$	$1 + 9 = 10$
2	$|+2 - (+4)|^2 = 4$	$|+2 + (+4)|^2 = 36$	$4 + 36 = 40$
3	$|+2 - (-1)|^2 = 9$	$|+2 + (-1)|^2 = 1$	$9 + 1 = 10$
4	$|+2 - (+2)|^2 = 0$	$|+2 + (+2)|^2 = 16$	$16 + 0 = 16$
5	$|+2 - (+5)|^2 = 9$	$|+2 + (+5)|^2 = 49$	$49 + 9 = 58$
6	$|+2 - (+1)|^2 = 1$	$|+2 + (+1)|^2 = 9$	$9 + 1 = 10$
7	$|+2 - (-2)|^2 = 16$	$|+2 + (-2)|^2 = 0$	$0 + 16 = 16$
8	$|+2 - (+4)|^2 = 4$	$|+2 + (+4)|^2 = 36$	$36 + 4 = 40$
9	$|+1 - (+4)|^2 = 9$	$|+1 + (+4)|^2 = 25$	$25 + 9 = 34$
10	$|+1 - (-1)|^2 = 4$	$|+1 + (-1)|^2 = 0$	$0 + 4 = 4$
11	$|+1 - (+2)|^2 = 1$	$|+1 + (+2)|^2 = 9$	$9 + 1 = 10$
12	$|+1 - (+5)|^2 = 16$	$|+1 + (+5)|^2 = 36$	$36 + 16 = 52$
13	$|+1 - (+1)|^2 = 0$	$|+1 + (+1)|^2 = 4$	$4 + 0 = 4$
14	$|+1 - (-2)|^2 = 9$	$|+1 + (-2)|^2 = 1$	$1 + 9 = 10$
15	$|+1 - (+4)|^2 = 9$	$|+1 + (+4)|^2 = 25$	$25 + 9 = 34$
16	$|+4 - (-1)|^2 = 25$	$|+4 + (-1)|^2 = 9$	$9 + 25 = 34$
17	$|+4 - (+2)|^2 = 4$	$|+4 + (+2)|^2 = 36$	$36 + 4 = 40$
18	$|+4 - (+5)|^2 = 1$	$|+4 + (+5)|^2 = 81$	$81 + 1 = 82$
19	$|+4 - (+1)|^2 = 9$	$|+4 + (+1)|^2 = 25$	$25 + 9 = 34$
20	$|+4 - (-2)|^2 = 36$	$|+4 + (-2)|^2 = 4$	$4 + 36 = 40$
21	$|+4 - (+4)|^2 = 0$	$|+4 + (+4)|^2 = 64$	$64 + 0 = 64$
22	$|-1 - (+2)|^2 = 9$	$|-1 + (+2)|^2 = 1$	$1 + 9 = 10$
23	$|-1 - (+5)|^2 = 36$	$|-1 + (+5)|^2 = 16$	$16 + 36 = 52$
24	$|-1 - (-1)|^2 = 4$	$|-1 + (-1)|^2 = 0$	$0 + 4 = 4$
25	$|-1 - (-2)|^2 = 1$	$|-1 + (-2)|^2 = 9$	$9 + 1 = 10$
26	$|-1 - (+4)|^2 = 25$	$|-1 + (+4)|^2 = 9$	$9 + 25 = 34$
27	$|+2 - (+5)|^2 = 9$	$|+2 + (+5)|^2 = 49$	$49 + 9 = 58$
28	$|+2 - (+1)|^2 = 1$	$|+2 + (+1)|^2 = 9$	$9 + 1 = 10$
29	$|+2 - (-2)|^2 = 16$	$|+2 + (-2)|^2 = 0$	$0 + 16 = 16$
30	$|+2 - (+4)|^2 = 4$	$|+2 + (+4)|^2 = 36$	$36 + 4 = 40$
31	$|+5 - (+1)|^2 = 16$	$|+5 + (+1)|^2 = 36$	$36 + 16 = 52$
32	$|+5 - (-2)|^2 = 49$	$|+5 + (-2)|^2 = 9$	$9 + 49 = 58$
33	$|+5 - (+4)|^2 = 1$	$|+5 + (+4)|^2 = 81$	$81 + 1 = 82$
34	$|+1 - (-2)|^2 = 9$	$|+1 + (-2)|^2 = 1$	$1 + 9 = 10$
35	$|+1 - (+4)|^2 = 9$	$|+1 + (+4)|^2 = 25$	$25 + 9 = 34$
36	$|-2 - (+4)|^2 = 36$	$|-2 + (+4)|^2 = 4$	$4 + 36 = 40$
Sum			1152

indicating a large effect size ($\hat{d} \geq 0.80$)[3] and Pearson's r^2 measure of effect size is

$$r^2 = \frac{t^2}{t^2 + N - 1} = \frac{(+1.8419)^2}{(+1.8419)^2 + 4 - 1} = 0.5307 \, ,$$

also indicating a large effect size ($r^2 \geq 0.25$).[4]

For Mielke and Berry's $\Re$ measure of effect size, the observed value of the permutation test statistic is $\delta = 17.8333$ and following Eq. (5.6) on p. 111, the exact expected value of test statistic δ under the Fisher–Pitman null hypothesis is

$$\mu_\delta = \frac{1}{M} \sum_{i=1}^{M} \delta_i = \frac{1272}{16} = 79.50 \, ,$$

where the sum,

$$\sum_{i=1}^{M} \delta_i = 1272 \, ,$$

is calculated in Table 5.1 on p. 107. Alternatively, following Eq. (5.7) on p. 111 the exact expected value of test statistic δ is

$$\mu_\delta = \frac{1}{N(N-1)} \sum_{i=1}^{N-1} \sum_{j=i+1}^{N} \left(|x_i - x_j|^2 + |x_i + x_j|^2 \right) = \frac{954}{4(4-1)} = 79.50 \, ,$$

where the six paired values for the example data are listed in Table 5.6 and yield the sum

$$\sum_{i=1}^{N-1} \sum_{j=i+1}^{N} \left(|x_i - x_j|^2 + |x_i + x_j|^2 \right) = 954 \, .$$

Then the observed chance-corrected measure of effect size is

$$\Re = 1 - \frac{\delta}{\mu_\delta} = 1 - \frac{17.8333}{79.50} = +0.7757 \, ,$$

---

[3]In general, $\hat{d}$ values equal to or less than $\hat{d} = 0.20$ are considered to be "small" effect sizes, $\hat{d}$ values greater than $\hat{d} = 0.20$ and less than $\hat{d} = 0.80$ are considered to be "medium" or "moderate" effect sizes, and $\hat{d}$ values equal to or greater than $\hat{d} = 0.80$ are considered to be "large" effect sizes.
[4]In general, r^2 values equal to or less than $r^2 = 0.09$ are considered to be "small" effect sizes, r^2 values greater than $r^2 = 0.09$ and less than $r^2 = 0.25$ are considered to be "medium" or "moderate" effect sizes, and r^2 values equal to or greater than $r^2 = 0.25$ are considered to be "large" effect sizes.

Table 5.6 Example calculations for $\sum_{i=1}^{N-1} \sum_{j=i+1}^{N} (|x_i - x_j|^2 + |x_i + x_j|^2)$, for example data 9, 7, 5, 2

Number	$|x_i - x_j|^2$	$|x_i + x_j|^2$	$|x_i - x_j|^2 + |x_i + x_j|^2$
1	$|9 - 7|^2 = 4$	$|9 + 7|^2 = 256$	260
2	$|9 - 5|^2 = 16$	$|9 + 5|^2 = 196$	212
3	$|9 - 2|^2 = 49$	$|9 + 2|^2 = 121$	170
4	$|7 - 5|^2 = 4$	$|7 + 5|^2 = 144$	148
5	$|7 - 2|^2 = 25$	$|7 + 2|^2 = 81$	106
6	$|5 - 2|^2 = 9$	$|5 + 2|^2 = 49$	58
Sum			954

indicating approximately 78% agreement among the $N = 4$ scores above what is expected by chance. In terms of Student's t test statistic, the observed chance-corrected measure of effect size is

$$\Re = \frac{t^2 + C - 1}{t^2 + C + N - 1} = \frac{(+1.8419)^2 + 11.4393 - 1}{(+1.8419)^2 + 11.4393 + 4 - 1} = +0.7757 \, ,$$

where C is an adjustment factor given by

$$C = \frac{\mu_x(2\bar{x} - \mu_x)}{s_{\bar{x}}^2} = \frac{3[2(5.75) - 3]}{(1.4930)^2} = 11.4393 \, .$$

5.5.1   Maximum and Minimum Values of $\Re$

Chance-corrected measures of effect size such as $\Re$ have much to commend them as they provide interpretations that are easily understood by the average reader. Positive values indicate an effect size greater than expected by chance, with a value of +1 indicating a perfect relationship among variables, negative values indicate an effect size less than expected by chance, and a value of zero indicates a chance effect size. The maximum and minimum values of the $\Re$ measure of effect size are integral to evaluating intermediate values. In the next section the $\Re$ measure of effect size is demonstrated to have a maximum value of +1. In the following section the $\Re$ measure of effect size is demonstrated to have a minimum value of $-1/(N - 1)$ for one-sample tests.

Maximum Value of $\Re$

In this section the $\Re$ measure of effect size is demonstrated to have a maximum value of $\Re = +1.00$ when there is perfect agreement among the N values; that is, all N values are identical. To illustrate, consider $N = 4$ values with $x_1 = x_2 = $

$x_3 = x_4 = 4$. For these data the sum of the $N = 4$ values is

$$\sum_{i=1}^{N} x_i = 4 + 4 + 4 + 4 = 16.00 ,$$

the sum of the $N = 4$ squared values is

$$\sum_{i=1}^{N} x_i^2 = 4^2 + 4^2 + 4^2 + 4^2 = 64.00 ,$$

the total sum-of-squares is

$$SS_{\text{Total}} = \sum_{i=1}^{N} x_i^2 - \left(\sum_{i=1}^{N} x_i \right)^2 \bigg/ N = 64.00 - (16.00)^2/4 = 0.00 ,$$

and the permutation test statistic is

$$\delta = \frac{2 SS_{\text{Total}}}{N - 1} = \frac{2(0.00)}{4 - 1} = 0.00 .$$

Table 5.7 details the required calculations for the expected value of test statistic δ. Given the preliminary calculations in Table 5.7, the exact expected value of test statistic δ under the Fisher–Pitman null hypothesis is

$$\mu_\delta = \frac{1}{N(N-1)} \sum_{i=1}^{N-1} \sum_{j=i+1}^{N} \left(|x_i - x_j|^2 + |x_i + x_j|^2 \right) = \frac{384}{4(4-1)} = 32.00$$

and the chance-corrected measure of effect size is

$$\Re = 1 - \frac{\delta}{\mu_\delta} = 1 - \frac{0.00}{32.00} = +1.00 ,$$

indicating perfect agreement among the $N = 4$ values.

Table 5.7 Example calculations for $\sum_{i=1}^{N-1} \sum_{j=i+1}^{N} (|x_i - x_j|^2 + |x_i + x_j|^2)$, for example data 4, 4, 4, 4

Number	$|x_i - x_j|^2$	$|x_i + x_j|^2$	$|x_i - x_j|^2 + |x_i + x_j|^2$
1	$|4 - 4|^2 = 0$	$|4 + 4|^2 = 64$	64
2	$|4 - 4|^2 = 0$	$|4 + 4|^2 = 64$	64
3	$|4 - 4|^2 = 0$	$|4 + 4|^2 = 64$	64
4	$|4 - 4|^2 = 0$	$|4 + 4|^2 = 64$	64
5	$|4 - 4|^2 = 0$	$|4 + 4|^2 = 64$	64
6	$|4 - 4|^2 = 0$	$|4 + 4|^2 = 64$	64
Sum			384

Minimum Value of $\mathfrak{R}$

In this section the $\mathfrak{R}$ measure of effect size is demonstrated to have a minimum value given by $-1/(N-1)$ for one-sample tests. To illustrate, consider $N = 4$ values with $x_1 = +4$, $x_2 = +4$, $x_3 = -4$, and $x_4 = -4$. For these data the sum of the $N = 4$ values is

$$\sum_{i=1}^{N} x_i = 4 + 4 - 4 - 4 = 0.00 \, ,$$

the sum of the $N = 4$ squared values is

$$\sum_{i=1}^{N} x_i^2 = +4^2 + 4^2 + (-4)^2 + (-4)^2 = 64.00 \, ,$$

the total sum-of-squares is

$$SS_{\text{Total}} = \sum_{i=1}^{N} x_i^2 - \left(\sum_{i=1}^{N} x_i\right)^2 \Big/ N = 64.00 - (0.00)^2/4 = 64.00 \, ,$$

and the permutation test statistic is

$$\delta = \frac{2SS_{\text{Total}}}{N - 1} = \frac{2(64.00)}{4 - 1} = 42.6667 \, .$$

Table 5.8 details the required calculations for the expected value of test statistic δ. Given the preliminary calculations in Table 5.8, the exact expected value of test statistic δ under the Fisher–Pitman null hypothesis is

$$\mu_\delta = \frac{1}{N(N-1)} \sum_{i=1}^{N-1} \sum_{j=i+1}^{N} \left(|x_i - x_j|^2 + |x_i + x_j|^2\right) = \frac{384}{4(4-1)} = 32.00$$

Table 5.8 Example calculations for $\sum_{i=1}^{N-1} \sum_{j=i+1}^{N} (|x_i - x_j|^2 + |x_i + x_j|^2)$, for example data 4, 4, −4, −4

Number	$|x_i - x_j|^2$	$|x_i + x_j|^2$	$|x_i - x_j|^2 + |x_i + x_j|^2$
1	$|(+4) - (+4)|^2 = 0$	$|(+4) + (+4)|^2 = 64$	64
2	$|(+4) - (-4)|^2 = 64$	$|(+4) + (-4)|^2 = 0$	64
3	$|(+4) - (-4)|^2 = 64$	$|(+4) + (-4)|^2 = 0$	64
4	$|(+4) - (-4)|^2 = 64$	$|(+4) + (-4)|^2 = 0$	64
5	$|(+4) - (-4)|^2 = 64$	$|(+4) + (-4)|^2 = 0$	64
6	$|(-4) - (-4)|^2 = 0$	$|(-4) + (-4)|^2 = 64$	64
Sum			384

and the chance-corrected measure of effect size is

$$\Re = 1 - \frac{\delta}{\mu_\delta} = 1 - \frac{42.6667}{32.00} = -0.3333 \,,$$

indicating less than chance agreement among the $N = 4$ values. More simply, the minimum value of $\Re$ is given by

$$\min(\Re) = \frac{-1}{N-1} = \frac{-1}{4-1} = -0.3333$$

for a one-sample test.

5.5.2 Comparisons of Effect Size Measures

For a one-sample test of means under the Neyman–Pearson population model, Student's t, Cohen's $\hat{d}$, Pearson's r^2, and Mielke and Berry's $\Re$ are interrelated. Any one of the measures can easily be derived from any of the other measures. The relationships between Student's t test statistic and Cohen's $\hat{d}$ measure of effect size are given by

$$t = \left(N\hat{d}^2\right)^{1/2} \quad \text{and} \quad \hat{d} = \left(\frac{t^2}{N}\right)^{1/2} , \tag{5.8}$$

the relationships between Student's t test statistic and Pearson's r^2 measure of effect size are given by

$$t = \left[\frac{r^2(N-1)}{1-r^2}\right]^{1/2} \quad \text{and} \quad r^2 = \frac{t^2}{t^2 + N - 1} , \tag{5.9}$$

the relationships between Student's t test statistic and Mielke and Berry's $\Re$ measure of effect size are given by

$$t = \left[\frac{\Re(N-1) + C(\Re-1) + 1}{1-\Re}\right]^{1/2} \quad \text{and} \quad \Re = \frac{t^2 + C - 1}{t^2 + C + N - 1} , \tag{5.10}$$

the relationships between Cohen's $\hat{d}$ measure of effect size and Pearson's r^2 measure of effect size are given by

$$\hat{d} = \left[\frac{r^2(N-1)}{N(1-r^2)}\right]^{1/2} \quad \text{and} \quad r^2 = \frac{N\hat{d}^2}{N(\hat{d}^2 + 1) - 1} , \tag{5.11}$$

the relationships between Cohen's $\hat{d}$ measure of effect size and Mielke and Berry's $\Re$ measure of effect size are given by

$$\hat{d} = \left[\frac{\Re(N-1) + C(\Re - 1) + 1}{N(1 - \Re)} \right]^{1/2}$$ (5.12)

and

$$\Re = \frac{N\hat{d}^2 + C - 1}{N(\hat{d}^2 + 1) + C - 1},$$ (5.13)

and the relationships between Pearson's r^2 measure of effect size and Mielke and Berry's $\Re$ measure of effect size are given by

$$r^2 = \frac{\Re(N + C - 1) - C + 1}{N + C(\Re - 1)} \quad \text{and} \quad \Re = \frac{r^2(N - C) + C - 1}{N + C - 1 + Cr^2}.$$ (5.14)

For the example data listed in Table 5.1 on p. 107 with $x_1 = 9$, $x_2 = 7$, $x_3 = 5$, and $x_4 = 2$, and following the expressions given in Eq. (5.8) for Student's t and Cohen's $\hat{d}$, the observed value of Student's t test statistic with respect to the observed value of Cohen's $\hat{d}$ measure of effect size is

$$t = \left(N\hat{d}^2 \right)^{1/2} = \left[4(0.9209)^2 \right]^{1/2} = \pm 1.8419$$

and the observed value of Cohen's $\hat{d}$ measure of effect size with respect to the observed value of Student's t test statistic is

$$\hat{d} = \left(\frac{t^2}{N} \right)^{1/2} = \left[\frac{(+1.8419)^2}{4} \right]^{1/2} = \pm 0.9209.$$

Following the expressions given in Eq. (5.9) for Student's t and Pearson's r^2, the observed value for Student's t test statistic with respect to the observed value of Pearson's r^2 measure of effect size is

$$t = \left[\frac{r^2(N - 1)}{1 - r^2} \right]^{1/2} = \left[\frac{0.5307(4 - 1)}{1 - 0.5307} \right]^{1/2} = \pm 1.8419$$

and the observed value for Pearson's r^2 measure of effect size with respect to the observed value of Student's t test statistic is

$$r^2 = \frac{t^2}{t^2 + N - 1} = \frac{(+1.8419)^2}{(+1.8419)^2 + 4 - 1} = 0.5307.$$

Following the expressions given in Eq. (5.10) for Student's t and Mielke and Berry's $\Re$, the observed value for Student's t test statistic with respect to the observed value of Mielke and Berry's $\Re$ measure of effect size is

$$
t = \left[\frac{\Re(N-1) + C(\Re - 1) + 1}{1 - \Re} \right]^{1/2}
$$

$$
= \left[\frac{+0.7757(4-1) + 11.4393(0.7757 - 1) + 1}{1 - 0.7757} \right]^{1/2} = \pm 1.8419
$$

and the observed value for Mielke and Berry's $\Re$ measure of effect size with respect to the observed value of Student's t test statistic is

$$
\Re = \frac{t^2 + C - 1}{t^2 + C + N - 1} = \frac{(+1.8419)^2 + 11.4393 - 1}{(+1.8419)^2 + 11.4393 + 4 - 1} = +0.7757 \;.
$$

Following the expressions given in Eq. (5.11) for Cohen's $\hat{d}$ and Pearson's r^2, the observed value for Cohen's $\hat{d}$ measure of effect size with respect to the observed value of Pearson's r^2 measure of effect size is

$$
\hat{d} = \left[\frac{r^2(N-1)}{N(1-r^2)} \right]^{1/2} = \left[\frac{0.5307(4-1)}{4(1-0.5307)} \right]^{1/2} = \pm 0.9209
$$

and the observed value for Pearson's r^2 measure of effect size with respect to the observed value of Cohen's $\hat{d}$ measure of effect size is

$$
r^2 = \frac{N\hat{d}^2}{N(\hat{d}^2 + 1) - 1} = \frac{4[(0.9209)^2]}{4[(0.9209)^2 + 1] - 1} = 0.5307 \;.
$$

Following the expressions given in Eqs. (5.12) and (5.13) for Cohen's $\hat{d}$ and Mielke and Berry's $\Re$, respectively, the observed value for Cohen's $\hat{d}$ measure of effect size with respect to the observed value of Mielke and Berry's $\Re$ measure of effect size is

$$
\hat{d} = \left[\frac{\Re(N-1) + C(\Re - 1) + 1}{N(1 - \Re)} \right]^{1/2}
$$

$$
= \left[\frac{+0.7757(4-1) + 11.4393(+0.7757 - 1) + 1}{4(1 - 0.7757)} \right]^{1/2} = \pm 0.9209
$$

and the observed value for Mielke and Berry's $\Re$ measure of effect size with respect to the observed value of Cohen's $\hat{d}$ measure of effect size is

$$
\Re = \frac{N\hat{d}^2 + C - 1}{N(\hat{d}^2 + 1) + C - 1} = \frac{4[(0.9209)^2] + 11.4393 - 1}{4[(0.9209)^2 - 1] + 11.4393 - 1} = +0.7757 \;.
$$

And following the expressions given in Eq. (5.14) for Pearson's r^2 and Mielke and Berry's $\Re$, the observed value for Pearson's r^2 measure of effect size with respect to the observed value of Mielke and Berry's $\Re$ measure of effect size is

$$r^2 = \frac{\Re(N + C - 1) - C + 1}{N + C(\Re - 1)}$$
$$= \frac{0.7757(4 + 11.4393 - 1) - 11.4393 + 1}{4 + 11.4393(0.7757 - 1)} = 0.5307$$

and the observed value for Mielke and Berry's $\Re$ measure of effect size with respect to the observed value of Pearson's r^2 measure of effect size is

$$\Re = \frac{r^2(N - C) + C - 1}{N + C - 1 + Cr^2}$$
$$= \frac{0.5307(4 - 11.4393) + 11.4393 - 1}{4 + 11.4393 - 1 - (11.4393)(0.5307)} = +0.7757 \ .$$

5.5.3   Interpretations of Effect Size Measures

While neither Cohen's $\hat{d}$ nor Pearson's r^2 measures of effect size lend themselves to meaningful interpretations, $\Re$ possesses an easy-to-understand chance-corrected interpretation. Positive values of $\Re$ indicate agreement among the subjects greater than expected by chance, negative values of $\Re$ indicate agreement among the subjects less than expected by chance, and a value of zero indicates chance agreement among the subjects.

Cohen's $\hat{d}$ measure of effect size norms between 0 and ∞ and provides an estimate of the magnitude of the effect size in standard deviation units. The benchmarks provided by Cohen are: if $\hat{d} \leq 0.20$ the effect size is considered "small," if $0.20 < \hat{d} < 0.80$ the effect size is considered "medium" or "moderate," and if $\hat{d} \geq 0.80$ the effect size is considered "large." In general, statisticians demand more precision than simply small, medium, and large. Also, Pearson's r^2 has not escaped criticism. As Howell noted:

> I am not happy with the r-family of measures simply because I don't think that they have a meaningful interpretation in most situations. ... I would suggest that you stay away from the older r-family measures unless you really have a good reason to use them [18, p. 157].

In like manner to Cohen's $\hat{d}$ measure of effect size, if $r^2 \leq 0.09$ the effect size is considered "small," if $0.09 < r^2 < 0.25$ the effect size is considered "medium" or "moderate," and if $r^2 \geq 0.25$ the effect size is considered "large."[5]

---

[5]The values for small, medium, and large effect sizes are not accepted by all researchers and have been in dispute for some time [24].

The use of Pearson's r^2 as a measure of effect size has been heavily criticized in the literature. McGrath and Meyer [24] and others have criticized the values put forward by Cohen [11, p. 22], recommending somewhat higher benchmarks. D'Andrade and Dart advocated the use of r instead of r^2, arguing that the usual interpretation of r^2 as "variance accounted for" is inappropriate since variance is a squared measure that no longer corresponds to the dimensionality of the original measurements [15, p. 47]. Kvålseth [23] and Ozer [26] demonstrated that for any model other than a linear model with an intercept, r^2 is inappropriate as a measure of effect size. Blalock [5] and Rosenthal and Rubin [29, 30] showed that values of r^2 underestimate the magnitudes of experimental effects, even though r^2 is biased upward. Finally, while r^2 is touted as varying between 0 and 1 with a clear interpretation, as is obvious in Eq. (5.4) on p. 111, r^2 approaches 1 only as t^2 approaches infinity and, thus, the only way that r^2 can possibly equal 1 for a one-sample t test is when there is only a single object for analysis; that is, with degrees of freedom equal to $N - 1 = 0$.

5.6 Example 3: Analyses with $v = 2$ and $v = 1$

For a third, more realistic example of a one-sample test under the Neyman–Pearson population model, consider the data on reaction times of $N = 12$ young children where the mean reaction time on a particular task has been reported as 1.7 s; that is, the null hypothesis is H_0: $\mu_x = 1.7$. The reaction-time data are listed in Table 5.9. For the reaction-time data given in Table 5.9 the sample mean is $\bar{x} = 1.4917$, the sample standard deviation is $s_x = 0.3502$, the standard error of $\bar{x}$ is

$$s_{\bar{x}} = \frac{s_x}{\sqrt{N}} = \frac{0.3502}{\sqrt{12}} = 0.1011 ,$$

and Student's t test statistic for the observed data listed in Table 5.9 is

$$t = \frac{\bar{x} - \mu_x}{s_{\bar{x}}} = \frac{1.4917 - 1.7}{0.1011} = -2.0603 .$$

Table 5.9 Recorded reaction times for $N = 12$ young children

Child	Time	Child	Time
A	1.4	G	1.5
B	1.8	H	2.0
C	1.1	I	1.4
D	1.3	J	1.9
E	1.6	K	1.8
F	0.8	L	1.3

Under the Neyman–Pearson null hypothesis, H_0: $\mu_x = 1.7$, test statistic t is asymptotically distributed as Student's t with $N - 1$ degrees of freedom. With $N - 1 = 12 - 1 = 11$ degrees of freedom the asymptotic two-tail probability value of $t = -2.0603$ is $P = 0.0638$, under the assumption of normality.

5.6.1   An Exact Analysis with $v = 2$

Under the Fisher–Pitman permutation model with $v = 2$ the observed value of test statistic δ is

$$\delta = \binom{N}{2}^{-1} \sum_{i=1}^{N-1} \sum_{j=i+1}^{N} |x_i - x_j|^2$$

$$= \binom{12}{2}^{-1} (16.1898) = \frac{2(16.1898)}{12(12 - 1)} = 0.2453 \;.$$

Alternatively, in terms of an analysis of variance model the permutation test statistic is

$$\delta = \frac{2SS_{\text{Total}}}{N - 1} = \frac{2(1.3492)}{12 - 1} = 0.2453 \;,$$

where the sum of the $N = 12$ values is

$$\sum_{i=1}^{N} x_i = 1.4 + 1.8 + 1.1 + 1.3 + 1.6 + 0.8 + 1.5$$

$$+ 2.0 + 1.4 + 1.9 + 1.8 + 1.3 = 17.90 \;,$$

the sum of the $N = 12$ squared values is

$$\sum_{i=1}^{N} x_i^2 = 1.4^2 + 1.8^2 + 1.1^2 + 1.3^2 + 1.6^2 + 0.8^2 + 1.5^2$$

$$+ 2.0^2 + 1.4^2 + 1.9^2 + 1.8^2 + 1.3^2 = 28.05 \;,$$

and the total sum-of-squares is

$$SS_{\text{Total}} = \sum_{i=1}^{N} x_i^2 - \left(\sum_{i=1}^{N} x_i \right)^2 \Big/ N = 28.05 - (17.90)^2/12 = 1.3492 \;.$$

To establish the exact permutation probability value of $\delta = 0.2453$ (or $t = -2.0603$), all possible arrangements of the observed data must be enumerated.

There are only

$$M = 2^N = 2^{12} = 4096$$

possible, equally-likely arrangements in the reference set of all permutations of the reaction-time data listed in Table 5.9. Under the Fisher–Pitman permutation model, the exact probability of an observed δ is the proportion of δ test statistic values calculated on all possible arrangements of the observed data that are equal to or less than the observed value of δ. There are only two δ test statistic values that are equal to or less than the observed value of $\delta = 0.2453$. If all M arrangements of the $N = 12$ observations listed in Table 5.9 occur with equal chance, the exact probability value computed on the $M = 4096$ possible arrangements of the observed data with $N = 12$ children preserved for each arrangement is

$$P(\delta \leq \delta_0) = \frac{\text{number of } \delta \text{ values } \leq \delta_0}{M} = \frac{2}{4096} = 0.4883 \times 10^{-3} \ ,$$

where δ_0 denotes the observed value of test statistic δ and M is the number of possible, equally-likely arrangements of the reaction-time data listed in Table 5.9.

Conversely, for test statistic t there are only two $|t|$ values that are equal to or greater than the observed value of $|t| = 2.0603$, yielding an exact two-tail probability value under the Fisher–Pitman null hypothesis of

$$P(|t| \geq |t_0|) = \frac{\text{number of } |t| \text{ values } \geq |t_0|}{M} = \frac{2}{4096} = 0.4883 \times 10^{-3} \ ,$$

where t_0 denotes the observed value of test statistic t. There is a substantial difference between the asymptotic probability value ($P = 0.0638$) and the exact permutation probability value ($P = 0.4883 \times 10^{-3}$); that is,

$$\Delta_P = 0.0638 - 0.4883 \times 10^{-3} = 0.0633 \ .$$

The difference is most likely due to the very small number of data points. A continuous mathematical function such as Student's t cannot be expected to provide a precise fit to just 12 observed values, of which only nine values are unique.

Conventional statistics, such as Student's one-sample t test, necessarily assume normality, where the density function of the standard normal distribution is given by

$$f(x) = \frac{1}{\sqrt{2\pi\sigma_x^2}} \exp\left[-\frac{(x - \mu_x)^2}{2\sigma_x^2}\right] \ . \tag{5.15}$$

As is evident in Eq. (5.15), the normal distribution is a two-parameter distribution where the two parameters are the population mean denoted by μ_x and the population variance denoted by σ_x^2. The remaining factors in Eq. (5.15) are constants; that is, 1,

$2, \pi = 3.1416$, and $e = 2.7183$. For Student's one-sample t test, the two population parameters are estimated by the sample mean—more accurately for these purposes, the unbiased estimated population mean—given by

$$\bar{x} = \frac{1}{N} \sum_{i=1}^{N} x_i$$

and the sample variance—more accurately, the unbiased estimated population variance—given by

$$s_x^2 = \frac{1}{N-1} \sum_{i=1}^{N} (x_i - \bar{x})^2 \,.$$

The sample mean is the point about which the sum of squared deviations is minimized and the sample variance is the average squared deviation about the sample mean. Thus because the t test assumes normality, squared differences among data values are an integral and necessary component of Student's one-sample t test statistic. On the other hand, statistical tests under the Fisher–Pitman permutation model are distribution-free, do not assume normality, and do not depend on squared differences among data values.

5.6.2 Congruent Data and Analysis Spaces

Permutation methods are distribution-free and, therefore, do not assume normality. Thus it is not necessary to measure differences among the data points in squared units—corresponding to $v = 2$ in Eq. (5.1) on p. 103. Indeed, any positive value for v could be considered. However, only ordinary Euclidean scaling, corresponding to $v = 1$ in Eq. (5.1), appears appropriate as it is congruent with the dimensionality of most data spaces. In addition, ordinary Euclidean scaling is the only function that is both a metric and satisfies the triangle inequality.

A scaling function is a metric if it satisfies three properties: (1) $\Delta(x, y) \geq 0$, and $\Delta(x, x) = 0$, that is, the difference is positive between two different points and the difference is equal to zero from any point to itself; (2) the difference is symmetric: $\Delta(x, y) = \Delta(y, x)$, that is, the difference between points x and y is the same in any direction; and (3) the triangle inequality is satisfied: $\Delta(x, y) \leq \Delta(x, z) + \Delta(y, z)$, that is, the difference between any two points is the shortest distance along any path.

The triangle inequality can be illustrated with some simple examples. Consider the three graphics in Fig. 5.1. The first (top) graphic in Fig. 5.1 depicts three values $(x, y,$ and $z)$ on the real number line. The second (middle) graphic in Fig. 5.1 assigns

Fig. 5.1 Graphic illustrations
for the triangle inequality

$$
\begin{array}{ccccc}
x \longleftrightarrow & y \longleftrightarrow & z \\
1 \longleftrightarrow & 2 \longleftrightarrow & 3 \\
1 \longleftrightarrow & 3 \longleftrightarrow & 5
\end{array}
$$

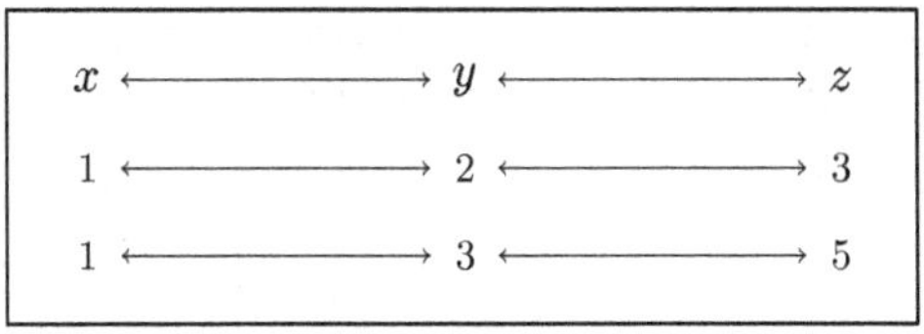

the three values 1, 2, and 3 to x, y, and z, respectively. For the second graphic,

$$
\begin{aligned}
\Delta(x, z) &= \Delta(1, 3) = 2 , \\
\Delta(x, y) &= \Delta(1, 2) = 1 , \\
\Delta(y, z) &= \Delta(2, 3) = 1 ,
\end{aligned}
$$

and $\Delta(x, z) \le \Delta(x, y) + \Delta(y, z)$; that is, $2 \le 1 + 1$. Thus, the triangle inequality holds for ordinary Euclidean scaling; that is, with $v = 1$. However, for squared Euclidean scaling with $v = 2$,

$$
\begin{aligned}
\Delta(x, z)^2 &= \Delta(1, 3)^2 = 2^2 = 4 , \\
\Delta(x, y)^2 &= \Delta(1, 2)^2 = 1^2 = 1 , \\
\Delta(y, z)^2 &= \Delta(2, 3)^2 = 1^2 = 1 ,
\end{aligned}
$$

and $\Delta(x, z)^2 \nleq \Delta(x, y)^2 + \Delta(y, z)^2$; that is, $4 \nleq 1 + 1$ and the triangle inequality fails.

Now consider the third (bottom) graphic in Fig. 5.1 where the values 1, 3, and 5 have been assigned to x, y, and z, respectively. For the third graphic,

$$
\begin{aligned}
\Delta(x, z) &= \Delta(1, 5) = 4 , \\
\Delta(x, y) &= \Delta(1, 3) = 2 , \\
\Delta(y, z) &= \Delta(3, 5) = 2 ,
\end{aligned}
$$

and $\Delta(x, z) \le \Delta(x, y) + \Delta(y, z)$; that is, $4 \le 2 + 2$. Thus, the triangle inequality holds for ordinary Euclidean scaling; that is, $v = 1$. However, for squared Euclidean scaling with $v = 2$,

$$
\begin{aligned}
\Delta(x, z)^2 &= \Delta(1, 5)^2 = 4^2 = 16 , \\
\Delta(x, y)^2 &= \Delta(1, 3)^2 = 2^2 = 4 , \\
\Delta(y, z)^2 &= \Delta(3, 5)^2 = 2^2 = 4 ,
\end{aligned}
$$

and $\Delta(x, z)^2 \nleq \Delta(x, y)^2 + \Delta(y, z)^2$; that is, $16 \nleq 4 + 4$ and the triangle inequality fails.

The importance of a metric space in statistical analysis cannot be overstated. Technically, for the permutation test statistic,

$$\delta = \binom{N}{2}^{-1} \sum_{i=1}^{N-1} \sum_{j=i+1}^{N} |x_i - x_j|^{\upsilon} \, ,$$

any positive value for $\upsilon \leq 1$ yields a metric analysis space. However, values of $\upsilon < 1$ are impossible to interpret and are, therefore, meaningless. Any value of $\upsilon > 1$ yields a non-metric analysis space. Thus, a metric analysis mandates $\upsilon = 1$. When $\upsilon = 2$, as is customary in conventional statistical analyses, the non-metric analysis space is not congruent with an ordinary Euclidean data space. The obvious solution is to set $\upsilon = 1$, ensuring that the analysis and data spaces are both metric and conform to each other.

5.6.3 An Exact Analysis with $\upsilon = 1$

Consider an analysis of the reaction-time data listed in Table 5.9 on p. 123 under the Fisher–Pitman permutation model with $\upsilon = 1$. It is a paradox of one-sample permutation tests that certain configurations of data yield the same exact probability value with either squared or ordinary Euclidean scaling; that is, $\upsilon = 2$ or $\upsilon = 1$, respectively. The data listed in Table 5.9 on p. 123 present one such configuration. For both $\upsilon = 2$ and $\upsilon = 1$, the exact probability value is $P = 0.4883 \times 10^{-3}$ under the Fisher–Pitman permutation model.

While the selection of $\upsilon = 2$ or $\upsilon = 1$ yields the same exact probability value for the reaction-time data in Table 5.9, the δ values differ and, consequently, the $\Re$ measures of effect size also differ. For squared Euclidean scaling with $\upsilon = 2$, the observed value of δ is $\delta = 0.2453$, the exact expected value of test statistic δ under the Fisher–Pitman null hypothesis is $\mu_\delta = 4.6750$, and the observed chance-corrected measure of effect size is

$$\Re = 1 - \frac{\delta}{\mu_\delta} = 1 - \frac{0.2453}{4.6750} = +0.9475 \, ,$$

indicating approximately 95% agreement among the $N = 12$ children above what is expected by chance. For comparison, Cohen's measure of effect size is

$$\hat{d} = \frac{|\bar{x} - \mu_x|}{s_x} = \frac{|1.4917 - 1.7|}{0.3502} = 0.5948 \, ,$$

indicating a medium or moderate effect size $(0.20 < \hat{d} < 0.80)$, and Pearson's measure of effect size is

$$r^2 = \frac{t^2}{t^2 + N - 1} = \frac{(1.4917)^2}{(1.4917)^2 + 12 - 1} = 0.1683 ,$$

also indicating a moderate effect size $(0.09 < r^2 < 0.25)$.

For ordinary Euclidean scaling with $v = 1$, the observed value of δ is $\delta = 0.4106$, the exact expected value of test statistic δ under the Fisher–Pitman null hypothesis is $\mu_\delta = 1.6970$, and the observed chance-corrected measure of effect size is

$$\Re = 1 - \frac{\delta}{\mu_\delta} = 1 - \frac{0.4106}{1.6970} = +0.7580 ,$$

indicating approximately 76% agreement among the $N = 12$ children above what is expected by chance. No comparisons are made with Cohen's $\hat{d}$ or Pearson's r^2 measures of effect size for a one-sample test as $\hat{d}$ and r^2 are undefined for ordinary Euclidean scaling.

5.6.4 Plus and Minus Data Configurations

The effects of various configurations of one-sample data can be illustrated with a small set of signed values, such as given in Table 5.10 with $N = 9$ objects arranged in three sets of paired columns. First, consider Columns A and B in Table 5.10 where the values are all positive (Column A) or all negative (Column B). For these two columns of data (A and B), the exact probability value with either $v = 2$ or $v = 1$ is $P = 0.3906 \times 10^{-2}$.

Second, consider Columns C and D in Table 5.10 where the values are all positive (Column C) or all negative (Column D), but extreme values have been added: for Object 9 the value $+5$ in Column A has been replaced by extreme value $+50$ in

Table 5.10 Example data illustrating $v = 2$ and $v = 1$ with and without extreme values ($+50$ and -50)

Object	A	B	C	D	E	F
1	+1	−1	+1	−1	−1	−1
2	+1	−1	+1	−1	+1	+1
3	+1	−1	+1	−1	+1	+1
4	+2	−2	+2	−2	−2	−2
5	+2	−2	+2	−2	+2	+2
6	+2	−2	+2	−2	+2	+2
7	+4	−4	+4	−4	+4	+4
8	+4	−4	+4	−4	+4	+4
9	+5	−5	+50	−50	+5	+50

Column C and the value -5 in Column B has been replaced by extreme value -50 in Column D. For these two columns of data (C and D), the exact probability value with either $v = 2$ or $v = 1$ is unchanged at $P = 0.3906 \times 10^{-2}$. The substitution of an extreme value for Object 9 does not affect the exact probability value for either $v = 2$ or $v = 1$ when all values in a given column are either positive or negative.

Finally, consider Columns E and F in Table 5.10, which have the same values as Columns C and D but where two of the values are negative (Objects 1 and 4) and the remaining seven values are positive. Here again, Column E does not contain an extreme value, but Column F does contain an extreme value for Object 9; that is, $+50$ in Column F has replaced $+5$ in Column E. For Column E, without an extreme value, the exact probability value with $v = 2$ is $P = 0.0781$ and the exact probability value with $v = 1$ is $P = 0.0898$. For Column F, with extreme value $+50$, the exact probability value with $v = 2$ is $P = 0.1563$—twice as large as $P = 0.0781$—and the exact probability value with $v = 1$ is unchanged at $P = 0.0898$.

Analyses based on ordinary Euclidean scaling functions with $v = 1$ are highly resistant to extreme values and are very robust when compared with analyses based on squared Euclidean scaling functions with $v = 2$. The term "robust" was coined by George Box while at the University of North Carolina in 1953 [6]. Box was concerned with how well standard statistical procedures held up when the assumptions behind the mathematical model were not quite correct [31, p. 88].[6]

5.7   Example 4: Exact and Monte Carlo Analyses

For a fourth, larger example of a one-sample test, consider the weight gain/loss data (in pounds) listed in Table 5.11 for $N = 28$ adult subjects. Because there are

$$M = 2^N = 2^{28} = 268{,}435{,}456$$

possible, equally-likely arrangements in the reference set of all permutations of the weight gain/loss data listed in Table 5.10, an exact permutation analysis is not practical. When the number of possible arrangements is very large, Monte Carlo permutation methods become necessary.

Monte Carlo permutation statistical methods generate a random sample of all possible arrangements of the observed data. The Monte Carlo probability value of an observed δ test statistic is the proportion of the δ test statistic values computed on the randomly-selected arrangements that are equal to or greater than the observed test statistic value. In general, a random sample of $L = 1{,}000{,}000$ arrangements

---

[6]George Edward Pelham Box is best remembered for his service at the University of Wisconsin–Madison where he founded the Department of Statistics in 1960 and served as Chair of the department for many years, retiring in 1992. Box passed away in March, 2013, shortly after publishing his memoirs [7].

Table 5.11 Example weight gain/loss data for a one-sample test with $N = 28$ subjects

Subject	Score	Subject	Score
1	+8.8	15	+6.5
2	−6.6	16	+8.7
3	+8.7	17	+6.0
4	−5.9	18	−8.6
5	+8.5	19	+5.5
6	−5.6	20	+8.5
7	+8.3	21	+5.2
8	−5.1	22	−8.1
9	+7.7	23	+5.1
10	+5.0	24	+7.7
11	+7.6	25	+5.1
12	+5.0	26	−7.4
13	+6.8	27	+5.0
14	−4.6	28	−6.7

ensures a probability value accurate to three decimal places, provided the probability value is not too small [19]. However, to ensure four decimal places of accuracy, an increase of two orders of magnitude is required; that is, $L = 100{,}000{,}000$.

For the weight gain/loss data listed in Table 5.11, assume H_0: $\mu_x = 0$; that is, the null hypothesis posits no expected gain or loss in weight. Then under the Neyman–Pearson population model the sample mean is $\bar{x} = 2.5393$, the sample standard deviation is $s_x = 6.5062$, the standard error of $\bar{x}$ is

$$ s_{\bar{x}} = \frac{s_x}{\sqrt{N}} = \frac{6.5062}{\sqrt{28}} = 1.2296 , $$

and Student's one-sample t test statistic for the observed data listed in Table 5.11 is

$$ t = \frac{\bar{x} - \mu_x}{s_{\bar{x}}} = \frac{2.5393 - 0}{1.2296} = +2.0652 . $$

Under the Neyman–Pearson null hypothesis, H_0: $\mu_x = 0$, test statistic t is asymptotically distributed as Student's t with $N - 1$ degrees of freedom. With $N - 1 = 28 - 1 = 27$ degrees of freedom the asymptotic two-tail probability value of $t = +2.0652$ is $P = 0.0486$, under the assumption of normality.

5.7.1 A Monte Carlo Analysis with $v = 2$

Now consider the weight gain/loss data listed in Table 5.11 under the Fisher–Pitman permutation model. Let $v = 2$, employing squared Euclidean differences between the paired scores for correspondence with Student's one-sample t test statistic. The observed value of test statistic δ is $\delta = 84.6612$, the exact expected value of test statistic δ under the Fisher–Pitman null hypothesis is $\mu_\delta = 94.5336$, and the Monte Carlo probability value based on a sample of $L = 1,000,000$ random arrangements of the observed data is

$$P(\delta \leq \delta_0 | H_0) = \frac{\text{number of } \delta \text{ values } \leq \delta_0}{L} = \frac{50,302}{1,000,000} = 0.0503 ,$$

where δ_0 denotes the observed value of test statistic δ and L is the number of randomly-selected, equally-likely arrangements of the $N = 28$ observations listed in Table 5.11.

Following Eq. (5.6) on p. 111, the exact expected value of the $M = 268,435,456$ δ test statistic values under the Fisher–Pitman null hypothesis is

$$\mu_\delta = \frac{1}{M} \sum_{i=1}^{M} \delta_i = \frac{25,376,170,023}{268,435,456} = 94.5336$$

and following Eq. (5.5) on p. 111, the observed chance-corrected measure of effect size is

$$\Re = 1 - \frac{\delta}{\mu_\delta} = 1 - \frac{84.6612}{94.5336} = +0.1044 ,$$

indicating approximately 10% agreement among the $N = 28$ scores above what is expected by chance. For comparison, Cohen's measure of effect size is

$$\hat{d} = \frac{|\bar{x} - \mu_x|}{s_x} = \frac{|2.5393 - 0|}{6.5062} = 0.3903 ,$$

indicating a medium or moderate effect size $(0.20 < \hat{d} < 0.80)$, and Pearson's measure of effect size is

$$r^2 = \frac{t^2}{t^2 + N - 1} = \frac{(2.0652)^2}{(2.0652)^2 + 28 - 1} = 0.1364 ,$$

also indicating a moderate effect size $(0.09 < r^2 < 0.25)$.

5.7.2   An Exact Analysis with $v = 2$

Although an exact permutation analysis may be impractical for the data listed in Table 5.11, it is not impossible. For an exact test of the data listed in Table 5.11 under the Fisher–Pitman permutation model with $v = 2$, the observed value of test statistic δ is $\delta = 84.6612$, the exact expected value of test statistic δ under the

Fisher–Pitman null hypothesis is $\mu_\delta = 94.5336$, and the exact probability value based on all $M = 268{,}435{,}456$ arrangements of the observed data is

$$P(\delta \leq \delta_0 | H_0) = \frac{\text{number of } \delta \text{ values } \leq \delta_0}{M} = \frac{13{,}500{,}360}{268{,}435{,}456} = 0.0503 \, ,$$

where δ_0 denotes the observed value of test statistic δ and M is the number of possible, equally-likely arrangements of the $N = 28$ observations listed in Table 5.11. In this example, the Monte Carlo probability value based on $L = 1{,}000{,}000$ random arrangements of the observed data ($P = 0.0503$) and the exact probability value ($P = 0.0503$) are identical to four decimal places, illustrating the accuracy of Monte Carlo permutation methods when the exact probability value is not too small. The difference between the Monte Carlo and exact probability values, when carried to six decimal places, is only

$$\Delta_P = 0.050302 - 0.050293 = 0.000009 \, .$$

Following Eq. (5.6) on p. 111, the exact expected value of the $M = 268{,}435{,}456$ δ test statistic values under the Fisher–Pitman null hypothesis is

$$\mu_\delta = \frac{1}{M} \sum_{i=1}^{M} \delta_i = \frac{25{,}376{,}170{,}023}{268{,}435{,}456} = 94.5336$$

and following Eq. (5.5) on p. 111, the observed chance-corrected measure of effect size is

$$\Re = 1 - \frac{\delta}{\mu_\delta} = 1 - \frac{84.6612}{94.5336} = +0.1044 \, ,$$

indicating approximately 10% agreement among the $N = 28$ scores above what is expected by chance.

5.7.3 A Monte Carlo Analysis with $v = 1$

Now consider the weight gain/loss data listed in Table 5.11 under the Fisher–Pitman permutation model with $v = 1$. The observed value of test statistic δ is $\delta = 6.9860$, the exact expected value of test statistic δ under the Fisher–Pitman null hypothesis is $\mu_\delta = 7.5685$, and the Monte Carlo probability value based on a sample of $L = 1{,}000{,}000$ random arrangements of the observed data is

$$P(\delta \leq \delta_0 | H_0) = \frac{\text{number of } \delta \text{ values } \leq \delta_0}{L} = \frac{53{,}971}{1{,}000{,}000} = 0.0540 \, ,$$

where δ_o denotes the observed value of test statistic δ and L is the number of randomly-selected, equally-likely arrangements of the $N = 28$ observations listed in Table 5.11. Following Eq. (5.6) on p. 111, the exact expected value of the $M = 268{,}435{,}456$ δ test statistic values under the Fisher–Pitman null hypothesis is

$$\mu_\delta = \frac{1}{M} \sum_{i=1}^{M} \delta_i = \frac{2{,}031{,}653{,}749}{268{,}435{,}456} = 7.5685$$

and following Eq. (5.5) on p. 111, the observed chance-corrected measure of effect size is

$$\Re = 1 - \frac{\delta}{\mu_\delta} = 1 - \frac{6.9860}{7.5685} = +0.0770 \,,$$

indicating approximately 8% agreement among the $N = 28$ scores above what is expected by chance. No comparisons are made with Cohen's $\hat{d}$ or Pearson's r^2 measures of effect size for one-sample tests as $\hat{d}$ and r^2 are undefined for ordinary Euclidean scaling.

5.7.4 An Exact Analysis with $v = 1$

For an exact test of the weight gain/loss data listed in Table 5.11 under the Fisher–Pitman permutation model with $v = 1$, the observed value of test statistic δ is $\delta = 6.9860$, the exact expected value of test statistic δ under the Fisher–Pitman null hypothesis is $\mu_\delta = 7.5685$, and the exact probability value based on all $M = 268{,}435{,}456$ arrangements of the observed data is

$$P(\delta \leq \delta_o | H_0) = \frac{\text{number of } \delta \text{ values} \leq \delta_o}{M} = \frac{14{,}487{,}686}{268{,}435{,}456} = 0.0540 \,,$$

where δ_o denotes the observed value of test statistic δ and M is the number of possible, equally-likely arrangements of the $N = 28$ observations listed in Table 5.11. Following Eq. (5.6) on p. 111, the exact expected value of the $M = 268{,}435{,}456$ δ test statistic values under the Fisher–Pitman null hypothesis is

$$\mu_\delta = \frac{1}{M} \sum_{i=1}^{M} \delta_i = \frac{2{,}031{,}653{,}749}{268{,}435{,}456} = 7.5685$$

and following Eq. (5.5) on p. 111, the observed chance-corrected measure of effect size is

$$\mathfrak{R} = 1 - \frac{\delta}{\mu_\delta} = 1 - \frac{6.9860}{7.5685} = +0.0770 \,,$$

indicating approximately 8% agreement among the $N = 28$ scores above what is expected by chance.

5.8   Example 5: Rank-Score Permutation Analyses

In conventional research it is sometimes necessary to analyze rank-score data. Two scenarios manifest themselves. First, the observed data are collected as ranks where, for example, experienced travelers are asked to rank preferences among airlines, airports, or cruise lines. Second, the raw data are converted to ranks because one or more of the assumptions for a one-sample t test cannot be satisfied. There is no need for the second scenario with permutation methods as the conventional assumptions underlying Student's t test are moot. The conventional approach to one-sample rank-score data under the population model is Wilcoxon's signed-ranks test [33].

5.8.1   The Wilcoxon Signed-Ranks Test

Consider a one-sample rank test for N univariate rank scores under the Neyman–Pearson population model. Wilcoxon's signed-ranks test statistic is the smaller of the sums of the like-signed ranks. An example set of $N = 18$ rank-score data is listed in Table 5.12, where a given task is predetermined to take 8 h and the difference columns listed in Table 5.11 represent the differences between the time actually taken and the hypothesized value of 8 h.

Table 5.12 Example rank-score data for the Wilcoxon signed-ranks test

Difference	Signed rank	Difference	Signed rank
−0 h 05 min	−1	+2 h 15 min	+10
−0 h 15 min	−2	−2 h 20 min	−11
+0 h 20 min	+3	+2 h 35 min	+12
−0 h 30 min	−4	−3 h 40 min	−13
+1 h 10 min	+5	+3 h 45 min	+14
+1 h 15 min	+6	+3 h 55 min	+15
+1 h 25 min	+7	+6 h 00 min	+16
+2 h 05 min	+8	+8 h 05 min	+17
+2 h 10 min	+9	+8 h 30 min	+18

The sums of the $(+)$ and $(-)$ signed ranks in Table 5.12 are

$$\sum(+) = 3 + 5 + 6 + 7 + 8 + 9 + 10 + 12$$

$$+ 14 + 15 + 16 + 17 + 18 = 140$$

and

$$\sum(-) = 1 + 2 + 4 + 11 + 13 = 31 ,$$

respectively. Then Wilcoxon's test statistic is $T = \sum(-) = 31$, the smaller of the two sums.

Test statistic T is asymptotically distributed $N(0, 1)$ under the Neyman–Pearson null hypothesis as $N \to \infty$. For the $N = 18$ rank scores listed in Table 5.12, the mean value of Wilcoxon's T is

$$\mu_T = \frac{N(N+1)}{4} = \frac{18(18+1)}{4} = 85.50 ,$$

the standard deviation of T is

$$\sigma_T = \left[\frac{N(N+1)(2N+1)}{24} \right]^{1/2} = \left\{ \frac{18(18+1)[2(18)+1]}{24} \right\}^{1/2} = 22.9619 ,$$

and the standard score of $T = 31$ is

$$z = \frac{T - \mu_T}{\sigma_T} = \frac{31 - 85.50}{22.9619} = -2.3735 ,$$

yielding an asymptotic $N(0, 1)$ two-tail probability value of $P = 0.0176$, under the assumption of normality. If a correction for continuity is applied,

$$z = \frac{T + 0.50 - \mu_T}{\sigma_T} = \frac{31 + 0.50 - 85.50}{22.9619} = -2.3517$$

and the two-tail probability value is increased slightly to $P = 0.0187$.

5.8.2   An Exact Analysis with $v = 2$

For an analysis of the one-sample rank-score data listed in Table 5.12 under the Fisher–Pitman permutation model let $v = 2$, employing squared Euclidean differences between the paired rank scores for correspondence with Wilcoxon's signed-ranks test. Let x_i denote the observed rank-score values for $i = 1, \ldots, N$, then the permutation test statistic is given by

$$\delta = \binom{N}{2}^{-1} \sum_{i=1}^{N-1} \sum_{j=i+1}^{N} |x_i - x_j|^v . \tag{5.16}$$

Following Eq. (5.16), for the rank-score data listed in Table 5.12 with $N = 18$ and $v = 2$, the observed value of the permutation test statistic is

$$\delta = \frac{2}{(18)(18-1)} \Big[|(-1) - (-2)|^2 + |(-1) - (+3)|^2$$
$$+ \cdots + |(+17) - (+18)|^2 \Big] = 170.4641 .$$

Because there are only

$$M = 2^N = 2^{18} = 262,144$$

possible, equally-likely arrangements in the reference set of all permutations of the rank-score data listed in Table 5.12, an exact permutation analysis is feasible. Under the Fisher–Pitman permutation model, the exact probability of an observed δ is the proportion of δ test statistic values calculated on all possible arrangements of the observed data that are equal to or less than the observed value of $\delta = 170.4641$. There are exactly 4176 δ test statistic values that are equal to or less than the observed value of $\delta = 170.4641$. If all M arrangements of the $N = 18$ rank scores listed in Table 5.12 occur with equal chance under the Fisher–Pitman null hypothesis, the exact probability value of $\delta = 170.4641$ computed on the $M = 262,144$ possible arrangements of the observed data with $N = 18$ observations preserved for each arrangement is

$$P(\delta \le \delta_0 | H_0) = \frac{\text{number of } \delta \text{ values } \le \delta_0}{M} = \frac{4176}{262,144} = 0.0159 ,$$

where δ_0 denotes the observed value of test statistic δ and M is the number of possible, equally-likely arrangements of the rank-score data listed in Table 5.12.

5.8.3   The Relationship Between Statistics T and δ

The functional relationships between test statistics T and δ are given by

$$\delta = \frac{N(N+1)(2N+1)}{3(N-1)} - \frac{[4T - N(N+1)]^2}{2N(N-1)} \tag{5.17}$$

and

$$T = \frac{N(N+1)}{4} - \left\{ \frac{N\left[N(N+1)(2N+1) - 3(N-1)\delta\right]}{24} \right\}^{1/2}. \tag{5.18}$$

Following Eq. (5.17), the observed value of test statistic δ with respect to the observed value of test statistic T for the rank-score data listed in Table 5.12 is

$$\delta = \frac{18(18+1)[2(18)+1]}{3(18-1)} - \frac{\left[4(31) - 18(18+1)\right]^2}{2(18)(18-1)}$$
$$= 248.1176 - 77.6536 = 170.4641$$

and following Eq. (5.18), the observed value of Wilcoxon's test statistic T with respect to the observed value of test statistic δ is

$$T = \frac{18(18+1)}{4}$$
$$- \left(\frac{18\{18(18+1)[2(18)+1] - 3(18-1)(170.4641)\}}{24} \right)^{1/2}$$
$$= 85.5 - 54.5 = 31 .$$

Because test statistics δ and T are equivalent under the Fisher–Pitman null hypothesis, the exact probability value of Wilcoxon's $T = 31$ is identical to the exact probability value of $\delta = 170.4641$; that is,

$$P(\delta \le \delta_0 | H_0) = \frac{\text{number of } \delta \text{ values} \le \delta_0}{M} = \frac{4176}{262{,}144} = 0.0159$$

and

$$P(T \ge T_0 | H_0) = \frac{\text{number of } T \text{ values} \ge T_0}{M} = \frac{4176}{262{,}144} = 0.0159 ,$$

where δ_0 and T_0 denote the observed values of test statistics δ and T, respectively, and M is the number of possible, equally-likely arrangements of the $N = 18$ rank scores listed in Table 5.12.

Following Eq. (5.6) on p. 111, the exact expected value of the $M = 262{,}144$ δ test statistic values under the Fisher–Pitman null hypothesis is

$$\mu_\delta = \frac{1}{M} \sum_{i=1}^{M} \delta_i = \frac{61{,}429{,}077}{262{,}144} = 234.3333$$

and following Eq. (5.5) on p. 111, the observed chance-corrected measure of effect size is

$$\Re = 1 - \frac{\delta}{\mu_\delta} = 1 - \frac{170.4641}{234.3333} = +0.2726,$$

indicating approximately 27% within-group agreement above what is expected by chance. No comparisons are made with Cohen's $\hat{d}$ or Pearson's r^2 measures of effect size for one-sample tests as $\hat{d}$ and r^2 are undefined for rank-score data.

5.8.4 An Exact Analysis with $v = 1$

Now consider an analysis of the rank-score data listed in Table 5.12 under the Fisher–Pitman permutation model with $v = 1$, employing ordinary Euclidean differences between the rank scores. The observed value of the permutation test statistic is

$$\delta = \binom{N}{2}^{-1} \sum_{i=1}^{N-1} \sum_{j=i+1}^{N} |x_i - x_j|^v$$

$$= \frac{2}{(18)(18-1)} \Big[\big|(-1) - (-2)\big|^1 + \big|(-1) - (+3)\big|^1$$

$$+ \cdots + \big|(+17) - (+18)\big|^1 \Big] = 10.6340.$$

Because there are only

$$M = 2^N = 2^{18} = 262,144$$

possible, equally-likely arrangements in the reference set of all permutations of the rank-score data listed in Table 5.12, an exact permutation analysis is feasible. Under the Fisher–Pitman permutation model, the exact probability of an observed δ is the proportion of δ test statistic values calculated on all possible arrangements of the observed data that are equal to or less than the observed value of $\delta = 10.6340$. There are exactly 4318 δ test statistic values that are equal to or less than the observed value of $\delta = 10.6340$. If all M arrangements of the $N = 18$ rank scores listed in Table 5.12 occur with equal chance under the Fisher–Pitman null hypothesis, the exact probability value of $\delta = 10.6340$ computed on the $M = 262,144$ possible arrangements of the observed data with $N = 18$ observations preserved for each arrangement is

$$P(\delta \le \delta_0 | H_0) = \frac{\text{number of } \delta \text{ values } \le \delta_0}{M} = \frac{4318}{262,144} = 0.0165,$$

where δ_o denotes the observed value of test statistic δ and M is the number of possible, equally-likely arrangements of the $N = 18$ rank scores listed in Table 5.12.

Following Eq. (5.6) on p. 111, the exact expected value of the $M = 262{,}144$ δ test statistic values under the Fisher–Pitman null hypothesis is

$$\mu_\delta = \frac{1}{M} \sum_{i=1}^{M} \delta_i = \frac{3{,}320{,}490}{262{,}144} = 12.6667$$

and following Eq. (5.5) on p. 111, the observed chance-corrected measure of effect size is

$$\Re = 1 - \frac{\delta}{\mu_\delta} = 1 - \frac{10.6340}{12.6667} = +0.1605 \; ,$$

indicating approximately 16% within-group agreement above what is expected by chance. No comparisons are made with Cohen's $\hat{d}$ or Pearson's r^2 measures of effect size for one-sample tests as $\hat{d}$ and r^2 are undefined for rank-score data.

5.8.5 The Sign Test

The sign test is the most elementary of all tests of differences and is so named because the test statistic is computed from data that have been reduced to simple plus (+) and minus (−) signs, representing positive and negative differences, respectively. The test statistic, denoted by the uppercase letter S, is the smaller of the number of (+) and (−) signs. Although generally not labeled as such, the popular sign test is in fact a permutation test as it follows the discrete binomial probability distribution.

To illustrate the sign test under the Neyman–Pearson population model, consider the sign data listed in Table 5.13 where $N = 16$ subjects attempted to recall as many words as possible out of a list of 25 words. The median value expected from previous trials was 15 words. For the sign data listed in Table 5.12, the column headed Words indicates the number of words recalled by each subject, the column headed Difference lists the differences between the number of words recalled and the predetermined value of 15 words, and the column headed Sign lists the signs of the differences. For the sign data listed in Table 5.13, there are 13 (+) signs and three (−) signs; thus, $S = 3$. Under the null hypothesis that the recall of words above and below the median of 15 words are equally likely, the sign test provides the exact probability of an arrangement with $S = 3$ (−) signs and $N - S = 13$ (+) signs or an arrangement more extreme.

Let p denote the probability of success on a single trial. The binomial results are asymptotically distributed $N(0, 1)$ under the Neyman–Pearson null hypothesis, $H_0\colon p = 0.50$, as $N \to \infty$. For the sign data listed in Table 5.13, the mean of the

Table 5.13 Number of
words correctly recalled for
$N = 16$ subjects

Subject	Words	Difference	Sign
1	14	-1	$-$
2	16	$+1$	$+$
3	18	$+3$	$+$
4	17	$+2$	$+$
5	18	$+3$	$+$
6	16	$+1$	$+$
7	17	$+2$	$+$
8	16	$+1$	$+$
9	19	$+4$	$+$
10	17	$+2$	$+$
11	19	$+4$	$+$
12	21	$+6$	$+$
13	14	-1	$-$
14	13	-2	$-$
15	17	$+2$	$+$
16	17	$+2$	$+$

binomial probability distribution with $N = 16$ and $p = 0.50$ is

$$\mu_b = Np = (16)(0.50) = 8.00 \, ,$$

the standard deviation of the binomial probability distribution is

$$\sigma_b = \sqrt{Np(1-p)} = \sqrt{(16)(0.50)(0.50)} = 2.00 \, ,$$

and the standard score of $S = 3$ is

$$z = \frac{S - \mu_b}{\sigma_b} = \frac{3 - 8.00}{2.00} = -2.50 \, ,$$

yielding an asymptotic $N(0, 1)$ two-tail probability value of $P = 0.0124$. Because $N = 16$ is a relatively small number, a correction for continuity should be applied. Thus,

$$z = \frac{S + 0.50 - \mu_b}{\sigma_b} = \frac{3 + 0.50 - 8}{2.00} = -2.25 \, ,$$

yielding an asymptotic $N(0, 1)$ two-tail probability value of $P = 0.0244$.

For comparison, the exact cumulative binomial probability value for any S is given by

$$P(S|N) = \sum_{i=0}^{S} \binom{N}{i} p^i (1-p)^{N-i} \, , \tag{5.19}$$

where p is the probability of success on a single trial. Since the null hypothesis for the sign test is simply that there is no difference expected between the number of $(+)$ and $(-)$ signs; that is, H_0: $p = 0.50$, Eq. (5.19) reduces to

$$P(S|N) = \sum_{i=0}^{S} \binom{N}{i} (0.50)^N .$$

For the sign data listed in Table 5.13 with $i = 0, 1, 2, 3$,

$$p(0|16) = \binom{16}{0} (0.50)^{16} = \frac{16!}{0! \, 16!} (0.50)^{16} = \frac{1}{65{,}536} = 0.1526 \times 10^{-4} ,$$

$$p(1|16) = \binom{16}{1} (0.50)^{16} = \frac{16!}{1! \, 15!} (0.50)^{16} = \frac{16}{65{,}536} = 0.2441 \times 10^{-3} ,$$

$$p(2|16) = \binom{16}{2} (0.50)^{16} = \frac{16!}{2! \, 14!} (0.50)^{16} = \frac{120}{65{,}536} = 0.1831 \times 10^{-2} ,$$

and

$$p(3|16) = \binom{16}{3} (0.50)^{16} = \frac{16!}{3! \, 13!} (0.50)^{16} = \frac{560}{65{,}536} = 0.8545 \times 10^{-2} .$$

Because the probability of success is $p = 0.50$, the binomial probability distribution is symmetrical and the exact two-tail probability value is

$$P = 2(0.1526 \times 10^{-4} + 0.2441 \times 10^{-3} + 0.1831 \times 10^{-2}$$
$$+ 0.8545 \times 10^{-2}) = 0.0213 .$$

5.8.6   An Exact Analysis with $v = 2$

For an analysis of the sign data listed in Table 5.13 under the Fisher–Pitman permutation model let $v = 2$, employing squared Euclidean differences between the signs, and let $x_i = \pm 1$ denote the observed signs for $i = 1, \ldots, N$. Then the permutation test statistic is given by

$$\delta = \binom{N}{2}^{-1} \sum_{i=1}^{N-1} \sum_{j=i+1}^{N} |x_i - x_j|^v . \tag{5.20}$$

Following Eq. (5.20) for the sign data listed in Table 5.13 with $N = 16$ and $v = 2$, the observed value of the permutation test statistic is

$$\delta = \frac{2}{(16)(16-1)}\left[\left|(-1)-(+1)\right|^2 + \left|(-1)-(+1)\right|^2\right.$$
$$\left. + \cdots + \left|(+1)-(+1)\right|^2\right] = 1.30 \,.$$

Because there are only

$$M = 2^N = 2^{16} = 65{,}536$$

possible, equally-likely arrangements in the reference set of all permutations of the sign data listed in Table 5.13, an exact permutation analysis is feasible. Under the Fisher–Pitman permutation model, the exact probability of an observed δ is the proportion of δ test statistic values calculated on all possible arrangements of the observed data that are equal to or less than the observed value of $\delta = 1.30$. There are exactly 1394 δ test statistic values that are equal to or less than the observed value of $\delta = 1.30$. If all M arrangements of the $N = 16$ signs listed in Table 5.13 occur with equal chance under the Fisher–Pitman null hypothesis, the exact probability value of $\delta = 1.30$ computed on the $M = 65{,}536$ possible arrangements of the observed signs with $N = 16$ observations preserved for each arrangement is

$$P(\delta \le \delta_0|H_0) = \frac{\text{number of } \delta \text{ values } \le \delta_0}{M} = \frac{1394}{65{,}536} = 0.0213 \,,$$

where δ_0 denotes the observed value of test statistic δ and M is the number of possible, equally-likely arrangements of the $N = 16$ signs listed in Table 5.13. Thus the exact permutation probability of $P = 0.0213$ is identical to the exact binomial probability of $P = 0.0213$.

Under the Neyman–Pearson null hypothesis, the relationships between test statistics δ and S are given by

$$\delta = \frac{2S(N-S)}{N(N-1)(0.5)^2} = \frac{8S(N-S)}{N(N-1)} \tag{5.21}$$

and

$$S = \frac{N}{2} \pm \frac{\sqrt{4N^2 - 2\delta N(N-1)}}{4}\,. \tag{5.22}$$

Following Eq. (5.21), the observed value of test statistic δ with respect to the observed value of test statistic S for the sign data listed in Table 5.13 is

$$\delta = \frac{(8)(3)(16-3)}{(16)(16-1)} = \frac{312}{240} = 1.30$$

and following Eq. (5.22), the observed value of test statistic S with respect to the observed value of test statistic δ is

$$S = \frac{16}{2} \pm \frac{\sqrt{4(16)^2 - 2(1.30)(16)(16-1)}}{4} = \frac{16}{2} \pm \frac{\sqrt{400}}{4} = 8 \pm 5 \, ,$$

where the two roots of the quadratic equation yield $8-5 = 3$ and $8+5 = 13$, which are the values for $S = 3$ $(-)$ signs and $N - S = 16 - 3 = 13$ $(+)$ signs, respectively.

Because test statistics δ and S are equivalent under the Fisher–Pitman null hypothesis, the exact probability value of $S = 3$ is identical to the probability value of $\delta = 1.30$; that is,

$$P(\delta \le \delta_0) = \frac{\text{number of } \delta \text{ values} \le \delta_0}{M} = \frac{1394}{65,536} = 0.0213$$

and

$$P(S \ge S_0) = \frac{\text{number of } S \text{ values} \ge S_0}{M} = \frac{1394}{65,536} = 0.0213 \, ,$$

where δ_0 and S_0 denote the observed values of δ and S, respectively, and M is the number of possible, equally-likely arrangements of the $N = 16$ signs listed in Table 5.13.

Following Eq. (5.6) on p. 111, the exact expected value of the $M = 65,536$ δ test statistic values under the Fisher–Pitman null hypothesis is

$$\mu_\delta = \frac{1}{M} \sum_{i=1}^{M} \delta_i = \frac{131,072}{65,536} = 2.00$$

and following Eq. (5.5) on p. 111, the observed chance-corrected measure of effect size is

$$\Re = 1 - \frac{\delta}{\mu_\delta} = 1 - \frac{1.30}{2.00} = +0.35 \, ,$$

indicating 35% within-group agreement above what is expected by chance. No comparisons are made with Cohen's $\hat{d}$ or Pearson's r^2 measures of effect size for one-sample tests as $\hat{d}$ and r^2 are undefined for simple sign data.

5.8.7 An Exact Analysis with $v = 1$

Consider an analysis of the sign data listed in Table 5.13 on p. 141 under the Fisher–Pitman permutation model with $v = 1$, employing ordinary Euclidean differences between the paired signs. The observed value of the permutation test statistic is

$$
\delta = \binom{N}{2}^{-1} \sum_{i=1}^{N-1} \sum_{j=i+1}^{N} |x_i - x_j|^v
$$

$$
= \frac{2}{(16)(16-1)} \Big[|(-1) - (+1)|^1 + |(-1) - (+1)|^1
$$

$$
+ \cdots + |(+1) - (+1)|^1 \Big] = 0.65 .
$$

Because there are only

$$
M = 2^N = 2^{16} = 65{,}536
$$

possible, equally-likely arrangements in the reference set of all permutations of the sign data listed in Table 5.13, an exact permutation analysis is possible. Under the Fisher–Pitman permutation model, the exact probability of an observed δ is the proportion of δ test statistic values calculated on all possible arrangements of the observed data that are equal to or less than the observed value of $\delta = 0.65$. There are exactly 1394 δ test statistic values that are equal to or less than the observed value of $\delta = 0.65$. If all M arrangements of the $N = 16$ signs listed in Table 5.13 occur with equal chance under the Fisher–Pitman null hypothesis, the exact probability value of $\delta = 0.65$ computed on the $M = 65{,}536$ possible arrangements of the observed data with $N = 16$ observations preserved for each arrangement is

$$
P(\delta \le \delta_0) = \frac{\text{number of } \delta \text{ values } \le \delta_0}{M} = \frac{1394}{65{,}536} = 0.0213 ,
$$

where δ_0 denotes the observed value of test statistic δ and M is the number of possible, equally-likely arrangements of the sign data listed in Table 5.13.

Following Eq. (5.6) on p. 111, the exact expected value of the $M = 65{,}536 \ \delta$ test statistic values under the Fisher–Pitman null hypothesis is

$$
\mu_\delta = \frac{1}{M} \sum_{i=1}^{M} \delta_i = \frac{65{,}536}{65{,}536} = 1.00
$$

and following Eq. (5.5) on p. 111, the observed chance-corrected measure of effect size is

$$
\Re = 1 - \frac{\delta}{\mu_\delta} = 1 - \frac{0.65}{1.00} = +0.35 ,
$$

indicating 35% within-group agreement above what is expected by chance. No comparisons are made with Cohen's $\hat{d}$ or Pearson's r^2 measures of effect size for the sign test as $\hat{d}$ and r^2 are undefined for simple sign data.

Because all the values for the sign test are either $+1$ or -1, the probability values for $v = 2$ and $v = 1$ are identical; that is, $P = 0.0213$. Also, the permutation test statistic value for $v = 2$ ($\delta = 1.30$) is exactly twice the value for $v = 1$ ($\delta = 0.65$) and the exact expected value of test statistic δ for $v = 2$ ($\mu_\delta = 2.00$) is exactly twice the value for $v = 1$ ($\mu_\delta = 1.00$). Consequently, the value for the measure of effect size based $v = 2$ ($\Re = +0.35$) is identical to the value based on $v = 1$; that is, $\Re = +0.35$.

5.9 Example 6: Multivariate Permutation Analyses

Permutation statistical methods applied to one-sample tests are not limited to univariate data and can easily accommodate multivariate data. Tests for multivariate data have found many applications in the biological and social sciences [27]. To illustrate the analysis of multivariate data in a one-sample test, consider the example data listed in Table 5.14 with $r = 3$ responses for each of $N = 9$ subjects. The responses are percentiles on three socioeconomic variables: income, occupation, and education. The advantage of a multivariate analysis is that the data are not reduced to a simple index with a concomitant loss of information. The usual approach for analyzing socioeconomic data is to average the income, occupation, and education values into a simplifying index of socioeconomic status (SES).[7] Thus a subject who is high on income, in the middle on occupation, and low on education will average about the same on SES as a subject who is low on income, in the middle on occupation, and high on education, although the profiles of the two subjects may differ greatly, as illustrated in Fig. 5.2.

A permutation test of multivariate one-sample data is easily defined [25, pp. 127–131]. Let x_{ik} denote the observed sample values for $i = 1, \ldots, N$ subjects and $k = 1, \ldots, r$ variates. The permutation test statistic is then given by

$$\delta = \binom{N}{2}^{-1} \sum_{i=1}^{N-1} \sum_{j=i+1}^{N} \sum_{k=1}^{r} |x_{ik} - x_{jk}|^v ,$$

where, typically, $v = 2$ or $v = 1$. For multivariate data, the exact expected value of test statistic δ under the Fisher–Pitman null hypothesis is given by

$$\mu_\delta = \frac{1}{M} \sum_{i=1}^{M} \delta_i$$

[7] Oftentimes a weighted average is used, providing different weights for the three variables: income, occupation, and education.

Table 5.14 Example
multivariate data on $N = 9$
subjects with percentile
scores on socioeconomic
variables: income (I),
occupation (O), education
(E), and socioeconomic
Status (SES)

Subject	I	O	E	SES
1	80	92	98	90
2	78	81	98	86
3	76	80	96	84
4	76	78	90	81
5	72	65	90	76
6	70	66	90	75
7	68	62	60	63
8	68	70	52	63
9	66	75	52	64

Fig. 5.2 Graphic comparing
two individuals (A and B)
scoring high, medium, low
and low, medium, high,
respectively, on income (I),
occupation (O), and
education (E)

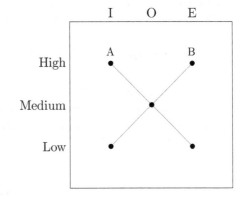

and the chance-corrected measure of effect size is given by

$$\Re = 1 - \frac{\delta}{\mu_\delta} \ .$$

5.9.1   An Exact Analysis with $v = 2$

Consider the socioeconomic data listed in Table 5.14 under the Fisher–Pitman permutation model with $v = 2$, employing squared Euclidean scaling. The observed value of the permutation test statistic is

$$\delta = \binom{N}{2}^{-1} \sum_{i=1}^{N-1} \sum_{j=i+1}^{N} \sum_{k=1}^{r} |x_{ik} - x_{jk}|^v$$

$$= \frac{2}{9(9-1)} \Big[|80 - 78|^2 + |92 - 81|^2 + |98 - 98|^2$$

$$+ \cdots + |68 - 66|^2 + |70 - 75|^2 + |52 - 52|^2 \Big] = 1024.50 \ .$$

Since there are only

$$M = 2^N = 2^9 = 256$$

possible, equally-likely arrangements in the reference set of all permutations of the multivariate socioeconomic data listed in Table 5.14, an exact analysis is possible.[8] The exact probability of an observed δ is the proportion of δ test statistic values calculated on all possible arrangements of the observed data that are equal to or less than the observed value of $\delta = 1024.50$. There is only one δ test statistic value that is equal to or less than the observed value of $\delta = 1024.50$. If all arrangements of the $N = 9$ values listed in Table 5.14 occur with equal chance under the Fisher–Pitman null hypothesis, the exact probability value of $\delta_0 = 1024.50$ based on all $M = 256$ arrangements of the observed data is

$$P(\delta \leq \delta_0 | H_0) = \frac{\text{number of } \delta \text{ values} \leq \delta_0}{M} = \frac{1}{256} = 0.3906 \times 10^{-2} ,$$

where δ_0 denotes the observed value of test statistic δ and M is the number of possible, equally-likely arrangements of the socioeconomic data listed in Table 5.14.

The exact expected value of test statistic δ under the Fisher–Pitman null hypothesis is

$$\mu_\delta = \frac{1}{M} \sum_{i=1}^{M} \delta_i = \frac{2,339,914.7520}{256} = 9,140.2920$$

and the observed chance-corrected measure of effect size is

$$\Re = 1 - \frac{\delta}{\mu_\delta} = 1 - \frac{1024.50}{9,140.2920} = +0.8879 ,$$

indicating approximately 89% agreement among the $N = 9$ subjects above what is expected by chance. No comparisons are made with Cohen's $\hat{d}$ or Pearson's r^2 measures of effect size as $\hat{d}$ and r^2 are undefined for multivariate data.

5.9.2 An Exact Analysis with $v = 1$

Permutation multivariate statistical methods are not confined to analyses with squared Euclidean differences; that is, $v = 2$. For the socioeconomic data listed in Table 5.14 with $v = 1$, employing ordinary Euclidean scaling, the observed value

---

[8]Note that the number of variates is not a factor in determining the number of possible arrangements of the observed data.

of the permutation test statistic is

$$\delta = \binom{N}{2}^{-1} \sum_{i=1}^{N-1} \sum_{j=i+1}^{N} \sum_{k=1}^{r} |x_{ik} - x_{jk}|^{v}$$

$$= \frac{2}{9(9-1)} \Big[|80 - 78|^{1} + |92 - 81|^{1} + |98 - 98|^{1}$$

$$+ \cdots + |68 - 66|^{1} + |70 - 75|^{1} + |52 - 52|^{1} \Big] = 39.2222 \, .$$

Since there are only

$$M = 2^{N} = 2^{9} = 256$$

possible, equally-likely arrangements in the reference set of all permutations of the multivariate socioeconomic data listed in Table 5.14, an exact analysis is possible. Under the Fisher–Pitman permutation model, the exact probability of an observed δ is the proportion of δ test statistic values calculated on all possible arrangements of the observed data that are equal to or less than the observed value of $\delta = 39.2222$. There is only one δ test statistic value that is equal to or less than the observed value of $\delta = 39.2222$. If all arrangements of the $N = 9$ values listed in Table 5.14 occur with equal chance under the Fisher–Pitman null hypothesis, the exact probability value of $\delta = 39.2222$ based on all $M = 256$ arrangements of the observed data is

$$P(\delta \leq \delta_0 | H_0) = \frac{\text{number of } \delta \text{ values } \leq \delta_0}{M} = \frac{1}{256} = 0.3906 \times 10^{-2} \, ,$$

where δ_0 denotes the observed value of δ and M is the number of possible, equally-likely arrangements of the multivariate socioeconomic data listed in Table 5.14.

The exact expected value of test statistic δ under the Fisher–Pitman null hypothesis is

$$\mu_\delta = \frac{1}{M} \sum_{i=1}^{M} \delta_i = \frac{18,714.5472}{256} = 73.1037 \, ,$$

and the observed chance-corrected measure of effect size is

$$\Re = 1 - \frac{\delta}{\mu_\delta} = 1 - \frac{39.2222}{73.1037} = +0.4635 \, ,$$

indicating approximately 46% agreement among the $N = 9$ subjects above what is expected by chance. No comparisons are made with Cohen's $\hat{d}$ or Pearson's r^2 measures of effect size as $\hat{d}$ and r^2 are undefined for multivariate data.

Because the values for income, occupation, and education in Table 5.14 are all positive, the probability values with $v = 2$ and $v = 1$ are identical under the Fisher–

Pitman null hypothesis. This is always true for one-sample tests: the probability values with either $v = 2$ and $v = 1$ are always the same whenever all the observed values are either positive or negative. In addition, extreme values do not affect the probability values under these conditions.

5.10   Summary

Under the Neyman–Pearson population model of statistical inference, this chapter examined one-sample tests where the null hypothesis typically posits a specified value other than zero for the population mean. The conventional one-sample test and two measures of effect size under the population model were described and illustrated: Student's one-sample t test and Cohen's $\hat{d}$ and Pearson's r^2 measures of effect size, respectively.

Under the Fisher–Pitman permutation model, test statistic δ and associated measure of effect size, $\mathfrak{R}$, were introduced and illustrated for one-sample tests. Test statistic δ was shown to have more flexibility than Student's t test statistic, incorporating either ordinary or squared Euclidean scaling with $v = 1$ and $v = 2$, respectively. Mielke and Berry's chance-corrected effect size measure $\mathfrak{R}$ was shown to be applicable to either $v = 1$ or $v = 2$ without modification and to have a more meaningful chance-corrected interpretation than either Cohen's $\hat{d}$ or Pearson's r^2 measures of effect size.

Six examples illustrated applications of test statistics δ and $\mathfrak{R}$. In the first example, a small sample of $N = 4$ values was utilized to describe and simplify the calculation of δ and $\mathfrak{R}$. The second example used a small sample of $N = 4$ values to develop a permutation-based measure of effect size, $\mathfrak{R}$, and related the permutation measure to various conventional measures of effect size; specifically, Cohen's $\hat{d}$ and Pearson's r^2. The third example with $N = 12$ values illustrated the effects of extreme values on various combinations of plus-and-minus values with both $v = 2$ and $v = 1$. The fourth example with $N = 28$ values compared exact and Monte Carlo probability procedures, showcasing the efficiency of Monte Carlo permutation methods. The fifth example with $N = 18$ values applied permutation statistical methods to univariate rank-score data, comparing permutation statistical methods to Wilcoxon's conventional signed-ranks test and the sign test. Finally, in the sixth example both δ and $\mathfrak{R}$ were extended to multivariate data with $N = 9$ subjects and $r = 3$ variates—something for which Student's t, Cohen's $\hat{d}$, and Pearson's r^2 are not suited. The Fisher–Pitman permutation model with test statistic δ and measure of effect size $\mathfrak{R}$ are not confined to one-sample tests and play important roles in the subsequent chapters.

Chapter 6 continues the presentation of permutation statistical methods, but examines research designs in which two independent samples are compared and contrasted. Because two-sample tests for differences constitute the classic control-treatment experimental design, two-sample tests are found in a wide variety of research areas. Two-sample tests are the simplest of the tests in a large class of completely-randomized tests of differences.

References

1. Benjamin, D.J., Berger, J.O., Johannesson, M., Nosek, B.A., Wagenmakers, E.J., Berk, R., et al.: Redefine statistical significance. Nat. Hum. Behav. **2**, 6–10 (2018)
2. Berry, K.J.: Algorithm 179: enumeration of all permutations of multi-sets with fixed repetition numbers. J. R. Stat. Soc. C Appl. **31**, 169–173 (1982)
3. Berry, K.J., Mielke, P.W., Johnston, J.E.: Permutation Statistical Methods: An Integrated Approach. Springer, Cham (2016)
4. Berry, K.J., Johnston, J.E., Mielke, P.W.: The Measurement of Association: A Permutation Statistical Approach. Springer, Cham (2018)
5. Blaug, M.: The myth of the old poor law and the making of the new. J. Econ. Hist. **23**, 151–184 (1963)
6. Box, G.E.P.: Non-normality and tests on variances. Biometrika **40**, 318–335 (1953)
7. Box, G.E.P.: An Accidental Statistician: The Life and Memories of George E. P. Box. Wiley, New York (2013). [Inscribed "With a little help from my friend, Judith L. Allen"]
8. Capraro, R.M., Capraro, M.M.: Treatments of effect sizes and statistical significance tests in textbooks. Educ. Psychol. Meas. **62**, 771–782 (2002)
9. Capraro, R.M., Capraro, M.M.: Exploring the APA fifth edition *Publication Manual's* impact on the analytic preferences of journal editorial board members. Educ. Psychol. Meas. **63**, 554–565 (2003)
10. Chawla, D.S.: *P*-value shake-up proposed. Nature **548**, 16–17 (2017)
11. Cohen, J.: Statistical Power Analysis for the Behavioral Sciences, 2nd edn. Erlbaum, Hillsdale (1988)
12. Cohen, J.: Things I have learned (so far). Am. Psychol. **45**, 1304–1312 (1990)
13. Cohen, J.: The earth is round ($p < .05$). Am. Psychol. **49**, 997–1003 (1994)
14. Cowles, M.: Statistics in Psychology: An Historical Perspective, 2nd edn. Lawrence Erlbaum, Mahwah (2001)
15. D'Andrade, R., Dart, J.: The interpretation of r versus r^2 or why percent of variance accounted for is a poor measure of size of effect. J. Quant. Anthro. **2**, 47–59 (1990)
16. Hess, B., Olejnik, S., Huberty, C.J.: The efficacy of two improvement-over-chance effect sizes for two-group univariate comparisons. Educ. Psychol. Meas. **61**, 909–936 (2001)
17. Hotelling, H., Pabst, M.R.: Rank correlation and tests of significance involving no assumption of normality. Ann. Math. Stat. **7**, 29–43 (1936)
18. Howell, D.C.: Statistical Methods for Psychology, 6th edn. Wadsworth, Belmont (2007)
19. Johnston, J.E., Berry, K.J., Mielke, P.W.: Permutation tests: precision in estimating probability values. Percept. Motor Skill. **105**, 915–920 (2007)
20. Kirk, R.E.: Experimental Design: Procedures for the Behavioral Sciences. Brooks/Cole, Belmont (1968)
21. Kirk, R.E.: Practical significance: a concept whose time has come. Educ. Psychol. Meas. **56**, 746–759 (1996)
22. Kline, R.B.: Beyond Significance Testing: Reforming Data Analysis Methods in Behavioral Research. American Psychological Association, Washington (2004)
23. Kvålseth, T.O.: Cautionary note about R^2. Am. Stat. **39**, 279–285 (1985)
24. McGrath, R.E., Meyer, G.J.: When effect sizes disagree: the case of r and d. Psychol. Methods **11**, 386–401 (2006)
25. Mielke, P.W., Berry, K.J.: Permutation Methods: A Distance Function Approach, 2nd edn. Springer, New York (2007)

26. Ozer, D.J.: Correlation and the coefficient of determination. Psychol. Bull. **97**, 307–315 (1985)
27. Reiss, P.T., Stevens, M.H.H., Shehzad, Z., Petkova, E., Milham, M.P.: On distance-based permutation tests for between-group comparisons. Biometrics **66**, 636–643 (2010)
28. Rosenthal, R.: Parametric measures of effect size. In: Cooper, H., Hedges, L.V. (eds.) The Handbook of Research Synthesis, pp. 231–234. Russell Sage, New York (1994)
29. Rosenthal, R., Rubin, D.B.: A note on percent variance explained as a measure of the importance of effects. J. Appl. Soc. Psychol. **9**, 395–396 (1979)
30. Rosenthal, R., Rubin, D.B.: A simple, general purpose display of magnitude of experimental effect. J. Educ. Psychol. **74**, 166–169 (1982)
31. Salsburg, D.S.: Errors, Blunders, and Lies: How to Tell the Difference. CRC Press, Boca Raton (2017)
32. Skipper, J.K., Guenther, A.L., Nass, G.: The sacredness of .05: a note concerning the uses of statistical levels of significance in social science. Am. Sociol. **2**, 16–18 (1967)
33. Wilcoxon, F.: Individual comparisons by ranking methods. Biometrics Bull. **1**, 80–83 (1945)
34. Wilkinson, L.: Statistical methods in psychology journals: guidelines and explanations. Am. Psychol. **54**, 594–604 (1999)

Chapter 6
Two-Sample Tests

Abstract This chapter introduces permutation methods for two-sample tests. Included in this chapter are six example analyses illustrating computation of exact permutation probability values for two-sample tests, calculation of measures of effect size for two-sample tests, the effect of extreme values on conventional and permutation two-sample tests, exact and Monte Carlo permutation procedures for two-sample tests, application of permutation methods to two-sample rank-score data, and analysis of two-sample multivariate data. Included in this chapter are permutation versions of Student's two-sample t test, the Wilcoxon–Mann–Whitney two-sample rank-sum test, Hotelling's multivariate T^2 test for two independent samples, and a permutation-based alternative for the four conventional measures of effect size for two-sample tests: Cohen's $\hat{d}$, Pearson's r^2, Kelley's ϵ^2, and Hays' $\hat{\omega}^2$.

This chapter presents exact and Monte Carlo permutation statistical methods for two-sample tests. Two-sample tests for experimental differences are of primary importance in basic research, whether that be in the behavioral, medical, biological, agricultural, or physical sciences. Statistical tests for differences between two samples are of two varieties. The first of the two varieties examines two sets of data obtained from two completely separate (independent) samples of subjects. For example, a study might seek to compare grades in an elementary statistics course for majors and non-majors, for female and male students, for transfer and non-transfer students, or for juniors and seniors. In a true experimental design with two independent samples a large pool of subjects is randomly assigned (randomized) to the treatments using a fair coin or a pseudo-random number generator.[1] More often than not, however, it is not possible to randomize subjects to treatments, especially in survey research. For example, it is not possible to randomly assign subjects to such

---

[1] For two treatments a fair coin works quite well with heads and tails. For three treatments, a fair die is often used with faces with one or two pips assigned to the first treatment, faces with 3 or 4 pips assigned to the second treatment, and faces with 5 or 6 pips assigned to the third treatment. For four treatments, a shuffled deck of cards works well with clubs (♣), diamonds (◇), hearts (♡), and spades (♠) assigned to Treatments 1, 2, 3, and 4, respectively.

© Springer Nature Switzerland AG 2019
K. J. Berry et al., *A Primer of Permutation Statistical Methods*,
https://doi.org/10.1007/978-3-030-20933-9_6

categories as gender, age, IQ, or educational level. The lack of random assignment to treatments can greatly compromise the results of two-sample tests.

The second variety of two-sample tests examines two sets of data obtained on the same or matched subjects. For example, a study might compare the same subjects at two different time periods, such as before and after an intervention, or matched subjects on two different diets: low- and high-carbohydrate. When compared with tests for two independent samples, matched-pairs tests generally have less variability between the two samples, provide more power with the same number of subjects, and because the sample sizes are the same for both treatments, matched-pairs tests produce larger test statistic values and smaller probability values than comparable tests for two independent samples, other factors being equal. Two-sample tests for independent samples are presented in this chapter. Matched-pairs tests for two related samples are presented in Chap. 7.[2]

6.1   Introduction

In this chapter permutation statistical methods for two-sample tests are illustrated with six example analyses. The first example utilizes a small set of data to illustrate the computation of exact permutation methods for two independent samples, wherein the permutation test statistic, δ, is developed and compared with Student's conventional t test for two independent samples. The second example develops a permutation-based measure of effect size as a chance-corrected alternative to the four conventional measures of effect size for two-sample tests: Cohen's $\hat{d}$, Pearson's r^2, Kelley's ϵ^2, and Hays' $\hat{\omega}^2$. The third example compares permutation methods based on ordinary and squared Euclidean scaling functions, emphasizing methods of analysis for data sets containing extreme values. The fourth example compares and contrasts exact and Monte Carlo permutation methods, demonstrating the accuracy and efficiency of Monte Carlo statistical methods. The fifth example illustrates the application of permutation statistical methods to univariate rank-score data, comparing permutation statistical methods with the conventional Wilcoxon–Mann–Whitney two-sample rank-sum test. The sixth example illustrates the application of permutation statistical methods to multivariate data, comparing permutation statistical methods with the conventional Hotelling's multivariate T^2 test for two independent samples.

One of the most familiar and popular two-sample tests looks at the mean difference between two independent treatment groups. This is the classic test for a difference between a control group and an experimental group. For example, a researcher might want to compare the number of trials on a specified task for two groups of rats—one raised under normal conditions and the other raised in semi-

---

[2]In some disciplines tests on two independent samples are known as between-subjects tests and tests for two dependent or related samples are known as within-subjects tests.

darkness. Or it might be of interest to examine the differences in performance between two groups of students—one in a section of a course taught in a face-to-face lecture format and the other in a section of the same course taught in an on-line distance-learning format by the same instructor.

The most popular univariate test for two independent samples under the Neyman–Pearson population model of inference is Student's two-sample t test wherein the null hypothesis (H_0) posits no mean difference between the two populations from which the samples are presumed to have been drawn; for example, H_0: $\mu_1 = \mu_2$. Alternatively, H_0: $\mu_1 - \mu_2 = 0$. The test does not determine whether the null hypothesis is true, but only provides the probability that, if the null hypothesis is true, the samples have been drawn from the specified population(s). Student's t test is the standard test for a mean difference between two independent samples and is taught in every introductory course.

6.1.1 The Student Two-Sample t Test

Consider two independent samples of sizes n_1 and n_2. Under the Neyman–Pearson null hypothesis, H_0: $\mu_1 = \mu_2$, Student's t test for two independent samples is given by

$$t = \frac{\bar{x}_1 - \bar{x}_2}{\left[s_p^2 \left(\dfrac{1}{n_1} + \dfrac{1}{n_2} \right) \right]^{1/2}} \, ,$$

where the unbiased pooled estimate of the population variance is given by

$$s_p^2 = \frac{(n_1 - 1)s_1^2 + (n_2 - 1)s_2^2}{N - 2} \, ,$$

the sample estimate of the population variance for the ith treatment group is given by

$$s_i^2 = \frac{1}{n_i - 1} \sum_{j=1}^{n_i} \left(x_{ij} - \bar{x}_i \right)^2 \, , \qquad i = 1, 2 \, ,$$

n_i denotes the number of objects in the ith of the two treatment groups,

$$N = \sum_{i=1}^{2} n_i$$

denotes the total number of objects in the two treatment groups, $\bar{x}_i$ denotes the arithmetic mean of the measurement scores for the ith of the two treatment groups, given by

$$\bar{x}_i = \frac{1}{n_i} \sum_{j=1}^{n_i} x_{ij}, \qquad i = 1, 2,$$

and x_{ij} is a measurement score for the jth object in the ith treatment group. Assuming independence, normality, and homogeneity of variance, test statistic t is asymptotically distributed as Student's t under the Neyman–Pearson null hypothesis with $N - 2$ degrees of freedom. The permissible probability of a type I error is denoted by α and if the observed value of t is more extreme than the critical values of $\pm t$ that define α, the null hypothesis is rejected with a probability of type I error equal to or less than α, under the assumptions of normality and homogeneity.

The assumptions underlying Student's t test for two independent samples are (1) the observations are independent, (2) the data are random samples from a well-defined population, (3) homogeneity of variance, that is $\sigma_1^2 = \sigma_2^2$, and (4) the target variable is normally distributed in the population. It should be noted that a number of textbooks have argued that what is important is that the sampling distribution of sample mean differences be normally distributed and not the target variable in the population. However, Student drew his random samples from populations of two sets of measurements on criminal anthropometry that had been published by William Robert Macdonell in *Biometrika* in 1902 [8]. Student's data consisted of two measurements obtained by Macdonell that were approximately normally distributed: (1) the height and (2) the length of the left middle finger of 3000 criminals over 20 years of age and serving sentences in the chief prisons of England and Wales. Moreover, Student proved in Sect. 2 of his 1908 paper that the mean and variance are independent and the normal distribution is the only distribution where this is always true, as noted by George Barnard [1, p. 169].[3]

6.2   A Permutation Approach

Now consider a test for two independent samples under the Fisher–Pitman permutation model of statistical inference. For the permutation model there is no null hypothesis specifying population parameters. Instead the null hypothesis is simply that all possible arrangements of the observed differences occur with equal chance [4]. Also, there is no alternative hypothesis under the permutation model and no specified α level. Moreover, there is no requirement of random sampling, no assumption of normality, and no assumption of homogeneity of variance. This is

---

[3] Also see a discussion by S.M. Stigler in *The Seven Pillars of Statistical Wisdom* [14, pp. 91–92].

not to say that the permutation model is unaffected by homogeneity of variance, but it is not a requirement as it is for Student's t test. Under the Neyman–Pearson null hypothesis, if the assumption of homogeneity is not met, t is no longer distributed as Student's t with $N - 2$ degrees of freedom.

A permutation alternative to the conventional test for two independent samples is easily defined. The permutation test statistic for two independent samples is given by

$$\delta = \sum_{i=1}^{2} C_i \xi_i , \tag{6.1}$$

where $C_i > 0$ is a positive treatment-group weight for $i = 1, 2$,

$$\xi_i = \binom{n_i}{2}^{-1} \sum_{j=1}^{N-1} \sum_{k=j+1}^{N} \Delta(j, k) \Psi_i(\omega_j) \Psi_i(\omega_k) \tag{6.2}$$

is the average distance-function value for all distinct pairs of objects in treatment group S_i for $i = 1, 2$,

$$\Delta(j, k) = |x_j - x_k|^v ,$$

is a symmetric distance-function value for paired objects j and k,

$$N = \sum_{i=1}^{2} n_i ,$$

and $\Psi(\cdot)$ is an indicator function given by

$$\Psi_i(\omega_j) = \begin{cases} 1 & \text{if } \omega_j \in S_i , \\ 0 & \text{otherwise} . \end{cases}$$

Under the Fisher–Pitman permutation model, the null hypothesis simply states that equal probabilities are assigned to each of the

$$M = \frac{(n_1 + n_2)!}{n_1! \, n_2!} \tag{6.3}$$

possible, equally-likely allocations of the N objects to the two treatment groups, S_1 and S_2. As noted in Chap. 5, it is imperative that the M possible arrangements of the observed data be generated systematically as expressed in Eq. (6.3), while preserving n_1 and n_2 for each arrangement. Only a systematic procedure guarantees M equally-likely arrangements. Simply shuffling values among the two treatment groups does not ensure the M possible, equally-likely arrangements mandated by the Fisher–Pitman permutation null hypothesis: all possible arrangements of the observed data occur with equal chance [4].

Under the Fisher–Pitman permutation model, the probability value associated with an observed value of δ, say δ_0, is the probability under the null hypothesis of observing a value of δ as extreme or more extreme than δ_0. Thus an exact probability value for δ_0 may be expressed as

$$P\left(\delta \leq \delta_0 | H_0\right) = \frac{\text{number of } \delta \text{ values } \leq \delta_0}{M} . \tag{6.4}$$

When M is large, an approximate probability value for δ may be obtained from a Monte Carlo procedure, where

$$P\left(\delta \leq \delta_0 | H_0\right) = \frac{\text{number of } \delta \text{ values } \leq \delta_0}{L}$$

and L denotes the number of randomly-sampled test statistic values. Typically, L is set to a large number to ensure accuracy; for example, $L = 1,000,000$ [6]. While $L = 1,000,000$ random arrangements does not guarantee that no two arrangements will be identical, the cycle lengths of modern pseudo-random number generators (PRNG) are sufficiently long that identical arrangements are either avoided or occur so rarely as to be inconsequential. For example, some pseudo-random generators utilize the expanded value of π where the cycle length is so long that it has yet to be determined. Older pseudo-random number generators had a cycle length of only

$$2^{32} - 1 = 4,294,967,295 .$$

The Mersenne twister is the current choice for a pseudo-random number generator and is by far the most widely-used general-purpose pseudo-random number generator, having been incorporated into a large number of computer statistical packages, including Microsoft Excel, GAUSS, GLib, Maple, MATLAB, Python, Stata, and the popular R statistical computing language. The cycle length for the Mersenne Twister is $2^{19937} - 1$, which is a very large number.

6.2.1   The Relationship Between Statistics t and δ

When the null hypothesis states H_0: $\mu_1 = \mu_2$, $v = 2$, and the treatment-group weights are given by

$$C_1 = \frac{n_1 - 1}{N - 2} \quad \text{and} \quad C_2 = \frac{n_2 - 1}{N - 2} ,$$

the functional relationships between test statistic δ and Student's t test statistic are given by

$$\delta = \frac{2SS_{\text{Total}}}{t^2 + N - 2} \quad \text{and} \quad t = \left[\frac{2SS_{\text{Total}}}{\delta} - N + 2\right]^{1/2}, \tag{6.5}$$

where

$$SS_{\text{Total}} = \sum_{i=1}^{N} x_i^2 - \left(\sum_{i=1}^{N} x_i\right)^2 \Big/ N$$

and x_i denotes a measurement score for the ith of N objects.

Because of the relationship between test statistic δ and Student's t test statistic, the exact probability values given by

$$P(\delta \leq \delta_o) = \frac{\text{number of } \delta \text{ values } \leq \delta_o}{M}$$

and

$$P(|t| \geq |t_o|) = \frac{\text{number of } |t| \text{ values } \geq |t_o|}{M}$$

are equivalent under the Fisher–Pitman null hypothesis, where δ_o and t_o denote the observed test statistic values of δ and t, respectively, and M is the number of possible, equally-likely arrangements of the observed data.

Also, given $v = 2$ and treatment-group weights

$$C_1 = \frac{n_1 - 1}{N - 2} \quad \text{and} \quad C_2 = \frac{n_2 - 1}{N - 2},$$

the two average distance-function values are related to the sample estimates of the population variance by

$$\xi_1 = 2s_1^2 \quad \text{and} \quad \xi_2 = 2s_2^2,$$

test statistic δ is related to the pooled estimate of the population variance by

$$\delta = 2s_p^2,$$

and the exact expected value of the M δ test statistic values is related to SS_{Total} by

$$\mu_\delta = \frac{2SS_{\text{Total}}}{N - 1}.$$

A chance-corrected measure of agreement among response measurement scores
is given by

$$\Re = 1 - \frac{\delta}{\mu_\delta} \, , \tag{6.6}$$

where μ_δ is the arithmetic average of the M δ test statistic values calculated on all
possible arrangements of the observed response measurement scores given by

$$\mu_\delta = \frac{1}{M} \sum_{i=1}^{M} \delta_i \, . \tag{6.7}$$

6.3   Example 1: Test Statistics t and δ

A small example will serve to illustrate the relationship between test statistics t and
δ. Consider a small set of data with $n_1 = 3$ female children in Group 1 and $n_2 = 4$
male children in Group 2, as given in Table 6.1, where the values indicate the ages
of the children. Under the Neyman–Pearson population model with null hypothesis
H_0: $\mu_1 = \mu_2$, $n_1 = 3$, $n_2 = 4$, $N = n_1 + n_2 = 3 + 4 = 7$, $\bar{x}_1 = 2.3333$, $\bar{x}_2 =$
5.25, $s_1^2 = 2.3333$, $s_2^2 = 2.9167$, the unbiased pooled estimate of the population
variance is

$$s_p^2 = \frac{(n_1 - 1)s_1^2 + (n_2 - 1)s_2^2}{N - 2}$$

$$= \frac{(3 - 1)(2.3333) + (4 - 1)(2.9167)}{7 - 2} = 2.6833 \, ,$$

and the observed value of Student's t test statistic is

$$t = \frac{\bar{x}_1 - \bar{x}_2}{\left[s_p^2 \left(\dfrac{1}{n_1} + \dfrac{1}{n_2} \right) \right]^{1/2}} = \frac{2.3333 - 5.25}{\left[2.6833 \left(\dfrac{1}{3} + \dfrac{1}{4} \right) \right]^{1/2}} = -2.3313 \, .$$

Table 6.1 Example data for
a test of two independent
samples with $N = 7$ subjects

Group 1		Group 2	
Females	Age	Males	Age
1	1	4	3
2	2	5	5
3	4	6	6
		7	7

Under the Neyman–Pearson null hypothesis, H_0: $\mu_1 = \mu_2$, test statistic t is asymptotically distributed as Student's t with $N - 2$ degrees of freedom. With $N - 2 = 7 - 2 = 5$ degrees of freedom, the asymptotic two-tail probability value of $t = -2.3313$ is $P = 0.0671$, under the assumptions of normality and homogeneity.

6.3.1   A Permutation Approach

Under the Fisher–Pitman permutation model, employing squared Euclidean scaling with $v = 2$ and treatment-group weights

$$C_1 = \frac{n_1 - 1}{N - 2} \quad \text{and} \quad C_2 = \frac{n_2 - 1}{N - 2}$$

for correspondence with Student's two-sample t test, the three symmetric distance-function values for Group 1 are

$$\Delta_{1,2} = |1 - 2|^2 = 1 , \quad \Delta_{1,3} = |1 - 4|^2 = 9 , \quad \Delta_{2,3} = |2 - 4|^2 = 4 ,$$

and the average distance-function value for Group 1 is

$$\xi_1 = \binom{n_1}{2}^{-1} (\Delta_{1,2} + \Delta_{1,3} + \Delta_{2,3}) = \binom{3}{2}^{-1} (1 + 9 + 4) = 4.6667 .$$

For Group 2 the six symmetric distance-function values are

$$\Delta_{4,5} = |3 - 5|^2 = 4 , \quad \Delta_{4,6} = |3 - 6|^2 = 9 , \quad \Delta_{4,7} = |3 - 7|^2 = 16 ,$$

$$\Delta_{5,6} = |5 - 6|^2 = 1 , \quad \Delta_{5,7} = |5 - 7|^2 = 4 , \quad \Delta_{6,7} = |6 - 7|^2 = 1 ,$$

and the average distance-function value for Group 2 is

$$\xi_2 = \binom{n_2}{2}^{-1} (\Delta_{4,5} + \Delta_{4,6} + \Delta_{4,7} + \Delta_{5,6} + \Delta_{5,7} + \Delta_{6,7})$$

$$= \binom{4}{2}^{-1} (4 + 9 + 16 + 1 + 4 + 1) = 5.8333 .$$

Then the observed permutation test statistic for the age data listed in Table 6.1 is

$$\delta = C_1 \xi_1 + C_2 \xi_2 = \left(\frac{3-1}{7-2}\right) (4.6667) + \left(\frac{4-1}{7-2}\right) (5.8333) = 5.3667 .$$

For the example data given in Table 6.1, the sum of the $N = 7$ observations is

$$\sum_{i=1}^{N} x_i = 1 + 2 + 4 + 3 + 5 + 6 + 7 = 28 ,$$

the sum of the $N = 7$ squared observations is

$$\sum_{i=1}^{N} x_i^2 = 1^2 + 2^2 + 4^2 + 3^2 + 5^2 + 6^2 + 7^2 = 140 ,$$

and the total sum-of-squares is

$$SS_{\text{Total}} = \sum_{i=1}^{N} x_i^2 - \left(\sum_{i=1}^{N} x_i\right)^2 \Big/ N = 140 - (28)^2/7 = 28.00 .$$

Then based on the expressions given in Eq. (6.5) on p. 159, the observed value for test statistic δ with respect to the observed value of Student's t statistic is

$$\delta = \frac{2SS_{\text{Total}}}{t^2 + N - 2} = \frac{2(28.00)}{(-2.3313)^2 + 7 - 2} = 5.3667$$

and the observed value for Student's t test statistic with respect to the observed value of test statistic δ is

$$t = \left(\frac{2SS_{\text{Total}}}{\delta} - N + 2\right)^{1/2} = \left[\frac{2(28.00)}{5.3667} - 7 + 2\right]^{1/2} = \pm 2.3313 .$$

Under the Fisher–Pitman permutation model there are exactly

$$M = \frac{(n_1 + n_2)!}{n_1! \, n_2!} = \frac{(3 + 4)!}{3! \, 4!} = 35$$

possible, equally-likely arrangements in the reference set of all permutations of the age data listed in Table 6.1 on p. 160. Since $M = 35$ is a relatively small number, it is possible to list the $M = 35$ arrangements in Table 6.2, along with the corresponding values for ξ_1, ξ_2, δ, and $|t|$, ordered by δ values from low ($\delta_1 = 2.8000$) to high ($\delta_{35} = 11.2000$) and by $|t|$ values from high ($t_1 = 3.8730$) to low ($t_{35} = 0.0000$).

Under the Fisher–Pitman permutation model, the exact probability of an observed δ is the proportion of δ test statistic values computed on all possible, equally-likely arrangements of the observed data that are equal to or less than the observed value of $\delta = 5.3667$. The observed permutation test statistic, $\delta = 5.3667$, obtained for the realized arrangement is unusual since 31 of the 35 δ test statistic values exceed the observed value and only four of the δ test statistic values are

Table 6.2 Arrangements of the observed data listed in Table 6.1 with corresponding ξ_1, ξ_2, δ, and $|t|$ values

Number	Arrangement	ξ_1	ξ_2	δ	$|t|$
1*	1, 2, 3 4, 5, 6, 7	2.0000	3.3333	2.8000	3.8730
2*	5, 6, 7 1, 2, 3, 4	2.0000	3.3333	2.8000	3.8730
3*	1, 2, 4 3, 5, 6, 7	4.6667	5.8333	5.3667	2.3313
4*	4, 6, 7 1, 2, 3, 5	4.6667	5.8333	5.3667	2.3313
5	1, 2, 5 3, 4, 6, 7	8.6667	6.6667	7.4667	1.5811
6	1, 3, 4 2, 5, 6, 7	4.6667	9.3333	7.4667	1.5811
7	4, 5, 7 1, 2, 3, 6	4.6667	9.3333	7.4667	1.5811
8	3, 6, 7 1, 2, 4, 5	8.6667	6.6666	7.4667	1.5811
9	1, 2, 6 3, 4, 5, 7	14.0000	5.8333	9.1000	1.0742
10	1, 3, 5 2, 4, 6, 7	8.0000	9.8333	9.1000	1.0742
11	2, 3, 4 1, 5, 6, 7	2.0000	13.8333	9.1000	1.0742
12	2, 6, 7 1, 3, 4, 5	14.0000	5.8333	9.1000	1.0742
13	3, 5, 7 1, 2, 4, 6	8.0000	9.8333	9.1000	1.0742
14	4, 5, 6 1, 2, 3, 7	2.0000	13.8333	9.1000	1.0742
15	1, 2, 7 3, 4, 5, 6	20.6667	3.3333	10.2667	0.6742
16	1, 3, 6 2, 4, 5, 7	12.6667	8.6667	10.2667	0.6742
17	1, 4, 5 2, 3, 6, 7	8.6667	11.3333	10.2667	0.6742
18	1, 6, 7 2, 3, 4, 5	20.6667	3.3333	10.2667	0.6742
19	2, 3, 5 1, 4, 6, 7	4.6667	14.0000	10.2667	0.6742
20	2, 5, 7 1, 3, 4, 6	12.6667	8.6667	10.2667	0.6742
21	3, 4, 7 1, 2, 5, 6	8.6667	11.3333	10.2667	0.6742
22	3, 5, 6 1, 2, 4, 7	4.6667	14.0000	10.2667	0.6742
23	3, 4, 6 1, 2, 5, 7	4.6667	15.1667	10.9667	0.3262
24	1, 3, 7 2, 4, 5, 6	18.6667	5.8333	10.9667	0.3262
25	1, 4, 6 2, 3, 5, 7	12.6667	9.8333	10.9667	0.3262
26	1, 5, 7 2, 3, 4, 6	18.6667	5.8333	10.9667	0.3262
27	2, 3, 6 1, 4, 5, 7	8.6667	12.5000	10.9667	0.3262
28	2, 4, 5 1, 3, 6, 7	4.6667	15.1667	10.9667	0.3262
29	2, 4, 7 1, 3, 5, 6	12.6667	9.8333	10.9667	0.3262
30	2, 5, 6 1, 3, 4, 7	8.6667	12.5000	10.9667	0.3262
31	1, 4, 7 2, 3, 5, 6	18.0000	6.6667	11.2000	0.0000
32	1, 5, 6 2, 3, 4, 7	14.0000	9.3333	11.2000	0.0000
33	2, 3, 7 1, 4, 5, 6	14.0000	9.3333	11.2000	0.0000
34	2, 4, 6 1, 3, 5, 7	8.0000	13.3333	11.2000	0.0000
35	3, 4, 5 1, 2, 6, 7	2.0000	17.3333	11.2000	0.0000
Sum				326.6667	

equal to or less than the observed value. The rows containing the lowest four δ test statistic values are indicated with asterisks in Table 6.2. If all M arrangements of the observed data occur with equal chance under the Fisher–Pitman null hypothesis, the exact probability value of $\delta = 5.3667$ computed on the $M = 35$ possible arrangements of the observed data with $n_1 = 3$ and $n_2 = 4$ preserved for each arrangement is

$$P(\delta \le \delta_o) = \frac{\text{number of } \delta \text{ values } \le \delta_o}{M} = \frac{4}{35} = 0.1143 ,$$

where δ_o denotes the observed value of test statistic δ and M is the number of possible, equally-likely arrangements of the $N = 7$ observations listed in Table 6.1.

Alternatively, there are only four $|t|$ test statistic values that are larger than the observed value of $|t| = 2.3313$. The rows containing the highest four $|t|$ values are indicated with asterisks in Table 6.2. Thus if all M arrangements of the observed data occur with equal chance, the exact probability value of $|t| = 2.3313$ under the Fisher–Pitman null hypothesis is

$$P(|t| \ge |t_o|) = \frac{\text{number of } |t| \text{ values } \ge |t_o|}{M} = \frac{4}{35} = 0.1143 ,$$

where t_o denotes the observed value of test statistic t. There is a considerable difference between the asymptotic probability value of $P = 0.0671$ and the exact probability value of $P = 0.1143$; that is,

$$\Delta_P = 0.1143 - 0.0671 = 0.0472 .$$

A continuous mathematical function such as Student's t cannot be expected to provide a precise fit to only $n_1 = 3$ and $n_2 = 4$ observed values.

For the example data listed in Table 6.1 on p. 160, the exact expected value of test statistic δ under the Fisher–Pitman null hypothesis is

$$\mu_\delta = \frac{1}{M} \sum_{i=1}^{M} \delta_i = \frac{326.6667}{35} = 9.3333 .$$

Alternatively, under an analysis of variance model the exact expected value of test statistic δ is

$$\mu_\delta = \frac{2 SS_{\text{Total}}}{N - 1} = \frac{2(28.00)}{7 - 1} = 9.3333 ,$$

where the sum of the $N = 7$ observations listed in Table 6.1 is

$$\sum_{i=1}^{N} x_i = 1 + 2 + 4 + 3 + 5 + 6 + 7 = 28 ,$$

the sum of the $N = 7$ squared observations is

$$\sum_{i=1}^{N} x_i^2 = 1^2 + 2^2 + 4^2 + 3^2 + 5^2 + 6^2 + 7^2 = 140 \, ,$$

and the total sum-of-squares is

$$SS_{\text{Total}} = \sum_{i=1}^{N} x_i^2 - \left(\sum_{i=1}^{N} x_i\right)^2 \bigg/ N = 140 - (28)^2/7 = 28.00 \, .$$

Then the observed chance-corrected measure of effect size is

$$\Re = 1 - \frac{\delta}{\mu_\delta} = 1 - \frac{5.3667}{9.3333} = +0.4250 \, ,$$

indicating approximately 42% within-group agreement above what is expected by chance.

6.4   Example 2: Measures of Effect Size

Measures of effect size express the practical or clinical significance of a difference between independent sample means, as contrasted with the statistical significance of a difference. Five measures of effect size are commonly used for determining the magnitude of treatment effects in conventional tests for two independent samples: Cohen's $\hat{d}$ measure of effect size given by

$$\hat{d} = \frac{|\bar{x}_1 - \bar{x}_2|}{\sqrt{s_p^2}} \, ,$$

Pearson's r^2 measure of effect size given by

$$r^2 = \frac{t^2}{t^2 + N - 2} \, ,$$

Kelley's ϵ^2 measure of effect size given by

$$\epsilon^2 = \frac{t^2 - 1}{t^2 + N - 2} \, ,$$

Hays' $\hat{\omega}^2$ measure of effect size given by

$$\hat{\omega}^2 = \frac{t^2 - 1}{t^2 + N - 1} ,$$

and Mielke and Berry's $\mathfrak{R}$ measure of effect size given by

$$\mathfrak{R} = 1 - \frac{\delta}{\mu_\delta} ,$$

where the permutation test statistic δ is defined in Eq. (6.1) on p. 157 and μ_δ is the exact expected value of test statistic δ under the Fisher–Pitman null hypothesis given by

$$\mu_\delta = \frac{1}{M} \sum_{i=1}^{M} \delta_i ,$$

where for a test of two independent samples, the number of possible arrangements of the observed data is given by

$$M = \frac{(n_1 + n_2)!}{n_1! \, n_2!} .$$

For the age data given in Table 6.1 on p. 160 for $N = 7$ subjects, Student's test statistic is $t = -2.3313$, Cohen's $\hat{d}$ measure of effect size is

$$\hat{d} = \frac{|\bar{x}_1 - \bar{x}_2|}{\sqrt{s_p^2}} = \frac{|2.3333 - 5.25|}{\sqrt{2.6833}} = 1.7805 ,$$

indicating a strong effect size ($\hat{d} \geq 0.80$); Pearson's r^2 measure of effect size is

$$r^2 = \frac{t^2}{t^2 + N - 2} = \frac{(-2.3313)^2}{(-2.3313)^2 + 7 - 2} = 0.5208 ,$$

also indicating a strong effect size ($r^2 \geq 0.25$); Kelley's ϵ^2 measure of effect size is

$$\epsilon^2 = \frac{t^2}{t^2 + N - 2} = \frac{(-2.3313)^2 - 1}{(-2.3313)^2 + 7 - 2} = 0.4250 ;$$

Hays' $\hat{\omega}^2$ measure of effect size is

$$\hat{\omega}^2 = \frac{t^2 - 1}{t^2 + N - 1} = \frac{(-2.3313)^2 - 1}{(-2.3313)^2 + 7 - 1} = 0.3878 ;$$

and Mielke and Berry's $\Re$ measure of effect size is

$$\Re = 1 - \frac{\delta}{\mu_\delta} = 1 - \frac{5.3667}{9.3333} = +0.4250 \,,$$

where δ is defined in Eq. (6.1) on p. 157, μ_δ is the exact expected value of δ under the Fisher–Pitman null hypothesis given by

$$\mu_\delta = \frac{1}{M} \sum_{i=1}^{M} \delta_i = \frac{326.6667}{35} = 9.3333 \,,$$

and the sum of the $M = 35$ δ test statistic values,

$$\sum_{i=1}^{M} \delta_i = 326.6667 \,,$$

is calculated in Table 6.2 on p. 163.

It is readily apparent that for a test of two independent samples, the five measures of effect size, $\hat{d}$, r^2, ϵ^2, $\hat{\omega}^2$, and $\Re$ provide similar results when $v = 2$,

$$C_1 = \frac{n_1 - 1}{N - 2} \,, \quad \text{and} \quad C_2 = \frac{n_2 - 1}{N - 2} \,,$$

and are directly related to each other and to Student's t test statistic for two independent samples. It can easily be shown that Kelley's ϵ^2 and Mielke and Berry's $\Re$ are identical measures of effect size for two independent samples under the Neyman–Pearson population model; that is,

$$\epsilon^2 = \Re = \frac{t^2 - 1}{t^2 + N - 2} = \frac{(-2.3313)^2 - 1}{(-2.3313)^2 + 7 - 2} = +0.4250 \,.$$

6.4.1 Efficient Calculation of μ_δ

Although the exact expected value of test statistic δ is defined as

$$\mu_\delta = \frac{1}{M} \sum_{i=1}^{M} \delta_i \,, \tag{6.8}$$

there is a more efficient way to calculate the expected value of δ than utilizing the expression given in Eq. (6.8) [11]. Because permutation methods are by their very nature computationally intensive methods, efficient calculation of the permutation test statistic δ and the exact expected value of δ is imperative. Define

$$\mu_\delta = \frac{(N-2)!}{N!} \sum_{i=1}^{N} \sum_{j=1}^{N} \Delta(i, j) , \tag{6.9}$$

where the symmetric distance function between paired objects i and j is given by $\Delta(i, j) = |x_i - x_j|^v$.

Table 6.3 illustrates the calculation of μ_δ for the example data listed in Table 6.1 with $v = 2$. Given the double sum,

$$\sum_{i=1}^{N} \sum_{j=1}^{N} \Delta(i, j) = 392$$

Table 6.3 Example data for a test of two independent samples with $N = 7$ subjects and $N^2 = 7^2 = 49$ possible values

Index	$\Delta(i, j)$	Index	$\Delta(i, j)$
1	$\Delta(1, 1) = \|1 - 1\|^2 = 0$	26	$\Delta(4, 5) = \|4 - 5\|^2 = 1$
2	$\Delta(1, 2) = \|1 - 2\|^2 = 1$	27	$\Delta(4, 6) = \|4 - 6\|^2 = 4$
3	$\Delta(1, 3) = \|1 - 3\|^2 = 9$	28	$\Delta(4, 7) = \|4 - 7\|^2 = 9$
4	$\Delta(1, 4) = \|1 - 3\|^2 = 4$	29	$\Delta(5, 1) = \|5 - 1\|^2 = 16$
5	$\Delta(1, 5) = \|1 - 5\|^2 = 16$	30	$\Delta(5, 2) = \|5 - 2\|^2 = 9$
6	$\Delta(1, 6) = \|1 - 6\|^2 = 25$	31	$\Delta(5, 3) = \|5 - 4\|^2 = 1$
7	$\Delta(1, 7) = \|1 - 7\|^2 = 36$	32	$\Delta(5, 4) = \|5 - 3\|^2 = 4$
8	$\Delta(2, 1) = \|2 - 1\|^2 = 1$	33	$\Delta(5, 5) = \|5 - 5\|^2 = 0$
9	$\Delta(2, 2) = \|2 - 2\|^2 = 0$	34	$\Delta(5, 6) = \|5 - 6\|^2 = 1$
10	$\Delta(2, 3) = \|2 - 4\|^2 = 4$	35	$\Delta(5, 7) = \|5 - 7\|^2 = 4$
11	$\Delta(2, 4) = \|2 - 3\|^2 = 1$	36	$\Delta(6, 1) = \|6 - 1\|^2 = 25$
12	$\Delta(2, 5) = \|2 - 5\|^2 = 9$	37	$\Delta(6, 2) = \|6 - 2\|^2 = 16$
13	$\Delta(2, 6) = \|2 - 6\|^2 = 16$	38	$\Delta(6, 3) = \|6 - 4\|^2 = 4$
14	$\Delta(2, 7) = \|1 - 2\|^2 = 25$	39	$\Delta(6, 4) = \|6 - 3\|^2 = 9$
15	$\Delta(3, 1) = \|3 - 1\|^2 = 4$	40	$\Delta(6, 5) = \|6 - 5\|^2 = 1$
16	$\Delta(3, 2) = \|3 - 2\|^2 = 1$	41	$\Delta(6, 6) = \|6 - 6\|^2 = 0$
17	$\Delta(3, 3) = \|3 - 4\|^2 = 1$	42	$\Delta(6, 7) = \|6 - 7\|^2 = 1$
18	$\Delta(3, 4) = \|3 - 3\|^2 = 0$	43	$\Delta(7, 1) = \|7 - 1\|^2 = 36$
19	$\Delta(3, 5) = \|3 - 5\|^2 = 4$	44	$\Delta(7, 2) = \|7 - 2\|^2 = 25$
20	$\Delta(3, 6) = \|3 - 6\|^2 = 9$	45	$\Delta(7, 3) = \|7 - 4\|^2 = 9$
21	$\Delta(3, 7) = \|3 - 7\|^2 = 16$	46	$\Delta(7, 4) = \|7 - 3\|^2 = 16$
22	$\Delta(4, 1) = \|4 - 1\|^2 = 9$	47	$\Delta(7, 5) = \|7 - 5\|^2 = 4$
23	$\Delta(4, 2) = \|4 - 2\|^2 = 4$	48	$\Delta(7, 6) = \|7 - 6\|^2 = 1$
24	$\Delta(4, 3) = \|4 - 4\|^2 = 0$	49	$\Delta(7, 7) = \|7 - 7\|^2 = 0$
25	$\Delta(4, 4) = \|4 - 3\|^2 = 1$		
Sum			392

calculated in Table 6.3,

$$\mu_\delta = \frac{(N-2)!}{N!} \sum_{i=1}^{N} \sum_{j=1}^{N} \Delta(i, j) = \frac{(7-2)!}{7!}(392) = \frac{47,040}{5,040} = 9.3333 \ .$$

Thus the actual computation of μ_δ involves only N^2 operations to obtain the exact expected value of test statistic δ. For example, if $n_1 = n_2 = 15$ there are

$$M = \frac{(n_1 + n_2)!}{n_1! \, n_2!} = \frac{(15+15)!}{15! \, 15!} = 155{,}117{,}520$$

δ test statistic values to be computed using the expression for μ_δ given in Eq. (6.8), but only $(15+15)^2 = 30^2 = 900 \, \Delta(i, j)$ values to be computed using the expression for μ_δ given in Eq. (6.9) for $i, j = 1, \ldots, N$—a much more efficient solution resulting in a substantial savings in computation time.

6.4.2   Comparisons of Effect Size Measures

The four measures of effect size and Student's t test statistic are all interrelated. Any one of the measures can be derived from any of the other measures. The functional relationships between Student's t test statistic and Mielke and Berry's $\Re$ measure of effect size for tests of two independent samples are given by

$$t = \left[\frac{\Re(N-2)+1}{1-\Re} \right]^{1/2} \quad \text{and} \quad \Re = \frac{t^2 - 1}{t^2 + N - 2} \ , \tag{6.10}$$

the relationships between Pearson's r^2 measure of effect size and Mielke and Berry's $\Re$ measure of effect size are given by

$$r^2 = \Re + \left(t^2 + N - 2\right)^{-1} \quad \text{and} \quad \Re = r^2 - \left(t^2 + N - 2\right)^{-1} , \tag{6.11}$$

the relationships between Hays' $\hat{\omega}^2$ measure of effect size and Mielke and Berry's $\Re$ measure of effect size are given by

$$\hat{\omega}^2 = \Re \left(\frac{t^2 + N - 2}{t^2 + N - 1} \right) \quad \text{and} \quad \Re = \hat{\omega}^2 \left(\frac{t^2 + N - 1}{t^2 + N - 2} \right) , \tag{6.12}$$

the relationships between Cohen's $\hat{d}$ measure of effect size and Mielke and Berry's $\Re$ measure of effect size are given by

$$\hat{d} = \left[\frac{\Re N(N-2) + N}{n_1 n_2 (1 - \Re)} \right]^{1/2} \quad \text{and} \quad \Re = \frac{n_1 n_2 \hat{d}^2 - N}{n_1 n_2 \hat{d}^2 + N(N-2)} , \tag{6.13}$$

the relationships between Cohen's $\hat{d}$ measure of effect size and Student's t test statistic are given by

$$\hat{d} = \left(\frac{Nt^2}{n_1 n_2}\right)^{1/2} \quad \text{and} \quad t = \left(\frac{n_1 n_2 \hat{d}^2}{N}\right)^{1/2}, \tag{6.14}$$

the relationships between Pearson's r^2 measure of effect size and Student's t test statistic are given by

$$r^2 = \frac{t^2}{t^2 + N - 2} \quad \text{and} \quad t = \left[\frac{r^2(N-2)}{1-r^2}\right]^{1/2}, \tag{6.15}$$

the relationships between Pearson's r^2 measure of effect size and Cohen's $\hat{d}$ measure of effect size are given by

$$r^2 = \frac{n_1 n_2 \hat{d}^2}{n_1 n_2 \hat{d}^2 + N(N-2)} \quad \text{and} \quad \hat{d} = \left[\frac{r^2 N(N-2)}{n_1 n_2 (1-r^2)}\right]^{1/2}, \tag{6.16}$$

the relationships between Pearson's r^2 measure of effect size and Hays' $\hat{\omega}^2$ measure of effect size are given by

$$r^2 = \frac{\hat{\omega}^2(N-1) + 1}{\hat{\omega}^2 + N - 1} \quad \text{and} \quad \hat{\omega}^2 = \frac{r^2(N-1) - 1}{N - (1 + r^2)}, \tag{6.17}$$

the relationships between Student's t test statistic and Hays' $\hat{\omega}^2$ measure of effect size are given by

$$t = \left[\frac{\hat{\omega}^2(N-1) + 1}{1 - \hat{\omega}^2}\right]^{1/2} \quad \text{and} \quad \hat{\omega}^2 = \frac{t^2 - 1}{t^2 + N - 1}, \tag{6.18}$$

and the relationships between Cohen's $\hat{d}$ measure of effect size and Hays' $\hat{\omega}^2$ measure of effect size are given by

$$\hat{d} = \left\{\frac{N[\hat{\omega}^2(N-1) + 1]}{n_1 n_2(1 - \hat{\omega}^2)}\right\}^{1/2} \quad \text{and} \quad \hat{\omega}^2 = \frac{n_1 n_2 \hat{d}^2 - N}{n_1 n_2 \hat{d}^2 + N(N-1)}. \tag{6.19}$$

It is important to note that the relationships between Student's t and Mielke and Berry's $\Re$, Pearson's r^2 and Mielke and Berry's $\Re$, Hays' $\hat{\omega}^2$ and Mielke and Berry's $\Re$, Cohen's $\hat{d}$ and Mielke and Berry's $\Re$, Cohen's $\hat{d}$ and Student's t, Pearson's r^2 and Student's t, Pearson's r^2 and Cohen's $\hat{d}$, Pearson's r^2 and Hays' $\hat{\omega}^2$, Student's t and Hays' $\hat{\omega}^2$, and Cohen's $\hat{d}$ and Hays' $\hat{\omega}^2$ hold only for Student's *pooled* two-sample t test. The measures of effect size, $\hat{d}$, r^2, and $\hat{\omega}^2$, all require homogeneity of variance and the relationships listed above do not hold for Student's non-pooled two-sample t test. On the other hand, $\mathfrak{R}$ does not require homogeneity of variance and is appropriate for both pooled and non-pooled two-sample tests [5].

6.4.3   Example Effect Size Comparisons

In this section, comparisons of Student's t, Cohen's $\hat{d}$, Mielke and Berry's $\mathfrak{R}$, Hays' $\hat{\omega}^2$, and Pearson's r^2 are illustrated with the example data listed in Table 6.1 on p. 160 with $n_1 = 3$, $n_2 = 4$, and $N = 7$ observations.

Given the age data listed in Table 6.1 and following the expressions given in Eq. (6.10) for Student's t test statistic and Mielke and Berry's $\mathfrak{R}$ measure of effect size, the observed value for Student's t test statistic with respect to the observed value of Mielke and Berry's $\mathfrak{R}$ measure of effect size is

$$t = \left[\frac{\mathfrak{R}(N-2)+1}{1-\mathfrak{R}} \right]^{1/2} = \left[\frac{0.4250(7-2)+1}{1-0.4250} \right]^{1/2} = \pm 2.3313$$

and the observed value for Mielke and Berry's $\mathfrak{R}$ measure of effect size with respect to the observed value of Student's t test statistic is

$$\mathfrak{R} = \frac{t^2-1}{t^2+N-2} = \frac{(-2.3313)^2-1}{(-2.3313)^2+7-2} = +0.4250 .$$

Following the expressions given in Eq. (6.11) for Pearson's r^2 measure of effect size and Mielke and Berry's $\mathfrak{R}$ measure of effect size, the observed value for Pearson's r^2 measure of effect size with respect to the observed value of Mielke and Berry's $\mathfrak{R}$ measure of effect size is

$$r^2 = \mathfrak{R} + \left(t^2 + N - 2 \right)^{-1} = 0.4250 + \left[(-2.3313)^2 + 7 - 2 \right]^{-1} = 0.5208$$

and the observed value for Mielke and Berry's $\mathfrak{R}$ measure of effect size with respect to the observed value of Pearson's r^2 measure of effect size is

$$\mathfrak{R} = r^2 - \left(t^2 + N - 2 \right)^{-1} = 0.5208 - \left[(-2.3313)^2 + 7 - 2 \right]^{-1} = +0.4250 .$$

Following the expressions given in Eq. (6.12) for Hays' $\hat{\omega}^2$ measure of effect size and Mielke and Berry's $\mathfrak{R}$ measure of effect size, the observed value for Hays' $\hat{\omega}^2$ measure of effect size with respect to the observed value of Mielke and Berry's $\mathfrak{R}$ measure of effect size is

$$\hat{\omega}^2 = \mathfrak{R} \left(\frac{t^2+N-2}{t^2+N-1} \right) = \left[\frac{(-2.3313)^2+7-2}{(-2.3313)^2+7-1} \right] = 0.3878$$

and the observed value for Mielke and Berry's $\mathfrak{R}$ measure of effect size with respect to the observed value of Hays' $\hat{\omega}^2$ measure of effect size is

$$\mathfrak{R} = \hat{\omega}^2 \left(\frac{t^2 + N - 1}{t^2 + N - 2} \right) = \left[\frac{(-2.3313)^2 + 7 - 1}{(-2.3313)^2 + 7 - 2} \right] = +0.4250 \,.$$

Following the expressions given in Eq. (6.13) for Cohen's $\hat{d}$ measure of effect size and Mielke and Berry's $\mathfrak{R}$ measure of effect size, the observed value for Cohen's $\hat{d}$ measure of effect size with respect to the observed value of Mielke and Berry's $\mathfrak{R}$ measure of effect size is

$$\hat{d} = \left[\frac{\mathfrak{R}N(N-2) + N}{n_1 n_2 (1 - \mathfrak{R})} \right]^{1/2} = \left[\frac{(0.4250)(7)(7-2) + 7}{(3)(4)(1 - 0.4250)} \right]^{1/2} = \pm 1.7805$$

and the observed value for Mielke and Berry's $\mathfrak{R}$ measure of effect size with respect to the observed value of Cohen's $\hat{d}$ measure of effect size is

$$\mathfrak{R} = \frac{n_1 n_2 \hat{d}^2 - N}{n_1 n_2 \hat{d}^2 + N(N-2)} = \frac{(3)(4)(1.7805)^2}{(3)(4)(1.7805)^2 + (7)(7-2)} = +0.4250 \,.$$

Following the expressions given in Eq. (6.14) for Cohen's $\hat{d}$ measure of effect size and Student's t test statistic, the observed value for Cohen's $\hat{d}$ measure of effect size with respect to the observed value of Student's t statistic is

$$\hat{d} = \left(\frac{Nt^2}{n_1 n_2} \right)^{1/2} = \left[\frac{7(-2.3313)^2}{(3)(4)} \right]^{1/2} = \pm 1.7805$$

and the observed value of Student's t test statistic with respect to the observed value of Cohen's $\hat{d}$ measure of effect size is

$$t = \left(\frac{n_1 n_2 \hat{d}^2}{N} \right)^{1/2} = \left[\frac{(3)(4)(1.7805)^2}{7} \right]^{1/2} = \pm 2.3313 \,.$$

Following the expressions given in Eq. (6.15) for Pearson's r^2 measure of effect size and Student's t test statistic, the observed value for Pearson's r^2 measure of effect size with respect to the observed value of Student's t statistic is

$$r^2 = \frac{t^2}{t^2 + N - 2} = \frac{(-2.3313)^2}{(-2.3313)^2 + 7 - 2} = 0.5208$$

and the observed value for Student's t test statistic with respect to the observed value of Pearson's r^2 measure of effect size is

$$t = \left[\frac{r^2(N-2)}{1-r^2}\right]^{1/2} = \left[\frac{0.5208(7-2)}{1-0.5208}\right]^{1/2} = \pm 2.3313 \, .$$

Following the expressions given in Eq. (6.16) for Pearson's r^2 measure of effect size and Cohen's $\hat{d}$ measure of effect size, the observed value for Pearson's r^2 measure of effect size with respect to the observed value of Cohen's $\hat{d}$ measure of effect size is

$$r^2 = \frac{n_1 n_2 \hat{d}^2}{n_1 n_2 \hat{d}^2 + N(N-2)} = \frac{(3)(4)(-1.7805)^2}{(3)(4)(-1.7805)^2 + 7(7-2)} = 0.5208$$

and the observed value for Cohen's $\hat{d}$ measure of effect size with respect to the observed value of Pearson's r^2 measure of effect size is

$$\hat{d} = \left[\frac{r^2 N(N-2)}{n_1 n_2 (1-r^2)}\right]^{1/2} = \left[\frac{(0.5208)(7)(7-2)}{(3)(4)(1-0.5208)}\right]^{1/2} = \pm 1.7805 \, .$$

Following the expressions given in Eq. (6.17) for Pearson's r^2 measure of effect size and Hays' $\hat{\omega}^2$ measure of effect size, the observed value for Pearson's r^2 measure of effect size with respect to the observed value of Hays' $\hat{\omega}^2$ measure of effect size is

$$r^2 = \frac{\hat{\omega}^2(N-1)+1}{\hat{\omega}^2 + N - 1} = \frac{(0.3878)(7-1)+1}{0.3878 + 7 - 1} = 0.5208$$

and the observed value for Hays' $\hat{\omega}^2$ measure of effect size with respect to the observed value of Pearson's r^2 measure of effect size is

$$\hat{\omega}^2 = \frac{r^2(N-1)-1}{N-(1+r^2)} = \frac{(0.5208)(7-1)-1}{7-(1+0.5208)} = 0.3878 \, .$$

Following the expressions given in Eq. (6.18) for Student's t test statistic and Hays' $\hat{\omega}^2$ measure of effect size, the observed value for Student's t statistic with respect to the observed value of Hays' $\hat{\omega}^2$ measure of effect size is

$$t = \left[\frac{\hat{\omega}^2(N-1)+1}{1-\hat{\omega}^2}\right]^{1/2} = \left[\frac{(0.3878)(7-1)+1}{1-0.3878}\right]^{1/2} = \pm 2.3313$$

and the observed value for Hays' $\hat{\omega}^2$ measure of effect size with respect to the observed value of Student's t test statistic is

$$\hat{\omega}^2 = \frac{t^2 - 1}{t^2 + N - 1} = \frac{(-2.3313)^2 - 1}{(-2.3313)^2 + 7 - 1} = 0.3878 \ .$$

And following the expressions given in Eq. (6.19) for Cohen's $\hat{d}$ measure of effect size and Hays' $\hat{\omega}^2$ measure of effect size, the observed value for Cohen's $\hat{d}$ measure of effect size with respect to the observed value of Hays' $\hat{\omega}^2$ measure of effect size is

$$\hat{d} = \left\{ \frac{N[\hat{\omega}^2(N-1)+1]}{n_1 n_2 (1 - \hat{\omega}^2)} \right\}^{1/2} = \left\{ \frac{7[0.3878(7-1)+1]}{(3)(4)(1-0.3878)} \right\}^{1/2} = \pm 1.7805$$

and the observed value for Hays' $\hat{\omega}^2$ measure of effect size with respect to the observed value of Cohen's $\hat{d}$ measure of effect size is

$$\hat{\omega}^2 = \frac{n_1 n_2 \hat{d}^2 - N}{n_1 n_2 \hat{d}^2 + N(N-1)} = \frac{(3)(4)(-1.7805)^2 - 7}{(3)(4)(-1.7805)^2 + 7(7-1)} = 0.3878 \ .$$

6.5 Example 3: Analyses with $v = 2$ and $v = 1$

For a third example of tests of differences for two independent samples, consider the error scores obtained for two groups of experimental animals running a maze under two different treatment conditions: treatment Group 1 without a reward and treatment Group 2 with a reward. The example data are given in Table 6.4.

Under the Neyman–Pearson population model with H_0: $\mu_1 = \mu_2$, $n_1 = 8$, $n_2 = 6$, $N = 14$, $\bar{x}_1 = 11.00$, $\bar{x}_2 = 8.00$, $s_1^2 = 57.7143$, $s_2^2 = 63.60$, the unbiased

Table 6.4 Example data for a test of two independent samples with $N = 14$ subjects

Group 1		Group 2	
Subject	Error	Subject	Error
1	16	9	20
2	9	10	5
3	4	11	1
4	23	12	16
5	19	13	2
6	10	14	4
7	5		
8	2		

pooled estimate of the population variance is

$$s_p^2 = \frac{(n_1 - 1)s_1^2 + (n_2 - 1)s_2^2}{N - 2}$$

$$= \frac{(8 - 1)(57.7143) + (6 - 1)(63.60)}{14 - 2} = 60.1667 ,$$

and the observed value of Student's t test statistic is

$$t = \frac{\bar{x}_1 - \bar{x}_2}{\left[s_p^2 \left(\frac{1}{n_1} + \frac{1}{n_2}\right)\right]^{1/2}} = \frac{11.00 - 8.00}{\left[60.1667 \left(\frac{1}{8} + \frac{1}{6}\right)\right]^{1/2}} = +0.7161 .$$

Under the Neyman–Pearson null hypothesis, H_0: $\mu_1 = \mu_2$, test statistic t is asymptotically distributed as Student's t with $N - 2$ degrees of freedom. With $N - 2 = 14 - 2 = 12$ degrees of freedom, the asymptotic two-tail probability value of $t = +0.7161$ is $P = 0.4876$, under the assumptions of normality and homogeneity.

6.5.1   An Exact Analysis with $v = 2$

Under the Fisher–Pitman permutation model, employing squared Euclidean scaling with $v = 2$ and treatment-group weights

$$C_1 = \frac{n_1 - 1}{N - 2} \quad \text{and} \quad C_2 = \frac{n_2 - 1}{N - 2}$$

for correspondence with Student's two-sample t test, the average distance-function values for treatment Groups 1 and 2 are

$$\xi_1 = 115.4286 \quad \text{and} \quad \xi_2 = 127.20 ,$$

respectively, and the observed permutation test statistic value is

$$\delta = \sum_{i=1}^{2} C_i \xi_i = \left(\frac{8 - 1}{14 - 2}\right)(115.4286) + \left(\frac{6 - 1}{14 - 2}\right)(127.20) = 120.3333 .$$

Alternatively, in terms of Student's t test statistic the average distance-function values are

$$\xi_1 = 2s_1^2 = 2(57.7143) = 115.4286 , \quad \xi_2 = 2s_2^2 = 2(63.60) = 127.20 ,$$

and the observed permutation test statistic value is

$$\delta = 2s_p^2 = 2(60.1667) = 120.3333 \ .$$

For the example data listed in Table 6.4, the sum of the $N = 14$ observations is

$$\sum_{i=1}^{N} x_i = 16 + 9 + 4 + 23 + 19 + 10 + 5$$

$$+ 2 + 20 + 5 + 1 + 16 + 2 + 4 = 136 \ ,$$

the sum of the $N = 14$ squared observations is

$$\sum_{i=1}^{N} x_i^2 = 16^2 + 9^2 + 4^2 + 23^2 + 19^2 + 10^2$$

$$+ 5^2 + 2^2 + 20^2 + 5^2 + 1^2 + 16^2 + 2^2 + 4^2 = 2074 \ ,$$

and the total sum-of-squares is

$$SS_{\text{Total}} = \sum_{i=1}^{N} x_i^2 - \left(\sum_{i=1}^{N} x_i \right)^2 \Big/ N = 2074 - (136)^2/14 = 752.8571 \ .$$

Then based on the expressions given in Eq. (6.5), the observed value for test statistic δ with respect to the observed value of Student's t test statistic is

$$\delta = \frac{2SS_{\text{Total}}}{t^2 + N - 2} = \frac{2(752.8571)}{(+0.7161)^2 + 14 - 2} = 120.3333$$

and the observed value for Student's t test statistic with respect to the observed value of test statistic δ is

$$t = \left(\frac{2SS_{\text{Total}}}{\delta} - N + 2 \right)^{1/2} = \left[\frac{2(752.8571)}{120.3333} - 14 + 2 \right]^{1/2} = \pm 0.7161 \ .$$

Under the Fisher–Pitman permutation model there are only

$$M = \frac{(n_1 + n_2)!}{n_1! \, n_2!} = \frac{(8 + 6)!}{8! \, 6!} = 3003$$

possible, equally-likely arrangements in the reference set of all permutations of the error data listed in Table 6.4, making an exact permutation analysis possible. Under the Fisher–Pitman permutation model, the exact probability of an observed δ is the proportion of δ test statistic values computed on all possible, equally-likely arrangements of the observed data that are equal to or less than the observed value of $\delta = 120.3333$. There are exactly 1487 δ test statistic values that are equal to or less than the observed value of $\delta = 120.3333$. If all M arrangements of the $N = 14$ observations listed in Table 6.4 occur with equal chance under the Fisher–Pitman null hypothesis, the exact probability value of $\delta = 120.3333$ computed on the $M = 3003$ possible arrangements of the observed data with $n_1 = 8$ and $n_2 = 6$ preserved for each arrangement is

$$P(\delta \leq \delta_0) = \frac{\text{number of } \delta \text{ values } \leq \delta_0}{M} = \frac{1487}{3003} = 0.5275 \,,$$

where δ_0 denotes the observed value of test statistic δ and M is the number of possible, equally-likely arrangements of the $N = 14$ observations listed in Table 6.4. Alternatively, the exact two-tail probability value of $|t| = 0.7161$ is

$$P(|t| \geq |t_0|) = \frac{\text{number of } |t| \text{ values } \geq |t_0|}{M} = \frac{1487}{3003} = 0.5275 \,,$$

where t_0 denotes the observed value of test statistic t.

6.5.2 Measures of Effect Size

For the example data listed in Table 6.4 on p. 174, Cohen's $\hat{d}$ measure of effect size is

$$\hat{d} = \frac{|\bar{x}_1 - \bar{x}_2|}{\sqrt{s_p^2}} = \frac{|11.00 - 8.00|}{\sqrt{60.1667}} = 0.3868 \,,$$

Pearson's r^2 measure of effect size is

$$r^2 = \frac{t^2}{t^2 + N - 2} = \frac{(+0.7161)^2}{(+0.7161)^2 + 14 - 2} = 0.0410 \,,$$

Kelley's ϵ^2 measure of effect size is

$$\epsilon^2 = \frac{t^2 - 1}{t^2 + N - 2} = \frac{(+0.7161)^2 - 1}{(+0.7161)^2 + 14 - 2} = -0.0389 \,, \tag{6.20}$$

Hays' $\hat{\omega}^2$ measure of effect size is

$$\hat{\omega}^2 = \frac{t^2 - 1}{t^2 + N - 1} = \frac{(+0.7161)^2 - 1}{(+0.7161)^2 + 14 - 1} = -0.0361 \,, \tag{6.21}$$

and Mielke and Berry's $\Re$ measure of effect size is

$$\Re = 1 - \frac{\delta}{\mu_\delta} = 1 - \frac{120.3333}{115.8242} = -0.0389 \,,$$

where, for the example data listed in Table 6.4, the exact expected value of test statistic δ under the Fisher–Pitman null hypothesis is

$$\mu_\delta = \frac{1}{M} \sum_{i=1}^{M} \delta_i = \frac{347,820}{3003} = 115.8242 \,.$$

Alternatively, under an analysis of variance model,

$$\mu_\delta = \frac{2 SS_{\text{Total}}}{N - 1} = \frac{2(752.8571)}{14 - 1} = 115.8242 \,,$$

where

$$SS_{\text{Total}} = \sum_{i=1}^{N} x_i^2 - \left(\sum_{i=1}^{N} x_i \right)^2 \bigg/ N = 2074 - (136)^2/14 = 752.8571 \,.$$

6.5.3 Chance-Corrected Measures of Effect Size

As is evident in Eqs. (6.20) and (6.21), some squared measures of effect size can be negative; in this case, Kelley's $\epsilon^2 = -0.0389$ and Hays' $\hat{\omega}^2 = -0.0361$. It is somewhat disconcerting, to say the least, to try to interpret squared coefficients with negative values. It is also important to recognize that negative values cannot simply be dismissed on theoretical grounds [10, p. 1000]. A number of authors have suggested that negative values be treated as zero [9]. It is not widely recognized that, like Mielke and Berry's $\Re$ measure of effect size, Kelley's ϵ^2 and Hays' $\hat{\omega}^2$ are chance-corrected measures of effect size. In fact $\Re$ and ϵ^2 are equivalent measures of effect size for tests of two independent samples. This places Kelley's ϵ^2 and Hays' $\hat{\omega}^2$ into the family of chance-corrected measures that includes such well-known members as Scott's π coefficient of inter-coder agreement [12], Cohen's κ coefficient of weighted agreement [2], Kendall and Babington Smith's u measure of agreement [7], and Spearman's footrule measure [13]. Negative values simply indicate that the magnitude of the differences between the two samples is less than expected by chance. It can easily be shown that, for the two-sample t test, the minimum value of $\Re$ and ϵ^2 is given by $-1/(N - 2)$. Thus, for the example data listed in Table 6.4,

$$\min(\Re) = \min(\epsilon^2) = \frac{-1}{N - 2} = \frac{-1}{14 - 2} = -0.0833 \,.$$

Incidentally, the minimum value for Hays' $\hat{\omega}^2$ measure of effect size is given by $-1/(N-1)$. Thus for the data listed in Table 6.4, the minimum value of Hays' $\hat{\omega}^2$ is $-1/(14-1) = -0.0769$.

6.5.4 An Exact Analysis with $v = 1$

Consider an analysis of the error data listed in Table 6.4 on p. 174 under the Fisher–Pitman permutation model with $v = 1$ and treatment-group weights given by

$$C_1 = \frac{n_1 - 1}{N - 2} \quad \text{and} \quad C_2 = \frac{n_2 - 1}{N - 2} \,.$$

For $v = 1$, the average distance-function values for the two treatment groups are

$$\xi_1 = 9.1429 \quad \text{and} \quad \xi_2 = 9.20 \,,$$

respectively, and the observed permutation test statistic is

$$\delta = \sum_{i=1}^{2} C_i \xi_i = \left(\frac{8 - 1}{14 - 2} \right) (9.1429) + \left(\frac{6 - 1}{14 - 2} \right) (9.20) = 9.1667 \,.$$

There are only

$$M = \frac{(n_1 + n_2)!}{n_1! \, n_2!} = \frac{(8 + 6)!}{8! \, 6!} = 3003$$

possible, equally-likely arrangements in the reference set of all permutations of the error data listed in Table 6.4, making an exact permutation analysis possible. Under the Fisher–Pitman permutation model, the exact probability of an observed δ is the proportion of δ test statistic values computed on all possible, equally-likely arrangements of the observed data that are equal to or less than the observed value of $\delta = 9.1667$. There are exactly 2114 δ test statistic values that are equal to or less than the observed value of $\delta = 9.1667$. If all M arrangements of the $N = 14$ observations listed in Table 6.4 occur with equal chance under the Fisher–Pitman null hypothesis, the exact probability value of $\delta = 9.1667$ computed on the $M = 3003$ possible arrangements of the observed data with $n_1 = 8$ and $n_2 = 6$ preserved for each arrangement is

$$P(\delta \leq \delta_o) = \frac{\text{number of } \delta \text{ values} \leq \delta_o}{M} = \frac{2114}{3003} = 0.7040 \,,$$

where δ_o denotes the observed value of test statistic δ and M is the number of possible, equally-likely arrangements of the $N = 14$ observations listed in Table 6.4.

No comparison is made with Student's t test statistic for two independent samples as Student's t is undefined for ordinary Euclidean scaling.

For the example data listed in Table 6.4, the exact expected value of test statistic δ under the Fisher–Pitman null hypothesis is

$$\mu_\delta = \frac{1}{M} \sum_{i=1}^{M} \delta_i = \frac{26,400}{3003} = 8.7912$$

and the observed chance-corrected measure of effect size is

$$\Re = 1 - \frac{\delta}{\mu_\delta} = 1 - \frac{9.1667}{8.7912} = -0.0427 \,,$$

indicating less than chance within-group agreement. No comparisons are made with Cohen's $\hat{d}$, Pearson's r^2, Kelley's ϵ^2, or Hays' $\hat{\omega}^2$ conventional measures of effect size for two independent samples as $\hat{d}$, r^2, ϵ^2, and $\hat{\omega}^2$ are undefined for ordinary Euclidean scaling.

6.5.5   The Effects of Extreme Values

For the example data listed in Table 6.4 on p. 174, the exact probability value employing squared Euclidean scaling with $v = 2$ is $P = 0.5275$ and the exact probability value employing ordinary Euclidean scaling with $v = 1$ is $P = 0.7040$. The difference between the two probability values of

$$\Delta_P = 0.7040 - 0.5275 = 0.1765$$

is entirely due to the squared and non-squared differences obtained with $v = 2$ and $v = 1$, respectively, under the Fisher–Pitman permutation model. Permutation test statistics employing squared Euclidean scaling with $v = 2$ are based on the sample mean ($\bar{x}$) and permutation test statistics employing ordinary Euclidean scaling with $v = 1$ are based on the sample median ($\tilde{x}$). Median-based statistics are highly resistant to extreme values and both treatment Group 1 and treatment Group 2 contain extreme values: $x_{14} = 23$ for Group 1 and $x_{21} = 20$ for Group 2. While these two values are not highly extreme, they are sufficiently removed from their respective mean values of $\bar{x}_1 = 11.00$ and $\bar{x}_2 = 8.00$ to strongly affect the probability value with $v = 2$. Incidentally, the median value for Group 1 is $\tilde{x} = 9.50$ and the median value for Group 2 is $\tilde{x} = 4.50$.

Extreme values are prevalent in applied research. Most variables are not even close to normally distributed and many are highly skewed, often positively. Some examples of positively-skewed variables are family income, net worth, prices of houses sold in a given month, age at first marriage, length of first marriage, and

Table 6.5 Raw-score observed values for two samples with $n_1 = n_2 = 13$ objects randomly assigned to each sample

Sample 1		Sample 2	
Object	Value	Object	Value
1	264.3	1	263.4
2	264.6	2	263.7
3	264.6	3	263.7
4	264.6	4	263.7
5	264.9	5	264.0
6	264.9	6	264.0
7	264.9	7	264.0
8	264.9	8	264.3
9	265.2	9	264.3
10	265.2	10	264.3
11	265.2	11	264.3
12	265.5	12	264.6
13	265.5	13	w

student debt. Consider the case of student debt: in 2017 upon graduation the average student debt was reported to be approximately \$34,000, while the median student debt was only approximately \$12,000. The mean is pulled higher than the median due to a small proportion of students with substantial debt. Graduate and professional students in veterinary medicine, dental school, law school, and medical school often graduate with hundreds of thousands of dollars in student debt.[4]

To demonstrate the difference between analyses based on squared Euclidean scaling with $v = 2$ and ordinary Euclidean scaling with $v = 1$, consider the two-sample data listed in Table 6.5. While the $n_1 = 13$ values in Sample 1 are fixed, one value in Sample 2, indicated by w, is allowed to vary in order to determine its effect on the exact probability values. Table 6.6 lists 21 values for w ranging from a low value of $w = 40$ up to a high value of $w = 988$, the exact permutation probability values with $v = 1$ and $v = 2$, and the two-tail probability values for Student's two-sample t test, under the usual assumptions of normality, homogeneity, and independence. Each of the exact probability values in Table 6.6 is based on

$$M = \frac{(n_1 + n_2)!}{n_1! \, n_2!} = \frac{(13 + 13)!}{13! \, 13!} = 10{,}400{,}600$$

possible, equally-likely arrangements of the $N = 26$ data values listed in Table 6.5, with the assigned value for w included. The two-tail probability values for the classical two-sample t test listed in Table 6.6 are based on Student's t distribution with $n_1 + n_2 - 2 = 13 + 13 - 2 = 24$ degrees of freedom.

---

[4]In 2017 the average student debt for law-school graduates was reported to be \$141,000 and the average student debt for medical-school graduates was reported to be \$192,000.

Table 6.6 Probability value comparisons for exact permutation tests with $v = 1$ and $v = 2$ and the classical Student two-sample t test for the data listed in Table 6.5

w	Exact permutation test $v = 1$	$v = 2$	Student's t test
40	0.4038×10^{-5}	0.4038×10^{-5}	0.3026
80	0.4038×10^{-5}	0.4038×10^{-5}	0.2975
120	0.4038×10^{-5}	0.4038×10^{-5}	0.2895
160	0.4038×10^{-5}	0.4038×10^{-5}	0.2759
200	0.4038×10^{-5}	0.4038×10^{-5}	0.2470
240	0.4038×10^{-5}	0.4038×10^{-5}	0.1481
258	0.4038×10^{-5}	0.4038×10^{-5}	0.8538×10^{-2}
261	0.4038×10^{-5}	0.4038×10^{-5}	0.2646×10^{-3}
264	0.4038×10^{-5}	0.4038×10^{-5}	0.5837×10^{-6}
267	0.9115×10^{-4}	0.0157	0.0159
270	0.9115×10^{-4}	0.4728	0.3455
273	0.9115×10^{-4}	0.9772	0.7459
276	0.9115×10^{-4}	1.0000	1.0000
288	0.9115×10^{-4}	1.0000	0.6222
388	0.9115×10^{-4}	1.0000	0.3753
488	0.9115×10^{-4}	1.0000	0.3533
588	0.9115×10^{-4}	1.0000	0.3451
688	0.9115×10^{-4}	1.0000	0.3409
788	0.9115×10^{-4}	1.0000	0.3382
888	0.9115×10^{-4}	1.0000	0.3365
988	0.9115×10^{-4}	1.0000	0.3352

As illustrated in Table 6.6, the exact probability values for the two-sample permutation test with $v = 1$ are stable, consistent, and relatively unaffected by the extreme values of w in either direction. The small change in the exact probability values from $P = 0.4038 \times 10^{-5}$ to $P = 0.9115 \times 10^{-4}$; that is,

$$\Delta_P = 0.9115 \times 10^{-4} - 0.4038 \times 10^{-5} = 0.8711 \times 10^{-4} \,,$$

with $v = 1$ occurs when w changes from $w = 264$ to $w = 267$ and passes the median value of $\tilde{x} = 264.9$. In contrast, the exact probability values for the two-sample permutation test with $v = 2$ range from $P = 0.4038 \times 10^{-5}$ for small values of w up to $P = 1.0000$ for large values of w, relative to the fixed values. Finally, the asymptotic two-tail probability values for the classical two-sample t test approach a common value as w becomes very small or very large, relative to the fixed values, and the classical t test is unable to detect the obvious differences in location between Samples 1 and 2.

6.5.6   Treatment-Group Weights

The treatment-group weighting functions with $N - 2$ degrees of freedom given by

$$C_1 = \frac{n_1 - 1}{N - 2} \quad \text{and} \quad C_2 = \frac{n_2 - 1}{N - 2}$$

are essential for Student's t test for two independent samples, but are not required for a permutation test, as degrees of freedom are irrelevant for nonparametric, distribution-free permutation methods.[5] For a reanalysis of the example data listed in Table 6.4 on p. 174, the treatment-group weighting functions are set to

$$C_1 = \frac{n_1}{N} \quad \text{and} \quad C_2 = \frac{n_2}{N} \,,$$

simply weighting each treatment group proportional to the number of observations in the group and setting $v = 1$, employing ordinary Euclidean difference between the pairs of values. For the example data listed in Table 6.4 on p. 174 the permutation test statistic is $\delta = 9.1673$.

Under the Fisher–Pitman permutation model, the exact probability of an observed δ is the proportion of δ test statistic values computed on all possible, equally-likely arrangements of the observed data that are equal to or less than the observed value of $\delta = 9.1673$. There are exactly 2127 δ test statistic values that are equal to or less than the observed value of $\delta = 9.1673$. If all M arrangements of the $N = 14$ observed values listed in Table 6.4 on p. 174 occur with equal chance under the Fisher–Pitman null hypothesis, the exact probability value of $\delta = 9.1673$ computed on the $M = 3003$ possible arrangements of the observed data with $n_1 = 8$ and $n_2 = 6$ preserved for each arrangement is

$$P\big(\delta \leq \delta_o\big) = \frac{\text{number of } \delta \text{ values } \leq \delta_o}{M} = \frac{2127}{3003} = 0.7083 \,,$$

where δ_o denotes the observed value of test statistic δ and M is the number of possible, equally-likely arrangements of the $N = 14$ observations listed in Table 6.4.

For comparison, the exact probability values based on squared Euclidean scaling with $v = 2$ and ordinary Euclidean scaling with $v = 1$ and

$$C_1 = \frac{n_1 - 1}{N - 2} \quad \text{and} \quad C_2 = \frac{n_2 - 1}{N - 2} \,,$$

---

[5] Degrees of freedom are not relevant for any nonparametric, distribution-free statistic. However, it is noteworthy that degrees of freedom may be required for a test statistic that is nonparametric but is not distribution-free, such as Pearson's χ^2 test statistics for goodness of fit and independence.

are $P = 0.5275$ and $P = 0.7040$, respectively. No comparison is made with Student's two-sample t test for two independent samples as Student's t is undefined for $C_i = n_i/N$, $i = 1, 2$.

The exact expected value of the $M = 3003$ δ test statistic values with $v = 1$ is

$$\mu_\delta = \frac{1}{M} \sum_{i=1}^{M} \delta_i = \frac{26{,}400}{3003} = 8.7912$$

and the observed chance-corrected measure of effect size is

$$\Re = 1 - \frac{\delta}{\mu_\delta} = 1 - \frac{9.1673}{8.7912} = -0.0428 \, ,$$

indicating less than chance within-group agreement. No comparisons are made with Cohen's $\hat{d}$, Pearson's r^2, Kelley's ϵ^2, or Hays' $\hat{\omega}^2$ conventional measures of effect size for two independent samples as $\hat{d}$, r^2, ϵ^2, and $\hat{\omega}^2$ are undefined for $C_i = n_i/N$, $i = 1, 2$.

6.6 Example 4: Exact and Monte Carlo Analyses

For a fourth, larger example of a test for two independent samples, consider the data on $N = 28$ subjects under the Neyman–Pearson population model, randomly divided into two groups of $n_1 = n_2 = 14$ subjects each and listed in Table 6.7. For the example data listed in Table 6.7, the null hypothesis is H_0: $\mu_1 = \mu_2$; that

Table 6.7 Example data for a test of two independent samples with $N = 28$ subjects

Group 1		Group 2	
Case	Value	Case	Value
1	72.87	15	72.92
2	72.78	16	72.86
3	72.61	17	72.85
4	72.55	18	72.80
5	72.53	19	72.74
6	72.50	20	72.73
7	72.47	21	72.69
8	72.47	22	72.66
9	72.44	23	72.66
10	72.42	24	72.62
11	72.38	25	72.57
12	72.31	26	72.51
13	72.17	27	72.36
14	72.14	28	72.25

is, no mean difference is expected between the two populations from which the samples are presumed to have been drawn. The two groups are of equal size with $n_1 = n_2 = 14$, the mean of treatment Group 1 is $\bar{x}_1 = 72.4743$, the mean of treatment Group 2 is $\bar{x}_2 = 72.6586$, the estimated population variance for Group 1 is $s_1^2 = 0.0402$, the estimated population variance for Group 2 is $s_2^2 = 0.0358$, the unbiased pooled estimate of the population variance is

$$
s_p^2 = \frac{(n_1 - 1)s_1^2 + (n_2 - 1)s_2^2}{N - 2}
$$

$$
= \frac{(14 - 1)(0.0402) + (14 - 1)(0.0358)}{28 - 2} = 0.0380 ,
$$

and the observed value of Student's t test statistic is

$$
t = \frac{\bar{x}_1 - \bar{x}_2}{\left[s_p^2 \left(\dfrac{1}{n_1} + \dfrac{1}{n_2} \right) \right]^{1/2}} = \frac{72.4743 - 72.6586}{\left[0.0380 \left(\dfrac{1}{14} + \dfrac{1}{14} \right) \right]^{1/2}} = -2.5011 .
$$

Under the Neyman–Pearson null hypothesis, test statistic t is asymptotically distributed as Student's t with $N - 2$ degrees of freedom. With $N - 2 = 28 - 2 = 26$ degrees of freedom, the asymptotic two-tail probability value of $t = -2.5011$ is $P = 0.0190$, under the assumptions of normality and homogeneity.

6.6.1 A Monte Carlo Analysis with $v = 2$

Under the Fisher–Pitman permutation model, employing squared Euclidean scaling with $v = 2$ and treatment-group weights

$$
C_1 = \frac{n_1 - 1}{N - 2} \quad \text{and} \quad C_2 = \frac{n_2 - 1}{N - 2}
$$

for correspondence with Student's two-sample t test, the average distance-function values for Groups 1 and 2 are

$$
\xi_1 = 0.0804 \quad \text{and} \quad \xi_2 = 0.0717 ,
$$

respectively, and the observed permutation test statistic is

$$
\delta = \sum_{i=1}^{2} C_i \xi_i = \left(\frac{14 - 1}{28 - 2} \right) (0.0804) + \left(\frac{14 - 1}{28 - 2} \right) (0.0717) = 0.0760 .
$$

Alternatively, in terms of Student's t test statistic,

$$\xi_1 = 2s_1^2 = 2(0.0402) = 0.0804 , \quad \xi_2 = 2s_2^2 = 2(0.0358) = 0.0717 ,$$

and

$$\delta = 2s_p^2 = 2(0.0380) = 0.0760 .$$

For the example data listed in Table 6.7, the sum of the $N = 28$ observations is

$$\sum_{i=1}^{N} x_i = 72.87 + 72.78 + \cdots + 72.36 + 72.25 = 2031.8600 ,$$

the sum of the $N = 28$ squared observations is

$$\sum_{i=1}^{N} x_i^2 = 72.87^2 + 72.78^2 + \cdots + 72.36^2 + 72.25^2 = 147{,}446.0494 ,$$

and the total sum-of-squares is

$$SS_{\text{Total}} = \sum_{i=1}^{N} x_i^2 - \left(\sum_{i=1}^{N} x_i \right)^2 \Big/ N$$

$$= 147{,}446.0494 - (2031.8600)^2/28 = 1.2258 .$$

Based on the expressions given in Eq. (6.5) on p. 159, the observed value for test statistic δ with respect to the observed value of Student's t statistic is

$$\delta = \frac{2SS_{\text{Total}}}{t^2 + N - 2} = \frac{2(1.2258)}{(-2.5011)^2 + 28 - 2} = 0.0760$$

and the observed value for Student's t statistic with respect to the observed value of test statistic δ is

$$t = \left(\frac{2SS_{\text{Total}}}{\delta} - N + 2 \right)^{1/2} = \left[\frac{2(1.2258)}{0.0760} - 28 + 2 \right]^{1/2} = \pm 2.5011 .$$

Under the Fisher–Pitman permutation model there are

$$M = \frac{(n_1 + n_2)!}{n_1! \, n_2!} = \frac{(14 + 14)!}{14! \, 14!} = 40{,}116{,}600$$

possible, equally-likely arrangements in the reference set of all permutations of the observed data listed in Table 6.7, making an exact permutation analysis impractical. Under the Fisher–Pitman permutation model, the Monte Carlo probability of an observed δ is the proportion of δ test statistic values computed on the randomly-selected, equally-likely arrangements of the observed data that are equal to or less than the observed value of $\delta = 0.0760$. Based on $L = 1{,}000{,}000$ random arrangements of the observed data, there are exactly 20,439 δ test statistic values that are equal to or less than the observed value of $\delta = 0.0760$. If all M arrangements of the $N = 28$ observations listed in Table 6.7 occur with equal chance under the Fisher–Pitman null hypothesis, the Monte Carlo probability value of $\delta = 0.0760$ computed on $L = 1{,}000{,}000$ random arrangements of the observed data with $n_1 = n_2 = 14$ preserved for each arrangement is

$$P\left(\delta \le \delta_o\right) = \frac{\text{number of } \delta \text{ values } \le \delta_o}{L} = \frac{20{,}439}{1{,}000{,}000} = 0.0204 \, ,$$

where δ_o denotes the observed value of test statistic δ and L is the number of randomly-selected, equally-likely arrangements of the $N = 28$ observations listed in Table 6.7. Alternatively, the Monte Carlo probability value of $|t| = 2.5011$ under the Fisher–Pitman null hypothesis is

$$P\left(|t| \ge |t_o|\right) = \frac{\text{number of } |t| \text{ values } \ge |t_o|}{L} = \frac{20{,}439}{1{,}000{,}000} = 0.0204 \, ,$$

where t_o denotes the observed value of test statistic t.

   For the example data listed in Table 6.7 the exact expected value of test statistic δ under the Fisher–Pitman null hypothesis is

$$\mu_\delta = \frac{1}{M} \sum_{i=1}^{M} \delta_i = \frac{3{,}642{,}715}{40{,}116{,}600} = 0.0908 \, .$$

Alternatively, in terms of an analysis of variance model the exact expected value of test statistic δ is

$$\mu_\delta = \frac{2SS_{\text{Total}}}{N-1} = \frac{2(1.2258)}{28-1} = 0.0908 \, ,$$

where

$$SS_{\text{Total}} = \sum_{i=1}^{N} x_i^2 - \left(\sum_{i=1}^{N} x_i\right)^2 \Bigg/ N$$

$$= 147{,}446.0494 - (2031.8600)/28 = 1.2258 \, .$$

Finally, the observed chance-corrected measure of effect size is

$$\Re = 1 - \frac{\delta}{\mu_\delta} = 1 - \frac{0.0760}{0.0908} = +0.1629 \, ,$$

indicating approximately 16% within-group agreement above what is expected by chance.

6.6.2   An Exact Analysis with $v = 2$

While an exact analysis may be impractical with $M = 40{,}116{,}600$ possible arrangements of the observed data, it is not impossible. For an exact test under the Fisher–Pitman permutation model with $v = 2$, the observed value of δ is still $\delta = 0.0760$, the exact expected value of δ under the Fisher–Pitman null hypothesis is $\mu_\delta = 0.0908$, there are exactly 815,878 δ test statistic values that are equal to or less than the observed value of $\delta = 0.0760$, and the exact probability value based on all $M = 40{,}116{,}600$ arrangements of the observed data under the Fisher–Pitman null hypothesis is

$$P\big(\delta \le \delta_0 | H_0\big) = \frac{\text{number of } \delta \text{ values} \le \delta_0}{M} = \frac{815{,}878}{40{,}116{,}600} = 0.0203 \, ,$$

where δ_0 denotes the observed value of test statistic δ and M is the number of possible, equally-likely arrangements of the $N = 28$ observations listed in Table 6.7.

Alternatively, the exact two-tail probability value of $|t| = 2.5011$ under the null hypothesis is

$$P\big(|t| \ge |t_0|\big) = \frac{\text{number of } |t| \text{ values} \ge |t_0|}{M} = \frac{815{,}878}{40{,}116{,}600} = 0.0203 \, ,$$

where t_0 denotes the observed value of test statistic t. The observed chance-corrected measure of effect size is unchanged at

$$\Re = 1 - \frac{\delta}{\mu_\delta} = 1 - \frac{0.0760}{0.0908} = +0.1629 \, ,$$

indicating approximately 16% within-group agreement above what is expected by chance.

6.6.3 Measures of Effect Size

For comparison, for the example data with $N = 28$ observations listed in Table 6.7 Cohen's $\hat{d}$ measure of effect size is

$$\hat{d} = \frac{|\bar{x}_1 - \bar{x}_2|}{\sqrt{s_p^2}} = \frac{|72.4743 - 72.6586|}{\sqrt{0.0380}} = 0.9454 \,,$$

Pearson's r^2 measure of effect size is

$$r^2 = \frac{t^2}{t^2 + N - 2} = \frac{(-2.5011)^2}{(-2.5011)^2 + 28 - 2} = 0.1939 \,,$$

Kelley's ϵ^2 measure of effect size is

$$\epsilon^2 = \frac{t^2 - 1}{t^2 + N - 2} = \frac{(-2.5011)^2 - 1}{(-2.5011)^2 + 28 - 2} = 0.1629 \,,$$

and Hays' $\hat{\omega}^2$ measure of effect size is

$$\hat{\omega}^2 = \frac{t^2 - 1}{t^2 + N - 1} = \frac{(-2.5011)^2 - 1}{(-2.5011)^2 + 28 - 2} = 0.1580 \,.$$

There is a considerable difference between the value for Cohen's measure of effect size ($\hat{d} = 0.9454$) and the other three measures (Pearson's $r^2 = 0.1939$, Kelley's $\epsilon^2 = 0.1629$, and Hays' $\hat{\omega}^2 = 0.1580$). In general, members of the r family, such as Pearson's r^2, Kelley's ϵ^2, and Hays' $\hat{\omega}^2$, produce measures of effect size that vary between the limits of 0 and 1, while members of the d family, such as Cohen's $\hat{d}$, produce measures of effect size in standard deviation units and, theoretically, can vary between 0 and ∞.

For comparison purposes, Cohen's $\hat{d}$ measure of effect size can be converted to the r family of measures of effect size. Cohen's $\hat{d}$ can then be compared with Pearson's r^2, Kelley's ϵ^2, and Hays' $\hat{\omega}^2$. Thus,

$$r^2 = \frac{n_1 n_2 \hat{d}^2}{n_1 n_2 \hat{d}^2 + N(N - 2)} = \frac{(14)(14)(0.9454)^2}{(14)(14)(0.9454)^2 + 28(28 - 2)} = 0.1939 \,,$$

which is similar to Kelley's $\epsilon^2 = 0.1629$ and Hays' $\hat{\omega}^2 = 0.1580$.

6.6.4   A Monte Carlo Analysis with $v = 1$

Consider an analysis of the error data listed in Table 6.7 under the Fisher–Pitman permutation model employing ordinary Euclidean scaling with $v = 1$, $N = 28$, and treatment-group weights

$$C_1 = \frac{n_1 - 1}{N - 2} \quad \text{and} \quad C_2 = \frac{n_2 - 1}{N - 2} .$$

For $v = 1$, the average distance-function values for treatment Groups 1 and 2 are

$$\xi_1 = 0.2288 \quad \text{and} \quad \xi_2 = 0.2167 ,$$

respectively, and the observed permutation test statistic is

$$\delta = \sum_{i=1}^{2} C_i \xi_i = \left(\frac{14 - 1}{28 - 2}\right) (0.2288) + \left(\frac{14 - 1}{28 - 2}\right) (0.2167) = 0.2227 .$$

There are exactly

$$M = \frac{(n_1 + n_2)!}{n_1! \, n_2!} = \frac{(14 + 14)!}{14! \, 14!} = 40,116,600$$

possible, equally-likely arrangements in the reference set of all permutations of the example data listed in Table 6.7. Under the Fisher–Pitman permutation model the Monte Carlo probability of an observed δ is the proportion of δ test statistic values computed on the randomly-selected, equally-likely arrangements of the observed data that are equal to or less than the observed value of $\delta = 0.2227$. Based on $L = 1,000,000$ random arrangements of the observed data, there are exactly 14,493 δ test statistic values that are equal to or less than the observed value of $\delta = 0.2227$. If all M arrangements of the $N = 28$ observations listed in Table 6.7 occur with equal chance under the Fisher–Pitman null hypothesis, the Monte Carlo probability value of $\delta = 0.2227$ computed on $L = 1,000,000$ random arrangements of the observed data with $n_1 = n_2 = 14$ preserved for each arrangement is

$$P(\delta \le \delta_0 | H_0) = \frac{\text{number of } \delta \text{ values} \le \delta_0}{L} = \frac{14,493}{1,000,000} = 0.0145 ,$$

where δ_0 denotes the observed value of test statistic δ and L is the number of randomly-selected, equally-likely arrangements of the $N = 28$ observations listed in Table 6.7. No comparison is made with Student's t test statistic for two independent samples as Student's t is undefined for ordinary Euclidean scaling.

For the data listed in Table 6.7, the exact expected value of test statistic δ under the Fisher–Pitman null hypothesis is

$$\mu_\delta = \frac{1}{M} \sum_{i=1}^{M} \delta_i = \frac{10{,}997{,}042}{40{,}116{,}600} = 0.2741 \ ,$$

and the observed chance-corrected measure of effect size is

$$\Re = 1 - \frac{\delta}{\mu_\delta} = 1 - \frac{0.2227}{0.2741} = +0.1875 \ ,$$

indicating approximately 19% within-group agreement above what is expected by chance. No comparisons are made with Cohen's $\hat{d}$, Pearson's r^2, Kelley's ϵ^2, or Hays' $\hat{\omega}^2$ measures of effect size for two independent samples as $\hat{d}$, r^2, ϵ^2, and $\hat{\omega}^2$ are undefined for ordinary Euclidean scaling.

6.6.5 An Exact Analysis with $v = 1$

For comparison, with $v = 1$ and treatment-group weights

$$C_1 = \frac{n_1 - 1}{N - 2} \quad \text{and} \quad C_2 = \frac{n_2 - 1}{N - 2} \ ,$$

the exact probability value of $\delta = 0.2227$ computed on the $M = 40{,}116{,}600$ possible arrangements of the observed data with $n_1 = n_2 = 14$ preserved for each arrangement is

$$P\left(\delta \le \delta_o\right) = \frac{\text{number of } \delta \text{ values } \le \delta_o}{M} = \frac{583{,}424}{40{,}116{,}600} = 0.0145 \ ,$$

where δ_o denotes the observed value of test statistic δ and M is the number of possible, equally-likely arrangements of the $N = 28$ observations listed in Table 6.7 on p. 184.

6.7 Example 5: Rank-Score Permutation Analyses

Oftentimes in conventional research it becomes necessary to analyze rank-score data, either because the observed data are collected as ranks or because the necessary parametric assumptions cannot be met and the raw data are subsequently converted to ranks. There is never any reason to convert raw scores to ranks with permutation statistical methods [3], so this example merely serves to demonstrate the relationship between a quotidian two-sample test of rank-score data and a permutation test of rank-score data. The conventional approach to rank-score data for two independent samples under the Neyman–Pearson population model is the Wilcoxon–Mann–Whitney (WMW) two-sample rank-sum test.

6.7.1 The Wilcoxon–Mann–Whitney Test

Consider a two-sample rank test for N univariate rank scores with n_1 and n_2 rank scores in the first and second samples, respectively. Under the Neyman–Pearson population model, the WMW two-sample rank-sum test is given by

$$W = \sum_{i=1}^{n_1} R_i \, ,$$

where R_i denotes the rank function of the ith response measurement and n_1 is, typically, the smaller of the two-sample sizes.

For an example analysis of rank-score data, consider the rank scores listed in Table 6.8, where for two samples, $n_1 = 8$, $n_2 = 12$, $N = n_1 + n_2 = 8 + 12 = 20$ total scores, and there are no tied rank scores. For this application, let $n_1 = 8$ denote the rank scores in Sample 1 and $n_2 = 12$ denote the rank scores in Sample 2.

The conventional Wilcoxon–Mann–Whitney two-sample rank-sum test on the $N = 20$ rank scores listed in Table 6.8 yields an observed test statistic value of

$$W = \sum_{i=1}^{n_1} R_i = 1 + 2 + 3 + 4 + 5 + 6 + 8 + 11 = 40 \, ,$$

Table 6.8 Example rank-score data for a conventional Wilcoxon–Mann–Whitney two-sample rank-sum test with $n_1 = 8$ and $n_2 = 12$ subjects

Sample 1		Sample 2	
Subject	Score	Subject	Score
1	1	9	7
2	2	10	9
3	3	11	10
4	4	12	12
5	5	13	13
6	6	14	14
7	8	15	15
8	11	16	16
		17	17
		18	18
		19	19
		20	20

where statistic W is asymptotically distributed $N(0, 1)$ under the Neyman–Pearson null hypothesis as $N \rightarrow \infty$. For the rank scores listed in Table 6.8, the mean value of test statistic W is

$$\mu_W = \frac{n_1(N+1)}{2} = \frac{8(20+1)}{2} = 84 ,$$

the variance of test statistic W is

$$\sigma_W^2 = \frac{n_1 n_2(N+1)}{12} = \frac{(8)(12)(20+1)}{12} = 168 ,$$

the standard score, corrected for continuity, is[6]

$$z = \frac{W + 0.5 - \mu_W}{\sqrt{\sigma_W^2}} = \frac{40 + 0.5 - 84}{\sqrt{168}} = -3.3561 ,$$

and the asymptotic two-tail $N(0, 1)$ probability value is $P = 0.3952 \times 10^{-3}$.

6.7.2 An Exact Analysis with $v = 2$

For an analysis of the rank-score data listed in Table 6.8 under the Fisher–Pitman permutation model let $v = 2$, employing squared Euclidean differences between the pairs of rank scores, and let the treatment-group weights be given by

$$C_1 = \frac{n_1 - 1}{N - 2} \quad \text{and} \quad C_2 = \frac{n_2 - 1}{N - 2}$$

for correspondence with the Wilcoxon–Mann–Whitney two-sample rank-sum test. Following Eq. (6.2) on p. 157, the average distance-function values for Samples 1 and 2 are

$$\xi_1 = 21.7143 \quad \text{and} \quad \xi_2 = 33.7576 ,$$

respectively, and the observed value of the permutation test statistic δ is

$$\delta = \sum_{i=1}^{2} C_i \xi_i = \left(\frac{8-1}{20-2} \right) (21.7143) + \left(\frac{12-1}{20-2} \right) (33.7576) = 29.0741 .$$

---

[6]When fitting a continuous mathematical function, such as the normal probability distribution, to a discrete permutation distribution, it is oftentimes necessary to correct the fit by adding or subtracting 0.5 to compensate for the discreteness of the distribution.

Although no self-respecting researcher would seriously consider calculating an estimated population variance on rank scores, since the WMW two-sample rank-sum test is directly derived from Student's two-sample t test, certain relationships still hold. Thus,

$$\xi_1 = 2s_1^2 = 2(10.8571) = 21.7143 , \quad \xi_2 = 2s_2^2 = 2(16.8788) = 33.7576 ,$$

and

$$\delta = 2s_p^2 = 2(14.5370) = 29.0741 ,$$

where $s_1^2 = 10.8571$ and $s_2^2 = 16.8788$ are calculated on the rank-score data listed in Table 6.8.

Because there are only

$$M = \frac{(n_1 + n_2)!}{n_1! \, n_2!} = \frac{(8 + 12)!}{8! \, 12!} = 125{,}970$$

possible, equally-likely arrangements in the reference set of all permutations of the $N = 20$ rank scores listed in Table 6.8, an exact permutation analysis is feasible. Under the Fisher–Pitman permutation model, the exact probability of an observed δ is the proportion of δ test statistic values computed on all possible, equally-likely arrangements of the observed data that are equal to or less than the observed value of $\delta = 29.0741$. There are exactly 24 δ test statistic values that are equal to or less than the observed value of $\delta = 29.0741$. If all M arrangements of the $N = 20$ rank scores listed in Table 6.8 occur with equal chance under the Fisher–Pitman null hypothesis, the exact probability value of $\delta = 29.0741$ computed on the $M = 125{,}970$ possible arrangements of the observed data with $n_1 = 8$ and $n_2 = 12$ preserved for each arrangement is

$$P(\delta \leq \delta_0 | H_0) = \frac{\text{number of } \delta \text{ values} \leq \delta_0}{M} = \frac{24}{125{,}970} = 0.1905 \times 10^{-3} ,$$

where δ_0 denotes the observed value of test statistic δ and M is the number of possible, equally-likely arrangements of the $N = 20$ observations listed in Table 6.8.

The functional relationships between test statistics δ and W are given by

$$\delta = \frac{2}{N(N-2)} \left[NT - S^2 - \frac{(NW - n_1 S)^2}{n_1 n_2} \right] \tag{6.22}$$

and

$$W = \frac{n_1 S}{N} - \left\{ \frac{n_1 n_2}{N^2} \left[NT - S^2 - \frac{N(N-2)\delta}{2} \right] \right\}^{1/2} , \tag{6.23}$$

where

$$S = \sum_{i=1}^{N} R_i \quad \text{and} \quad T = \sum_{i=1}^{N} R_i^2 \ .$$

In the absence of any tied rank scores, it is well known that S and T may simply be expressed as

$$S = \sum_{i=1}^{N} i = \frac{N(N+1)}{2} \quad \text{and} \quad T = \sum_{i=1}^{N} i^2 = \frac{N(N+1)(2N+1)}{6} \ .$$

The relationships between test statistics δ and W are confirmed as follows. For the $N = 20$ rank scores listed in Table 6.8 with no tied values, the observed value of S is

$$S = \sum_{i=1}^{N} i = \frac{N(N+1)}{2} = \frac{20(20+1)}{2} = 210$$

and the observed value of T is

$$T = \sum_{i=1}^{N} i^2 = \frac{N(N+1)(2N+1)}{6} = \frac{20(20+1)[2(20)+1]}{6} = 2870 \ .$$

Then following Eq. (6.22), the observed value of test statistic δ with respect to the observed value of test statistic W for the rank scores listed in Table 6.8 is

$$\delta = \frac{2}{N(N-2)} \left[NT - S^2 - \frac{(NW - n_1 S)^2}{n_1 n_2} \right]$$

$$= \frac{2}{20(20-2)} \left\{ 20(2,870) - (210)^2 - \frac{[20(40) - 8(210)]^2}{(8)(12)} \right\}$$

$$= \frac{2}{360} \left(13,300 - \frac{774,400}{96} \right) = 29.0741$$

and following Eq. (6.23), the observed value of test statistic W with respect to the observed value of test statistic δ is

$$W = \frac{n_1 S}{N} - \left\{ \frac{n_1 n_2}{N^2} \left[NT - S^2 - \frac{N(N-2)\delta}{2} \right] \right\}^{1/2}$$

$$= \frac{(8)(210)}{20} - \left\{ \frac{(8)(12)}{20^2} \left[(20)(2870) - (210)^2 - \frac{20(20-2)(29.0741)}{2} \right] \right\}$$

$$= 84 - \left[(0.24)(8,066.6667) \right]^{1/2} = 40 \ .$$

Because of the relationship between test statistics δ and W, the exact probability of $W = 40$ is the same as the exact probability of $\delta = 29.0741$. Thus,

$$P\left(\delta \le \delta_0 | H_0\right) = \frac{\text{number of } \delta \text{ values } \le \delta_0}{M} = \frac{24}{125{,}970} = 0.1905 \times 10^{-3}$$

and

$$P\left(W \ge W_0 | H_0\right) = \frac{\text{number of } W \text{ values } \ge W_0}{M}$$

$$= \frac{24}{125{,}970} = 0.1905 \times 10^{-3} \,,$$

where δ_0 and W_0 denote the observed values of test statistics δ and W, respectively, and M is the number of possible, equally-likely arrangements of the $N = 20$ rank scores listed in Table 6.8.

Following Eq. (6.7) on p. 160, the exact expected value of the $M = 125{,}970$ δ test statistic values under the Fisher–Pitman null hypothesis is

$$\mu_\delta = \frac{1}{M} \sum_{i=1}^{M} \delta_i = \frac{8{,}817{,}900}{125{,}970} = 70.00$$

and following Eq. (6.6) on p. 160, the observed chance-corrected measure of effect size is

$$\Re = 1 - \frac{\delta}{\mu_\delta} = 1 - \frac{29.0741}{70.00} = +0.5847 \,,$$

indicating approximately 58% within-group agreement above what is expected by chance. No comparisons are made with Cohen's $\hat{d}$, Pearson's r^2, Kelley's ϵ^2, or Hays' $\hat{\omega}^2$ measures of effect size for two independent samples as $\hat{d}$, r^2, ϵ^2, and $\hat{\omega}^2$ are undefined for rank-score data.

6.7.3 An Exact Analysis with $v = 1$

For a reanalysis of the rank-score data listed in Table 6.8 on p. 192 under the Fisher–Pitman permutation model let $v = 1$ instead of $v = 2$, employing ordinary Euclidean differences between the pairs of rank scores, and let the treatment-group weights be given by

$$C_1 = \frac{n_1 - 1}{N - 2} \quad \text{and} \quad C_2 = \frac{n_2 - 1}{N - 2} \,.$$

Following Eq. (6.2) on p. 157, the average distance-function values for Samples 1 and 2 are

$$\xi_1 = 3.9286 \quad \text{and} \quad \xi_2 = 4.9091 \, ,$$

respectively, and the observed value of test statistic δ is

$$\delta = \sum_{i=1}^{2} C_i \xi_i = \left(\frac{8-1}{20-2} \right) (3.9286) + \left(\frac{12-1}{20-2} \right) (4.9091) = 4.5278 \, .$$

Because there are only

$$M = \frac{(n_1 + n_2)!}{n_1! \, n_2!} = \frac{(8+12)!}{8! \, 12!} = 125{,}970$$

possible, equally-likely arrangements in the reference set of all permutations of the $N = 20$ rank scores listed in Table 6.8, an exact permutation analysis is feasible. Under the Fisher–Pitman permutation model, the exact probability of an observed δ is the proportion of δ test statistic values computed on all possible, equally-likely arrangements of the observed data that are equal to or less than the observed value of $\delta = 4.5278$. There are exactly 24 δ test statistic values that are equal to or less than the observed value of $\delta = 4.5278$. If all M arrangements of the $N = 20$ rank scores listed in Table 6.8 occur with equal chance under the Fisher–Pitman null hypothesis, the exact probability value of $\delta = 4.5278$ computed on the $M = 125{,}970$ possible arrangements of the observed data with $n_1 = 8$ and $n_2 = 12$ preserved for each arrangement is

$$P\left(\delta \le \delta_0 | H_0 \right) = \frac{\text{number of } \delta \text{ values} \le \delta_0}{M} = \frac{24}{125{,}970} = 0.1905 \times 10^{-3} \, ,$$

where δ_0 denotes the observed value of test statistic δ and M is the number of possible, equally-likely arrangements of the $N = 20$ observations listed in Table 6.8. For comparison, the exact probability value based on $v = 2$, $M = 125{,}970$, and treatment-group weights

$$C_1 = \frac{n_1 - 1}{N - 2} \quad \text{and} \quad C_2 = \frac{n_2 - 1}{N - 2}$$

in the previous analysis was also $P = 0.1905 \times 10^{-3}$. No comparison is made with the conventional Wilcoxon–Mann–Whitney two-sample rank-sum test as the WMW test is undefined for ordinary Euclidean scaling.

Following Eq. (6.7) on p. 160, the exact expected value of the $M = 125{,}970\ \delta$ test statistic values under the Fisher–Pitman null hypothesis is

$$\mu_\delta = \frac{1}{M} \sum_{i=1}^{M} \delta_i = \frac{881{,}790}{125{,}970} = 7.00$$

and, following Eq. (6.6) on p. 160, the observed chance-corrected measure of effect size is

$$\Re = 1 - \frac{\delta}{\mu_\delta} = 1 - \frac{4.5278}{7.00} = +0.3532 \, ,$$

indicating approximately 35% within-group agreement above what is expected by chance. No comparisons are made with Cohen's $\hat{d}$, Pearson's r^2, Kelley's ϵ^2, or Hays' $\hat{\omega}^2$ measures of effect size for two independent samples as $\hat{d}$, r^2, ϵ^2, and $\hat{\omega}^2$ are undefined for rank-score data.

Finally, it should be noted that for the example data listed in Table 6.8 the observed ξ_1 and ξ_2 values differ for $v = 2$ ($\xi_1 = 21.7143$ and $\xi_2 = 33.7576$) and $v = 1$ ($\xi_1 = 3.9286$ and $\xi_2 = 4.9091$), the observed δ values differ for $v = 2$ ($\delta = 29.0741$) and $v = 1$ ($\delta = 4.5278$), and the exact values for μ_δ also differ for $v = 2$ ($\mu_\delta = 70.00$) and $v = 1$ ($\mu_\delta = 7.00$). However, the probability values for $v = 2$ ($P = 0.1905 \times 10^{-3}$) and $v = 1$ ($P = 0.1905 \times 10^{-3}$) do not differ. This is always true for two-sample tests of rank scores under the Fisher–Pitman permutation model. Unlike two-sample tests of raw (interval-level) values, there is never any difference in probability values for $v = 2$ and $v = 1$ with rank-score (ordinal-level) data.

6.8   Example 6: Multivariate Permutation Analyses

Oftentimes a research design calls for a test of difference between two independent treatment groups when $r \geq 2$ response measurements have been obtained for each subject. The conventional approach to such a research design under the Neyman–Pearson population model is Hotelling's multivariate T^2 test for two independent samples given by

$$T^2 = \frac{n_1 n_2}{N} (\bar{y}_2 - \bar{y}_2) \mathbf{S}^{-1} (\bar{y}_1 - \bar{y}_2) \, , \tag{6.24}$$

where $\bar{y}_1$ and $\bar{y}_2$ denote vectors of mean differences between treatment Groups 1 and 2, respectively, n_1 and n_2 are the number of multivariate measurement scores in treatment Groups 1 and 2, respectively, $N = n_1 + n_2$, and $\mathbf{S}$ is a variance–covariance matrix given by

$$
\begin{bmatrix}
\dfrac{1}{N} \displaystyle\sum_{I=1}^{N} (y_{1I} - \bar{y}_1)^2 & \cdots & \dfrac{1}{N} \displaystyle\sum_{I=1}^{N} (y_{1I} - \bar{y}_1)(y_{rI} - \bar{y}_r) \\
\vdots & & \vdots \\
\dfrac{1}{N} \displaystyle\sum_{I=1}^{N} (y_{rI} - \bar{y}_r)(y_{1I} - \bar{y}_1) & \cdots & \dfrac{1}{N} \displaystyle\sum_{I=1}^{N} (y_{rI} - \bar{y}_r)^2
\end{bmatrix} .
$$

The observed value of Hotelling's T^2 is conventionally transformed into an F test statistic by

$$
F = \frac{N - r - 1}{r(N - 2)} T^2 ,
$$

which is asymptotically distributed as Snedecor's F under the Neyman–Pearson null hypothesis with $v_1 = r$ and $v_2 = N - r - 1$ degrees of freedom.

6.8.1 The Hotelling Two-Sample T^2 Test

To illustrate a conventional multivariate analysis under the Neyman–Pearson population model, consider the multivariate measurement scores listed in Table 6.9, where $r = 2$, $n_1 = 4$, $n_2 = 6$, and $N = n_1 + n_2 = 4 + 6 = 10$.

A conventional two-sample Hotelling T^2 test of the $N = 10$ multivariate measurement scores listed in Table 6.9 yields

$$
\bar{y}_{11} = 2.7750 ,
$$
$$
s_{11}^2 = 3.1092 ,
$$
$$
\bar{y}_{12} = 4.5250 ,
$$
$$
s_{12}^2 = 5.1892 ,
$$

Table 6.9 Example multivariate response measurement scores with $r = 2$, $n_1 = 4$, $n_2 = 6$, and $N = n_1 + n_2 = 10$

Treatment	
1	2
(1.2, 3.1)	(3.7, 6.1)
(2.9, 6.8)	(6.1, 8.3)
(1.8, 2.1)	(6.2, 7.9)
(5.2, 6.1)	(4.8, 9.7)
	(5.1, 9.9)
	(4.2, 7.8)

$$\text{cov}(1, 2)_1 = +2.9042 ,$$

$$\bar{y}_{21} = 5.0167$$

$$s_{21}^2 = 1.0057 ,$$

$$\bar{y}_{22} = 8.2833 ,$$

$$s_{22}^2 = 1.9537 ,$$

and

$$\text{cov}(1, 2)_2 = +0.5323 .$$

Then the vector of mean differences for treatment Group 1 is

$$\bar{y}_1 = \bar{y}_{11} - \bar{y}_{21} = 2.7550 - 5.0167 = -2.2417$$

and the vector of mean differences for treatment Group 2 is

$$\bar{y}_2 = \bar{y}_{12} - \bar{y}_{22} = 4.5250 - 8.2833 = -3.7583 .$$

The variance–covariance matrices for Treatments 1 and 2 are

$$\hat{\boldsymbol{\Sigma}}_1 = \begin{bmatrix} 3.1092 & +2.9042 \\ +2.9042 & 5.1892 \end{bmatrix} \quad \text{and} \quad \hat{\boldsymbol{\Sigma}}_2 = \begin{bmatrix} 1.0057 & +0.5323 \\ +0.5323 & 1.9537 \end{bmatrix} ,$$

respectively, and the pooled variance–covariance matrix and its inverse are

$$\mathbf{S} = \begin{bmatrix} 1.7945 & +1.4218 \\ +1.4218 & 3.1670 \end{bmatrix} \quad \text{and} \quad \mathbf{S}^{-1} = \begin{bmatrix} +0.8649 & -0.3883 \\ -0.3883 & +0.4901 \end{bmatrix} ,$$

respectively.

Following Eq. (6.24) on p. 198, the observed value of Hotelling's T^2 is

$$T^2 = \frac{n_1 n_2}{N} (\bar{y}_1 - \bar{y}_2)' \mathbf{S}^{-1} (\bar{y}_1 - \bar{y}_2)$$

$$= \frac{(4)(6)}{10} \begin{bmatrix} -2.2417 & -3.7583 \end{bmatrix} \begin{bmatrix} +0.8649 & -0.3883 \\ -0.3883 & +0.4901 \end{bmatrix} \begin{bmatrix} -2.2417 \\ -3.7583 \end{bmatrix}$$

$$= (2.40)(4.7260) = 11.3423$$

and the F test statistic for Hotelling's T^2 is

$$F = \frac{N - r - 1}{r(N - 2)} T_0^2 = \frac{10 - 2 - 1}{2(10 - 2)} (11.3423) = 4.9623 \, ,$$

where T_0^2 denotes the observed value of Hotelling's T^2.

Assuming independence, normality, homogeneity of variance, and homogeneity of covariance, Hotelling's F test statistic is asymptotically distributed as Snedecor's F with $\nu_1 = r = 2$ and $\nu_2 = N - r - 1 = 10 - 2 - 1 = 7$ degrees of freedom. Under the Neyman–Pearson null hypothesis, the observed value of $F = 4.9623$ yields an asymptotic probability value of $P = 0.0455$.

6.8.2 An Exact Analysis with $v = 2$

For an analysis under the Fisher–Pitman permutation model let $v = 2$, employing squared Euclidean differences between pairs of measurement scores and let the treatment-group weights be given by

$$C_1 = \frac{n_1 - 1}{N - 2} \quad \text{and} \quad C_2 = \frac{n_2 - 1}{N - 2}$$

for correspondence with Hotelling's T^2 test for two independent samples. Since there are only

$$M = \frac{(n_1 + n_2)!}{n_1! \, n_2!} = \frac{(4 + 6)!}{4! \, 6!} = 210$$

possible, equally-likely arrangements in the reference set of all permutations of the $N = 10$ multivariate measurement scores listed in Table 6.9, an exact permutation analysis is feasible. The multivariate measurement scores listed in Table 6.9 yield average distance-function values for Treatments 1 and 2 of

$$\xi_1 = 0.4862 \quad \text{and} \quad \xi_2 = 0.2737 \, ,$$

respectively, and the observed permutation test statistic is

$$\delta = \sum_{i=1}^{2} C_i \xi_i = \left(\frac{4 - 1}{10 - 2} \right) (0.4862) + \left(\frac{6 - 1}{10 - 2} \right) (0.2737) = 0.3534 \, .$$

If all M arrangements of the $N = 10$ observed multivariate measurement scores listed in Table 6.9 occur with equal chance under the Fisher–Pitman null hypothesis, the exact probability value of $\delta = 0.3534$ computed on the $M = 210$ possible arrangements of the observed data with $n_1 = 4$ and $n_2 = 6$ scores preserved for each arrangement is

$$P(\delta \le \delta_0 | H_0) = \frac{\text{number of } \delta \text{ values } \le \delta_0}{M} = \frac{12}{210} = 0.0571 \ ,$$

where δ_0 denotes the observed value of test statistic δ and M is the number of possible, equally-likely arrangements of the $N = 10$ multivariate observations listed in Table 6.9.

Following Eq. (6.7) on p. 160, the exact expected value of the $M = 210$ δ test statistic values under the Fisher–Pitman null hypothesis is

$$\mu_\delta = \frac{1}{M} \sum_{i=1}^{M} \delta_i = \frac{93.3333}{210} = 0.4444$$

and following Eq. (6.6) on p. 160, the observed chance-corrected measure of effect size is

$$\Re = 1 - \frac{\delta}{\mu_\delta} = 1 - \frac{0.3534}{0.4444} = +0.2049 \ ,$$

indicating approximately 20% within-group agreement above what is expected by chance. No comparisons are made with Cohen's $\hat{d}$, Pearson's r^2, Kelley's ϵ^2, or Hays' $\hat{\omega}^2$ measures of effect size for two-sample tests as $\hat{d}$, r^2, ϵ^2, and $\hat{\omega}^2$ are undefined for multivariate data.

The identity relating Hotelling's two-sample T^2 test and the permutation test statistic is given by

$$\delta = \frac{2[r - V^{(s)}]}{N - 2} \ , \tag{6.25}$$

where

$$V^{(s)} = \frac{T^2}{T^2 + N - 2} \tag{6.26}$$

and $s = \min(g - 1, r)$; in this case with $g - 1 = 2 - 1 = 1$ and $r = 2$, $s = \min(2 - 1, 2) = 1$. Thus, following Eqs. (6.25) and (6.26), the observed value of $V^{(1)}$ is

$$V^{(1)} = \frac{T^2}{T^2 + N - 2} = \frac{11.3423}{11.3423 + 10 - 2} = \frac{11.3423}{19.3423} = 0.5864$$

and the observed value of δ is

$$\delta = \frac{2(r - V^{(s)})}{N - g} = \frac{2(2 - 0.5864)}{10 - 2} = \frac{2.8272}{8} = 0.3534 \ .$$

6.8.3   An Exact Analysis with $v = 1$

Under the Fisher–Pitman permutation model, it is not necessary to set $v = 2$, thereby illuminating the squared differences between pairs of measurement scores. For a reanalysis of the measurement scores listed in Table 6.9 on p. 199, let the treatment-group weights be given by

$$C_1 = \frac{n_1 - 1}{N - 2} \quad \text{and} \quad C_2 = \frac{n_2 - 1}{N - 2}$$

as in the previous example, but set $v = 1$ instead of $v = 2$, employing ordinary Euclidean differences between pairs of measurement scores. Following Eq. (6.2) on p. 157, the average distance-function values for Treatments 1 and 2 are

$$\xi_1 = 3.7865 \quad \text{and} \quad \xi_2 = 2.2200 ,$$

respectively, and following Eq. (6.1) on p. 157, the observed value of the permutation test statistic is

$$\delta = \sum_{i=1}^{2} C_i \xi_i = \left(\frac{4 - 1}{10 - 2} \right) (3.7865) + \left(\frac{6 - 1}{10 - 2} \right) (2.2200) = 2.8074 .$$

If all M arrangements of the $N = 10$ observed multivariate measurement scores listed in Table 6.9 occur with equal chance under the Fisher–Pitman null hypothesis, the exact probability value of $\delta = 2.8074$ computed on the $M = 210$ possible arrangements of the observed data with $n_1 = 4$ and $n_2 = 6$ measurement scores preserved for each arrangement is

$$P\left(\delta \le \delta_0 | H_0 \right) = \frac{\text{number of } \delta \text{ values } \le \delta_0}{M} = \frac{4}{210} = 0.0190 ,$$

where δ_0 denotes the observed value of test statistic δ and M is the number of possible, equally-likely arrangements of the $N = 10$ multivariate observations listed in Table 6.9. For comparison, the exact probability value based on $v = 2$, $M = 210$, and treatment-group weights

$$C_1 = \frac{n_1 - 1}{N - 2} \quad \text{and} \quad C_2 = \frac{n_2 - 1}{N - 2}$$

in the previous example is $P = 0.0571$. No comparison is made with Hotelling's multivariate two-sample T^2 test as T^2 is undefined for ordinary Euclidean scaling.

Following Eq. (6.7) on p. 160, the exact expected value of the $M = 210$ δ test statistic values under the Fisher–Pitman null hypothesis is

$$\mu_\delta = \frac{1}{M} \sum_{i=1}^{M} \delta_i = \frac{790.1880}{210} = 3.7628$$

and, following Eq. (6.6) on p. 160, the observed chance-corrected measure of effect size is

$$\Re = 1 - \frac{\delta}{\mu_\delta} = 1 - \frac{2.8074}{3.7628} = +0.2539 \, ,$$

indicating approximately 25% within-group agreement above what is expected by chance. No comparisons are made with Cohen's $\hat{d}$, Pearson's r^2, Kelley's ϵ^2, or Hays' $\hat{\omega}^2$ measures of effect size for two-sample tests as $\hat{d}$, r^2, ϵ^2, and $\hat{\omega}^2$ are undefined for multivariate data.

6.9 Summary

This chapter examined tests for two independent samples where the null hypothesis under the Neyman–Pearson population model typically posits no difference between the means of two populations; that is, H_0: $\mu_1 = \mu_2$. The conventional tests for two independent samples and four measures of effect size under the Neyman–Pearson population model were described and illustrated: Student's two-sample t test and Cohen's $\hat{d}$, Pearson's r^2, Kelley's ϵ^2, and Hays' $\hat{\omega}^2$ measures of effect size, respectively.

Under the Fisher–Pitman permutation model, test statistic δ and associated measure of effect size $\Re$ were introduced and illustrated for tests of two independent samples. Test statistic δ was related to Student's t test statistic and shown to be flexible enough to incorporate either ordinary or squared Euclidean scaling with $v = 1$ and $v = 2$, respectively. Effect-size measure $\Re$ was shown to be applicable to either $v = 1$ or $v = 2$ without modification and to have a clear and meaningful chance-corrected interpretation.

Six examples illustrated permutation statistics δ and $\Re$. In the first example, a small sample of $N = 7$ values was utilized to describe and illustrate the calculations of δ and $\Re$ for two independent samples. The second example demonstrated the permutation-based, chance-corrected measure of effect size, $\Re$, and related $\Re$ to the four conventional measures of effect size for two independent samples: Cohen's $\hat{d}$, Pearson's r^2, Kelley's ϵ^2, and Hays' $\hat{\omega}^2$. The third example with $N = 14$ values was designed to illustrate the effects of extreme values on both conventional and permutation tests for two independent samples. The fourth example utilized a larger sample with $N = 28$ observations to compare and contrast exact and Monte Carlo permutation tests for two independent samples. The fifth example applied permutation methods to univariate rank-score data and compared the permutation results with conventional results from the Wilcoxon–Mann–Whitney two-sample rank-sum test. Finally, the sixth example illustrated the application of permutation methods to multivariate data and compared the permutation results with conventional results from Hotelling's T^2 test for two independent samples.

Chapter 7 continues the presentation of permutation statistical methods for two samples, but examines research designs in which the subjects in the two samples have been matched on specific characteristics; that is to say, not independent. Research designs that posit no mean difference between two matched treatment groups in which univariate measurements have been obtained are ubiquitous in the statistical literature. Matched-pairs tests are the simplest of the tests in an extensive class of randomized-blocks tests and are taught in every introductory course.

References

1. Barnard, G.A.: 2 × 2 tables. A note on E. S. Pearson's paper. Biometrika **34**, 168–169 (1947)
2. Cohen, J.: Weighted kappa: nominal scale agreement with provision for scaled disagreement or partial credit. Psychol. Bull. **70**, 213–220 (1968)
3. Feinstein, A.R.: Clinical biostatistics XXIII: the role of randomization in sampling, testing, allocation, and credulous idolatry (Part 2). Clin. Pharmacol. Ther. **14**, 898–915 (1973)
4. Hotelling, H., Pabst, M.R.: Rank correlation and tests of significance involving no assumption of normality. Ann. Math. Stat. **7**, 29–43 (1936)
5. Johnston, J.E., Berry, K.J., Mielke, P.W.: A measure of effect size for experimental designs with heterogeneous variances. Percept. Motor Skill. **98**, 3–18 (2004)
6. Johnston, J.E., Berry, K.J., Mielke, P.W.: Permutation tests: precision in estimating probability values. Percept. Motor Skill. **105**, 915–920 (2007)
7. Kendall, M.G., Babington Smith, B.: On the method of paired comparisons. Biometrika **31**, 324–345 (1940)
8. Macdonell, W.R.: On criminal anthropometry and the identification of criminals. Biometrika **1**, 177–227 (1902)
9. Maxwell, S.E., Camp, C.J., Arvey, R.D.: Measures of strength of association: a comparative examination. J. Appl. Psychol. **66**, 525–534 (1981)
10. McHugh, R.B., Mielke, P.W.: Negative variance estimates and statistical dependence in nested sampling. J. Am. Stat. Assoc. **63**, 1000–1003 (1968)
11. Mielke, P.W., Berry, K.J., Johnson, E.S.: Multi-response permutation procedures for a priori classifications. Commun. Stat. Theor. Methods **5**, 1409–1424 (1976)
12. Scott, W.A.: Reliability of content analysis: the case of nominal scale coding. Public Opin. Quart. **19**, 321–325 (1955)
13. Spearman, C.E.: 'Footrule' for measuring correlation. Brit. J. Psychol. **2**, 89–108 (1906)
14. Stigler, S.M.: The Seven Pillars of Statistical Wisdom. Harvard University Press, Cambridge (2016)

Chapter 7
Matched-Pairs Tests

Abstract This chapter introduces permutation methods for matched-pairs tests. Included in this chapter are six example analyses illustrating computation of exact permutation probability values for matched-pairs tests, calculation of measures of effect size for matched-pairs tests, the effect of extreme values on conventional and permutation matched-pairs tests, exact and Monte Carlo permutation procedures for matched-pairs tests, application of permutation methods to matched-pairs rank-score data, and analysis of matched-pairs multivariate data. Included in this chapter are permutation versions of Student's matched-pairs t test, Wilcoxon's signed-ranks test, the sign test, Hotelling's multivariate T^2 test for two matched samples, and a permutation-based alternative for the two conventional measures of effect size for matched pairs: Cohen's $\hat{d}$ and Pearson's r^2.

This chapter presents exact and Monte Carlo permutation statistical methods for two matched or otherwise related samples, commonly called matched-pairs tests under the Neyman–Pearson population model of statistical inference. As noted in Chap. 6, statistical tests for differences between two samples are of two varieties. The first examines two independent samples, such as in control- and treatment-group designs. The second variety examines two matched samples, such as in before-and-after research designs. Two-sample tests for independent samples were presented in Chap. 6. Matched-pairs tests for two related samples are presented in this chapter.

Two-sample tests of experimental differences between matched samples are the backbone of research in such diverse fields as psychology, education, biology, and horticulture. As in Chaps. 5 and 6, six example analyses illustrate permutation methods for matched-pairs tests. The first example utilizes a small set of data to illustrate the computation of exact permutation statistical methods for two matched samples, wherein the permutation test statistic, δ, is developed and compared with Student's conventional matched-pairs t test statistic. The second example develops a permutation-based measure of effect size as a chance-corrected alternative to the two conventional measures of effect size for matched-pairs tests: Cohen's $\hat{d}$ and Pearson's r^2. The third example compares permutation statistical methods based

© Springer Nature Switzerland AG 2019   207
K. J. Berry et al., *A Primer of Permutation Statistical Methods*,
https://doi.org/10.1007/978-3-030-20933-9_7

on ordinary and squared Euclidean scaling functions, emphasizing methods of analysis for data sets containing extreme values. The fourth example compares exact permutation statistical methods with Monte Carlo permutation statistical methods, demonstrating the accuracy, efficiency, and practicality of Monte Carlo statistical methods. The fifth example illustrates the application of permutation statistical methods to univariate rank-score data, comparing permutation statistical methods to Wilcoxon's conventional signed-ranks test and the sign test. The sixth example illustrates the application of permutation statistical methods to multivariate data, comparing permutation statistical methods to Hotelling's conventional multivariate T^2 test for two matched samples.

7.1 Introduction

Consider Student's conventional matched-pairs t test where variables x_1 and x_2 denote univariate observations taken on two sets of matched subjects, such as twins, or observations on the same subjects at two time periods—before and after an intervention, treatment, or administration of a test stimulus. Matched-pairs tests go by a variety of names in addition to matched pairs: repeated measures, within-subjects, randomized-blocks, or dependent samples, but they all indicate tests on the same or matched sets of subjects.[1]

Given two sets of values obtained from matched subjects denoted by x_{i1} and x_{i2} for $i = 1, \ldots, N$ pairs of subjects, the most popular matched-pairs test is Student's t test wherein the null hypothesis (H_0) posits no difference between the means of two populations; for example, H_0: $\mu_1 = \mu_2$ or H_0: $\mu_d = 0$, where $\mu_d = \mu_1 - \mu_2$. Matched-pairs tests have become extremely popular in biology, animal husbandry, and horticulture where cloning and embryo transplants produce closely matched subjects.[2]

There are four advantages to matched-pairs tests under the Neyman–Pearson population model when compared with tests for two independent samples under the same model. First, because the variability between treatments has been reduced by matching, matched-pairs tests generally provide either more power than a test for two independent samples with the same number of subjects or the same power with fewer subjects, where power is defined as the probability of rejecting a false null hypothesis. In addition, permutation statistical methods are efficient alternatives for

---

[1]When the same, not matched, subjects are observed at two time periods, the test is often called repeated-measures, within-subjects, subject-is-own-control, or a before-and-after test.

[2]It should be emphasized that cloning does not produce identical offspring. All the inherited information is not carried in the genes of a cell's nucleus. A very small number of genes are carried by intracellular bodies, the mitochondria. When an egg cell has its nucleus removed to make room for the genes of the donor cell, the egg cell has not had its mitochondria removed. The result of the egg fusion is then a mixture of the nucleus genes from the donor and the mitochondrial genes from the recipient.

matched-pairs tests where the two samples are comprised of only a few observations and where the approximating function may be a poor fit to the underlying discrete sampling distribution.

Second, matched-pairs tests always have the same number of subjects in each treatment. Tests for two independent samples often have different numbers of subjects in each treatment—oftentimes wildly different numbers of subjects, especially in survey research. Unequal numbers of subjects always yield a reduction in power. Moreover, when the smaller of the two samples has the greater variance, there is the risk of an increase in type I or α error: incorrectly rejecting a true null hypothesis. On the other hand, when the larger of the two samples has the greater variance, there is increased risk of type II or β error: failure to reject a false null hypothesis. The problems are largely moot with matched-pairs tests as the sample sizes are always equal.

Third, matched-pairs tests utilize the same or matched subjects in both treatment conditions. Consequently, there is little risk that the subjects in one treatment group differ substantially from the subjects in the other treatment group. With an independent two-sample test there is always the possibility that the results are biased because the subjects in one treatment are systematically different from the subjects in the other treatment; for example, smarter, older, taller, richer, more educated, bigger, faster, and so on.

Fourth, an underlying assumption of tests for two independent samples is homogeneity of variance; that is, $\sigma_1^2 = \sigma_2^2$. As Alvan Feinstein observed many years ago, it is usually known that the variances of the two samples are not remotely similar for a test of two independent samples [2]. When, for a test of two independent samples the variances are unequal, then strictly speaking the t statistic is not distributed as Student's t with $N - 2$ degrees of freedom. This is generally recognized as the Behrens–Fisher problem. When the variances are unequal test statistic t is, in fact, distributed as Student's t, but the degrees of freedom are known with certitude only within defined limits; that is,

$$\min(n_1 - 1, n_2 - 1) \le df \le n_1 + n_2 - 2 ,$$

and need to be approximated, typically using either a procedure given by Satterthwaite [6]

$$\widehat{df} = \frac{\left(s_1^2/n_1 + s_2^2/n_2\right)^2}{\left(s_1^2/n_1\right)^2/(n_1 - 1) + \left(s_2^2/n_2\right)^2/(n_2 - 1)}$$

or Welch [7]

$$\widehat{df} = \frac{\left(s_1^2/n_1 + s_2^2/n_2\right)^2}{\left(s_1^2/n_1\right)^2/(n_1 + 1) + \left(s_2^2/n_2\right)^2/(n_2 + 1)} - 2 ,$$

where n_1 and n_2 denote the sample sizes for samples 1 and 2, respectively, and s_1^2 and s_2^2 denote the sample-estimated population variances for samples 1 and 2, respectively.

Especially problematic is the combination of unequal variances and unequal sample sizes, which often occurs in survey research. In general, homogeneity of variance is not of concern with a matched-pairs t test as the two samples are either matched or identical, except for exposure to a test stimulus or an experimental intervention.

The primary disadvantage to matched-pairs designs whenever the same subjects are used before and after a treatment or intervention is that factors other than the treatment effect might cause a subject's score to change from the first treatment to the second. While the other factors might be the subject's mood, health, stress, and so on, the largest concern is carry-over or order effects, where participation in the first treatment may influence the subject's responses in the second treatment. Subjects are quite often sensitized to information after exposure to the first treatment. For example, a subject might gain experience in the first treatment that helps the subject improve on the second treatment. In such cases, the difference in the scores might not be due to the treatment, but might be due to practice. One way to control for carry-over or order effects is to counterbalance the order of presentation of treatments. Thus, half the subjects receive treatment 1 followed by treatment 2 and the other half receive treatment 2 followed by treatment 1, but this is not possible in many applications.

The most common test for two matched samples under the Neyman–Pearson population model of inference is a test wherein the null hypothesis (H_0) posits no mean difference between the two populations; for example, H_0: $\mu_d = 0$, where $\mu_d = \mu_1 - \mu_2$. Student's t test is the most popular test for the mean difference between two matched samples and is presented in every introductory textbook.[3]

Under the Neyman–Pearson population model with null hypothesis, H_0: $\mu_d = 0$, Student's t test for two matched samples is given by

$$t = \frac{\bar{d} - \mu_d}{s_{\bar{d}}} = \frac{\bar{d} - 0}{s_{\bar{d}}} \, ,$$

where $\bar{d}$ is the arithmetic mean of the differences between variables x_1 and x_2 given by

$$\bar{d} = \frac{1}{N} \sum_{i=1}^{N} d_i \, ,$$

---

[3]Technically, when $d_i = x_{i_1} - x_{i_2}$ for $i = 1, \ldots, N$, Student's t test for two matched samples is simply a one-sample test and is treated as such in many introductory textbooks.

d_i denotes the ith of N observed differences between x_{i_1} and x_{i_2} for $i = 1, \ldots, N$, $s_{\bar{d}}$ is the sample-estimated standard error of $\bar{d}$ given by

$$s_{\bar{d}} = \frac{s_d}{\sqrt{N}} \, ,$$

and s_d denotes the sample-estimated population standard deviation of variable d given by

$$s_d = \left[\frac{1}{N-1} \sum_{i=1}^{N} (d_i - \bar{d})^2 \right]^{1/2} .$$

Assuming independence and normality, test statistic t is asymptotically distributed as Student's t under the Neyman–Pearson null hypothesis with $N - 1$ degrees of freedom. The permissible probability of a type I error is denoted by α and if the observed value of t is more extreme than the critical values of $\pm t$ that define α, the null hypothesis is rejected with a probability of type I error equal to or less than α for Student's t distribution with $N - 1$ degrees of freedom, under the assumption of normality.

The assumptions underlying Student's matched-pairs t test are (1) the observations are independent within variables x_1 and x_2, (2) the data are random samples from a well-defined population, and (3) variables x_1 and x_2 are normally distributed in the population.

7.2 A Permutation Approach

Consider a matched-pairs test under the permutation model. Under the Fisher–Pitman permutation model there is no null hypothesis specifying a population parameter. Instead the null hypothesis is simply that all possible arrangements of the observed differences occur with equal chance [4]. Furthermore, there is no alternative hypothesis under the permutation model, no degrees of freedom, and no specified α level. Moreover, there is no requirement of random sampling and no assumption of normality.

A permutation alternative to the conventional matched-pairs t test is easily defined [1]. Let $d_i = x_{i_1} - x_{i_2}$ denote the observed sample differences for $i = 1, \ldots, N$. The permutation matched-pairs test statistic is given by

$$\delta = \binom{N}{2}^{-1} \sum_{i=1}^{N-1} \sum_{j=i+1}^{N} |d_i - d_j|^v , \tag{7.1}$$

where for correspondence with Student's matched-pairs t test, $v = 2$.

Under the Fisher–Pitman permutation model, the exact probability of an observed δ is the proportion of δ test statistic values calculated on all possible, equally-likely arrangements of the observed differences that are equal to or less than the observed value of δ; that is,

$$P(\delta \leq \delta_0 | H_0) = \frac{\text{number of } \delta \text{ values } \leq \delta_0}{M} ,$$

where δ_0 denotes the observed value of δ and $M = 2^N$ is the number of possible, equally-likely arrangements of the N observed differences.

7.2.1 The Relationship Between Statistics t and δ

Under the Neyman–Pearson null hypothesis, H_0: $\mu_d = 0$, the functional relationships between test statistics δ and t are given by

$$\delta = \frac{2 \sum_{i=1}^{N} d_i^2}{t^2 + N - 1} \quad \text{and} \quad t = \left(\frac{2}{\delta} \sum_{i=1}^{N} d_i^2 - N + 1 \right)^{1/2} , \tag{7.2}$$

where $d_i = x_{i_1} - x_{i_2}$ for $i = 1, \ldots, N$.

7.3 Example 1: Test Statistics t and δ

An example will serve to illustrate the relationships between test statistics t and δ. As in previous chapters, consider a small set of data with $N = 5$ matched subjects, as given in Table 7.1. For the example data listed in Table 7.1, $N = 5$, $d_1 = +9$, $d_2 = +7$, $d_3 = +6$, $d_4 = +5$, $d_5 = +3$, and let H_0: $\mu_d = 0$. Under the Neyman–Pearson population model the sample mean is $\bar{d} = 6.00$, the sample

Table 7.1 Example data for a matched-pairs test with $N = 5$ subjects

Subject	x_1	x_2	d
1	27	18	+9
2	24	17	+7
3	26	20	+6
4	24	19	+5
5	25	22	+3

standard deviation of the differences is $s_d = 2.2361$, the standard error of $\bar{d}$ is

$$s_{\bar{d}} = \frac{s_d}{\sqrt{N}} = \frac{2.2361}{\sqrt{5}} = 1.00 \,,$$

and the observed value of Student's t test statistic is

$$t = \frac{\bar{d} - \mu_d}{s_{\bar{d}}} = \frac{6.00 - 0}{1.00} = +6.00 \,.$$

Under the Neyman–Pearson null hypothesis, H_0: $\mu_d = 0$, test statistic t is asymptotically distributed as Student's t with $N - 1$ degrees of freedom. With $N - 1 = 5 - 1 = 4$ degrees of freedom, the asymptotic two-tail probability value of $t = +6.00$ is $P = 0.3883 \times 10^{-2}$, under the assumption of normality.

7.3.1 An Exact Analysis with $v = 2$

Under the Fisher–Pitman permutation model, employing squared Euclidean scaling with $v = 2$ for correspondence with Student's matched-pairs t test, the sum of the squared differences between all pairs of differences is

$$\sum_{i=1}^{N-1} \sum_{j=i+1}^{N} |d_i - d_j|^2 = |9 - 7|^2 + |9 - 6|^2 + |9 - 5|^2 + |9 - 3|^2$$

$$+ |7 - 6|^2 + |7 - 5|^2 + |7 - 3|^2 + |6 - 5|^2 + |6 - 3|^2 + |5 - 3|^2 = 100$$

and following Eq. (7.1) with $v = 2$, the observed value of test statistic δ is

$$\delta = \binom{N}{2}^{-1} \sum_{i=1}^{N-1} \sum_{j=i+1}^{N} |d_i - d_j|^2 = \binom{5}{2}^{-1} (100) = \frac{2(100)}{5(5-1)} = 10.00 \,.$$

Alternatively, the observed value of test statistic δ is

$$\delta = 2s_d^2 = 2(2.2361)^2 = 10.00 \,.$$

Following the expressions given in Eq. (7.2) for the functional relationships between test statistics δ and t, the observed value of test statistic δ with respect to the observed value of Student's t test statistic is

$$\delta = \frac{2 \sum_{i=1}^{N} d_i^2}{t^2 + N - 1} = \frac{2(9^2 + 7^2 + 6^2 + 5^2 + 3^2)}{(6.00)^2 + 5 - 1} = 10.00$$

and the observed value of Student's t test statistic with respect to the observed value of test statistic δ is

$$
t = \left(\frac{2}{\delta} \sum_{i=1}^{N} d_i^2 - N + 1 \right)^{1/2}
$$

$$
= \left[\frac{2(9^2 + 7^2 + 6^2 + 5^2 + 3^2)}{10.00} - 5 + 1 \right]^{1/2} = \pm 6.00 \, .
$$

Because of the functional relationship between test statistics δ and t, the exact probability values given by

$$
P(\delta \leq \delta_o) = \frac{\text{number of } \delta \text{ values } \leq \delta_o}{M}
$$

and

$$
P(|t| \geq |t_o|) = \frac{\text{number of } |t| \text{ values } \geq |t_o|}{M}
$$

are equivalent under the Fisher–Pitman null hypothesis, where δ_o and t_o denote the observed values of δ and t, respectively, and M is the number of possible, equally-likely arrangements of the $N = 5$ matched pairs listed in Table 7.1.

To establish the exact permutation probability of $\delta = 10.00$ (or $t = \pm 6.00$) under the Fisher–Pitman permutation model, it is necessary to completely enumerate all possible arrangements of the observed data, of which there are only

$$
M = 2^N = 2^5 = 32
$$

possible, equally-likely arrangements in the reference set of all permutations of the matched-pairs data listed in Table 7.1. Let $y_i = d_i z_i$ denote the transformed d_i values for $i = 1, \ldots, N$ where z_i is either plus or minus one. Since $M = 32$ is a small number, it is possible to list the z, y, δ, and $|t|$ values in Table 7.2. Under the Fisher–Pitman permutation model, the exact probability of an observed δ is the proportion of δ test statistic values calculated on all possible, equally-likely arrangements of the $N = 5$ matched pairs listed in Table 7.1 that are equal to or less than the observed value of δ. For test statistic δ there are only two δ test statistic values that are equal to or less than the observed value of $\delta = 10.00$ (numbers 1 and 32 marked with asterisks) in Table 7.2. If all M arrangements of the $N = 10$ observations listed in Table 7.1 occur with equal chance under the Fisher–Pitman null hypothesis, the exact probability value computed on all $M = 32$ possible arrangements of the observed data with $N = 5$ subjects preserved for each

Table 7.2 Calculation of δ and $|t|$ values for differences $d_1 = +9$, $d_2 = +7$, $d_3 = +6$, $d_4 = +5$, and $d_5 = +3$

Number	z	y	δ	$|t|$
1*	$+1 +1 +1 +1 +1$	$+9 +7 +6 +5 +3$	10.00	6.0000
2	$+1 +1 +1 +1 -1$	$+9 +7 +6 +5 -3$	42.40	2.3311
3	$+1 +1 +1 -1 +1$	$+9 +7 +6 -5 +3$	60.00	1.6330
4	$+1 +1 -1 +1 +1$	$+9 +7 -6 +5 +3$	67.60	1.3846
5	$+1 -1 +1 +1 +1$	$+9 -7 +6 +5 +3$	74.40	1.1732
6	$-1 +1 +1 +1 +1$	$-9 +7 +6 +5 +3$	85.60	0.8203
7	$+1 +1 +1 -1 -1$	$+9 +7 +6 -5 -3$	80.40	0.9875
8	$+1 +1 -1 -1 +1$	$+9 +7 -6 -5 +3$	93.60	0.5230
9	$+1 -1 -1 +1 +1$	$+9 -7 -6 +5 +3$	98.40	0.2550
10	$-1 -1 +1 +1 +1$	$-9 -7 +6 +5 +3$	99.60	0.1267
11	$+1 +1 -1 +1 -1$	$+9 +7 -6 +5 -3$	85.60	0.8203
12	$+1 -1 +1 -1 +1$	$+9 -7 +6 -5 +3$	96.40	0.3865
13	$-1 +1 -1 +1 +1$	$-9 +7 -6 +5 +3$	100.00	0.0000
14	$+1 -1 +1 +1 -1$	$+9 -7 +6 +5 -3$	90.00	0.6667
15	$-1 +1 +1 -1 +1$	$-9 +7 +6 -5 +3$	99.60	0.1267
16	$-1 +1 +1 +1 -1$	$-9 +7 +6 +5 -3$	96.40	0.3865
17	$-1 -1 -1 +1 +1$	$-9 -7 -6 +5 +3$	80.40	0.9875
18	$-1 -1 +1 +1 -1$	$-9 -7 +6 +5 -3$	93.60	0.5230
19	$-1 +1 +1 -1 -1$	$-9 +7 +6 -5 -3$	98.40	0.2550
20	$+1 +1 -1 -1 -1$	$+9 +7 -6 -5 -3$	99.60	0.1267
21	$-1 -1 +1 -1 +1$	$-9 -7 +6 -5 +3$	85.60	0.8203
22	$-1 +1 -1 +1 -1$	$-9 +7 -6 +5 -3$	96.40	0.3865
23	$+1 -1 +1 -1 -1$	$+9 -7 +6 -5 -3$	100.00	0.0000
24	$-1 +1 -1 -1 +1$	$-9 +7 -6 -5 +3$	90.00	0.6667
25	$+1 -1 -1 +1 -1$	$+9 -7 -6 +5 -3$	99.60	0.1267
26	$+1 -1 -1 -1 +1$	$+9 -7 -6 -5 +3$	96.40	0.3865
27	$-1 -1 -1 -1 +1$	$-9 -7 -6 -5 +3$	42.40	2.3311
28	$-1 -1 -1 +1 -1$	$-9 -7 -6 +5 -3$	60.00	1.6330
29	$-1 -1 +1 -1 -1$	$-9 -7 +6 -5 -3$	67.60	1.3846
30	$-1 +1 -1 -1 -1$	$-9 +7 -6 -5 -3$	74.40	1.1732
31	$+1 -1 -1 -1 -1$	$+9 -7 -6 -5 -3$	85.60	0.8203
32*	$-1 -1 -1 -1 -1$	$-9 -7 -6 -5 -2$	10.00	6.0000
Sum			2560.00	

arrangement is

$$P(\delta \leq \delta_o) = \frac{\text{number of } \delta \text{ values } \leq \delta_o}{M} = \frac{2}{32} = 0.0625 \ ,$$

where δ_o denotes the observed value of test statistic δ and M is the number of possible, equally-likely arrangements of the $N = 5$ matched pairs listed in Table 7.1.

Alternatively, for test statistic t there are exactly two $|t|$ values that are equal to or greater than the observed value of $|t| = 6.00$ (numbers 1 and 32 marked with asterisks) in Table 7.2. If all $M = 32$ arrangements of the observed data listed in Table 7.1 occur with equal chance, the exact probability value is

$$P(|t| \geq |t_o|) = \frac{\text{number of } |t| \text{ values} \geq |t_o|}{M} = \frac{2}{32} = 0.0625 \, ,$$

where t_o denotes the observed value of test statistic t.

Finally, for computational efficiency it should be noted that the δ and $|t|$ values in Table 7.2 possess duplicate values; for example, $\delta_1 = \delta_{32} = 10.00$, $\delta_2 = \delta_{27} = 42.40$, $\delta_3 = \delta_{28} = 60.00$, and so on. Therefore, it is only necessary to generate

$$M = 2^{N-1} = 2^{5-1} = 16 \quad \text{instead of} \quad M = 2^N = 2^5 = 32$$

equally-likely arrangements of the observed data. Table 7.3 lists the $M = 16$ non-duplicated values ordered by the δ values from low ($\delta_1 = 10.00$) to high ($\delta_{16} = 100.00$) and by the $|t|$ values from high ($t_1 = 6.0000$) to low ($t_{16} = 0.0000$).

In this example analysis there is a considerable difference between the asymptotic probability value ($P = 0.3883 \times 10^{-2}$) and the exact permutation probability value ($P = 0.0625$); the actual difference between the two probability values is

$$\Delta_P = 0.0625 - 0.0039 = 0.0586 \, .$$

Table 7.3 Calculation of δ and $|t|$ values for $x_1 = 9$, $x_2 = 7$, $x_3 = 5$, and $x_4 = 2$

Number	z	y	δ	$|t|$
1	+1 +1 +1 +1 +1	+9 +7 +6 +5 +3	10.00	6.0000
2	+1 +1 +1 +1 −1	+9 +7 +6 +5 −3	42.40	2.3311
3	+1 +1 +1 −1 +1	+9 +7 +6 −5 +3	60.00	1.6330
4	+1 +1 −1 +1 +1	+9 +7 −6 +5 +3	67.60	1.3846
5	+1 −1 +1 +1 +1	+9 −7 +6 +5 +3	74.40	1.1732
7	+1 +1 +1 −1 −1	+9 +7 +6 −5 −3	80.40	0.9875
6	−1 +1 +1 +1 +1	−9 +7 +6 +5 +3	85.60	0.8203
8	+1 +1 −1 +1 −1	+9 +7 −6 +5 −3	85.60	0.8203
9	+1 −1 +1 +1 −1	+9 −7 +6 +5 −3	90.00	0.6667
10	+1 +1 −1 −1 +1	+9 +7 −6 −5 +3	93.60	0.5230
11	+1 −1 +1 −1 +1	+9 −7 +6 −5 +3	96.40	0.3865
12	−1 +1 +1 +1 −1	−9 +7 +6 +5 −3	96.40	0.3865
13	+1 −1 −1 +1 +1	+9 −7 −6 +5 +3	98.40	0.2550
14	−1 −1 +1 +1 +1	−9 −7 +6 +5 +3	99.60	0.1267
15	−1 +1 +1 −1 +1	−9 +7 +6 −5 +3	99.60	0.1267
16	−1 +1 −1 +1 +1	−9 +7 −6 +5 +3	100.00	0.0000

In general, asymptotic tests are not appropriate for samples as small as $N = 5$, while exact permutation tests are ideally suited for small samples. Fitting a continuous mathematical function such as Student's t to a discrete distribution with only $M = 16$ data points of which only 13 values are different often results in a poor fit to the discrete probability distribution. A larger example in Sect. 7.6 on p. 230 with $N = 30$ observations and $M = 1,073,741,824$ possible arrangements better illustrates the differences in probability values produced by a conventional matched-pairs t test and a permutation matched-pairs test with $v = 2$.

7.4 Example 2: Measures of Effect Size

Measures of effect size express the practical or clinical significance of a difference between sample means, as contrasted with the statistical significance of the difference. The usual measures of effect size for a conventional matched-pairs t test are Cohen's $\hat{d}$ given by

$$\hat{d} = \frac{|\bar{d} - \mu_d|}{s_d} \, ,$$

Pearson's r^2 given by

$$r^2 = \frac{t^2}{t^2 + N - 1} \, ,$$

and Mielke and Berry's $\Re$ given by

$$\Re = 1 - \frac{\delta}{\mu_\delta} \, , \tag{7.3}$$

where δ is defined in Eq. (7.1) on p. 211 and μ_δ is the exact expected value of test statistic δ under the Fisher–Pitman null hypothesis given by

$$\mu_\delta = \frac{1}{M} \sum_{i=1}^{M} \delta_i \, , \tag{7.4}$$

where for a matched-pairs test $M = 2^N$. For calculation purposes the exact expected value of test statistic δ is given by

$$\mu_\delta = \frac{1}{N(N-1)} \sum_{i=1}^{N-1} \sum_{j=i+1}^{N} \left(|d_i - d_j|^2 + |d_i + d_j|^2 \right) . \tag{7.5}$$

Alternatively, in terms of an analysis of variance model the expected value of test statistic δ is given by

$$\mu_\delta = \frac{2SS_{\text{Total}}}{N(1 - r^2)} \, ,$$

where the total sum-of-squares is given by

$$SS_{\text{Total}} = \sum_{i=1}^{N} (d_i - \bar{d})^2 \, ,$$

the mean of the N differences is given by

$$\bar{d} = \frac{1}{N} \sum_{i=1}^{N} d_i \, ,$$

and Pearson's r^2 measure of effect size is given by

$$r^2 = \frac{t^2}{t^2 + N - 1} \, .$$

For the example data with $N = 5$, $d_1 = +9$, $d_2 = +7$, $d_3 = +6$, $d_4 = +5$, $d_5 = +3$, and H_0: $\mu_d = 0$, Cohen's $\hat{d}$ measure of effect size is

$$\hat{d} = \frac{|\bar{d} - \mu_d|}{s_d} = \frac{|6.00 - 0|}{2.2361} = 2.6833 \, ,$$

indicating a large effect size ($\hat{d} \geq 0.80$) and Pearson's r^2 measure of effect size is

$$r^2 = \frac{t^2}{t^2 + N - 1} = \frac{(6.00)^2}{(6.00)^2 + 5 - 1} = 0.90 \, ,$$

also indicating a large effect size ($r^2 \geq 0.25$).[4]

For Mielke and Berry's $\mathfrak{R}$ measure of effect size, the observed value of test statistic δ is $\delta = 10.00$ and following Eq. (7.4), the exact expected value of test

---

[4]Given the relationships between Cohen's $\hat{d}$ and Pearson's r^2 and given the wide range of values defining "small," "medium," and "large" effect sizes, the results for $\hat{d}$ and r^2 often agree, but occasionally will disagree.

statistic δ under the Fisher–Pitman null hypothesis is

$$\mu_\delta = \frac{1}{M} \sum_{i=1}^{M} \delta_i = \frac{2560}{32} = 80.00 \,,$$

where the sum,

$$\sum_{i=1}^{M} \delta_i = 2560 \,,$$

is calculated in Table 7.2 on p. 215. Alternatively, following Eq. (7.4) the exact expected value of test statistic δ under the Fisher–Pitman null hypothesis is

$$\mu_\delta = \frac{1}{N(N-1)} \sum_{i=1}^{N-1} \sum_{j=i+1}^{N} \left(|d_i - d_j|^2 + |d_i + d_j|^2 \right) = \frac{1600}{5(5-1)} = 80.00 \,,$$

where the sum,

$$\sum_{i=1}^{N-1} \sum_{j=i+1}^{N} \left(|d_i - d_j|^2 + |d_i + d_j|^2 \right) = 1600 \,,$$

is calculated in Table 7.4 on the

$$\frac{N(N-1)}{2} = \frac{5(5-1)}{2} = 10$$

Table 7.4 Example calculation of $\sum_{i=1}^{N-1} \sum_{j=i+1}^{N} \left(|d_i - d_j|^2 + |d_i + d_j|^2 \right)$

Number	$|d_i - d_j|^2$	$|d_i + d_j|^2$	$|d_i - d_j|^2 + |d_i + d_j|^2$
1	$|9 - 7|^2 = 4$	$|9 + 7|^2 = 256$	260
2	$|9 - 6|^2 = 9$	$|9 + 6|^2 = 225$	234
3	$|9 - 5|^2 = 16$	$|9 + 5|^2 = 196$	212
4	$|9 - 3|^2 = 36$	$|9 + 3|^2 = 144$	180
5	$|7 - 6|^2 = 1$	$|7 + 6|^2 = 169$	170
6	$|7 - 5|^2 = 4$	$|7 + 5|^2 = 144$	148
7	$|7 - 3|^2 = 16$	$|7 + 3|^2 = 100$	116
8	$|6 - 5|^2 = 1$	$|6 + 5|^2 = 121$	122
9	$|6 - 3|^2 = 9$	$|6 + 3|^2 = 81$	90
10	$|5 - 3|^2 = 4$	$|5 + 3|^2 = 64$	68
Sum			1600

pairs of squared differences. Then the observed chance-corrected measure of effect size is

$$\Re = 1 - \frac{\delta}{\mu_\delta} = 1 - \frac{10.00}{80.00} = +0.8750 \,,$$

indicating approximately 87% agreement above what is expected by chance.

7.4.1   Relationships Among Measures of Effect Size

For a matched-pairs test, Student's t, Cohen's $\hat{d}$, Pearson's r^2, and Mielke and Berry's $\Re$ are all interrelated. Any one of the measures can be derived from any of the other measures. The relationships between Student's t test statistic and Cohen's $\hat{d}$ measure of effect size are given by

$$t = \hat{d}\sqrt{N} \quad \text{and} \quad \hat{d} = \frac{t}{\sqrt{N}} \,, \tag{7.6}$$

the relationships between Student's t test statistic and Pearson's r^2 measure of effect size are given by

$$t = \left[\frac{r^2(N-1)}{1-r^2} \right]^{1/2} \quad \text{and} \quad r^2 = \frac{t^2}{t^2 + N - 1} \,, \tag{7.7}$$

the relationships between Student's t test statistic and Mielke and Berry's $\Re$ measure of effect size are given by

$$t = \left[\frac{\Re(N-1)+1}{1-\Re} \right]^{1/2} \quad \text{and} \quad \Re = \frac{t^2 - 1}{t^2 + N - 1} \,, \tag{7.8}$$

the relationships between Cohen's $\hat{d}$ measure of effect size and Pearson's r^2 measure of effect size are given by

$$\hat{d} = \left[\frac{r^2(N-1)}{N(1-r^2)} \right]^{1/2} \quad \text{and} \quad r^2 = \frac{N\hat{d}^2}{N(\hat{d}^2+1)-1} \,, \tag{7.9}$$

the relationships between Cohen's $\hat{d}$ measure of effect size and Mielke and Berry's $\Re$ measure of effect size are given by

$$\hat{d} = \left[\frac{\Re(N-1)+1}{N(1-\Re)} \right]^{1/2} \quad \text{and} \quad \Re = \frac{N\hat{d}^2 - 1}{N(\hat{d}^2+1)-1} \,, \tag{7.10}$$

and the relationships between Pearson's r^2 measure of effect size and Mielke and Berry's $\Re$ measure of effect size are given by

$$r^2 = 1 - \frac{(1 - \Re)(N - 1)}{N} \quad \text{and} \quad \Re = 1 - \frac{N(1 - r^2)}{N - 1}. \tag{7.11}$$

For the example data listed in Table 7.1 on p. 212 and following the expressions given in Eq. (7.6) for Student's t test statistic and Cohen's $\hat{d}$ measure of effect size, the observed value for Student's t test statistic with respect to the observed value of Cohen's $\hat{d}$ measure of effect size is

$$t = \hat{d}\sqrt{N} = 2.6833\sqrt{5} = \pm6.00$$

and the observed value for Cohen's $\hat{d}$ measure of effect size with respect to the observed value of Student's t test statistic is

$$\hat{d} = \frac{t}{\sqrt{N}} = \frac{\pm6.00}{\sqrt{5}} = \pm2.6833.$$

Following the expressions given in Eq. (7.7) for Student's t test statistic and Pearson's r^2 measure of effect size, the observed value for Student's t test statistic with respect to the observed value of Pearson's r^2 measure of effect size is

$$t = \left[\frac{r^2(N - 1)}{1 - r^2}\right]^{1/2} = \left[\frac{0.90(5 - 1)}{1 - 0.90}\right]^{1/2} = \pm6.00$$

and the observed value of Pearson's r^2 measure of effect size with respect to the observed value of Student's t test statistic is

$$r^2 = \frac{t^2}{t^2 + N - 1} = \frac{(6.00)^2}{(6.00)^2 + 5 - 1} = 0.90.$$

Following the expressions given in Eq. (7.8) for Student's t test statistic and Mielke and Berry's $\Re$ measure of effect size, the observed value for Student's t test statistic with respect to the observed value of Mielke and Berry's $\Re$ measure of effect size is

$$t = \left[\frac{\Re(N - 1) + 1}{1 - \Re}\right]^{1/2} = \left[\frac{0.8750(5 - 1) + 1}{1 - 0.8750}\right]^{1/2} = \pm6.00$$

and the observed value of Mielke and Berry's $\Re$ measure of effect size with respect to the observed value of Student's t test statistic is

$$\Re = \frac{t^2 - 1}{t^2 + N - 1} = \frac{(6.00)^2 - 1}{(6.00)^2 + 5 - 1} = +0.8750.$$

Following the expressions given in Eq. (7.9) for Cohen's $\hat{d}$ measure of effect size and Pearson's r^2 measure of effect size, the observed value for Cohen's $\hat{d}$ measure of effect size with respect to the observed value of Pearson's r^2 measure of effect size is

$$\hat{d} = \left[\frac{r^2(N-1)}{N(1-r^2)}\right]^{1/2} = \left[\frac{0.90(5-1)}{5(1-0.90)}\right]^{1/2} = \pm 2.6833$$

and the observed value of Pearson's r^2 measure of effect size with respect to the observed value of Cohen's $\hat{d}$ measure of effect size is

$$r^2 = \frac{N\hat{d}^2}{N(\hat{d}^2+1)-1} = \frac{5(2.6833)^2}{5[(2.6833)^2+1]-1} = 0.90 \ .$$

Following the expressions given in Eq. (7.10) for Cohen's $\hat{d}$ measure of effect size and Mielke and Berry's $\mathfrak{R}$ measure of effect size, the observed value of Cohen's $\hat{d}$ measure of effect size with respect to the observed value of Mielke and Berry's $\mathfrak{R}$ measure of effect size is

$$\hat{d} = \left[\frac{\mathfrak{R}(N-1)+1}{N(1-\mathfrak{R})}\right]^{1/2} = \left[\frac{0.8750(5-1)+1}{5(1-0.8750)}\right]^{1/2} = \pm 2.6833$$

and the observed value of Mielke and Berry's $\mathfrak{R}$ measure of effect size with respect to the observed value of Cohen's $\hat{d}$ measure of effect size is

$$\mathfrak{R} = \frac{N\hat{d}^2-1}{N(\hat{d}^2+1)-1} = \frac{5(2.6833)^2-1}{5[(2.6833)^2+1]-1} = +0.8750 \ .$$

And following the expressions given in Eq. (7.11) for Pearson's r^2 measure of effect size and Mielke and Berry's $\mathfrak{R}$ measure of effect size, the observed value for Pearson's r^2 measure of effect size with respect to the observed value of Mielke and Berry's $\mathfrak{R}$ measure of effect size is

$$r^2 = 1 - \frac{(1-\mathfrak{R})(N-1)}{N} = 1 - \frac{(1-0.8750)(5-1)}{5} = 0.90$$

and the observed value of Mielke and Berry's $\mathfrak{R}$ measure of effect size with respect to the observed value of Pearson's r^2 measure of effect size is

$$\mathfrak{R} = 1 - \frac{N(1-r^2)}{N-1} = 1 - \frac{5(1-0.90)}{5-1} = +0.8750 \ .$$

7.5 Example 3: Analyses with $v = 2$ and $v = 1$

For a third example of a matched-pairs test under the Neyman–Pearson population model, consider the data on $N = 9$ subjects listed in Table 7.5. For the example data listed in Table 7.5, the null hypothesis is H_0: $\mu_d = 0$; that is, no difference is expected between the treatments. The sample mean is $\bar{d} = -2.00$, the sample standard deviation of the differences is $s_d = 2.00$, the standard error of $\bar{d}$ is

$$s_{\bar{d}} = \frac{s_d}{\sqrt{N}} = \frac{2.00}{\sqrt{9}} = 0.6667 \,,$$

and the observed value of Student's matched-pairs t test statistic is

$$t = \frac{\bar{d} - \mu_d}{s_{\bar{d}}} = \frac{-2.00 - 0}{0.6667} = -3.00 \,.$$

Under the Neyman–Pearson null hypothesis, H_0: $\mu_d = 0$, test statistic t is asymptotically distributed as Student's t with $N - 1$ degrees of freedom. With $N - 1 = 9 - 1 = 8$ degrees of freedom, the asymptotic two-tail probability value of $t = -3.00$ is $P = 0.0171$, under the assumption of normality.

7.5.1 An Exact Analysis with $v = 2$

Under the Fisher–Pitman permutation model, employing squared Euclidean scaling with $v = 2$ for correspondence with Student's conventional matched-pairs t test, the observed value of test statistic δ is

$$\delta = \binom{N}{2}^{-1} \sum_{i=1}^{N-1} \sum_{j=i+1}^{N} |d_i - d_j|^v = \binom{9}{2}^{-1} (288) = \frac{2(288)}{9(9-1)} = 8.00 \,.$$

Table 7.5 Example data for a matched-pairs test with $N = 9$ subjects

Subject	x_1	x_2	d	d^2
1	9	7	−2	4
2	8	7	−1	1
3	7	3	−4	16
4	7	8	+1	1
5	8	6	−2	4
6	9	4	−5	25
7	7	6	−1	1
8	7	7	0	0
9	8	4	−4	16
Sum			−18	68

Following the expressions given in Eq. (7.2) on p. 212 for the relationships between test statistics δ and t, the observed value of test statistic δ with respect to the observed value of Student's t test statistic is

$$\delta = \frac{2\sum_{i=1}^{N} d_i^2}{t^2 + N - 1} = \frac{2(68)}{(-3.00)^2 + 9 - 1} = 8.00 \ .$$

Alternatively, the observed value of test statistic δ is

$$\delta = 2s_d^2 = 2(2.00)^2 = 8.00 \ ,$$

or in terms of an analysis of variance model,

$$\delta = \frac{2SS_{\text{Total}}}{N - 1} = \frac{2(32)}{9 - 1} = 8.00 \ ,$$

where for the example data listed in Table 7.5, the sum of the $N = 9$ differences is

$$\sum_{i=1}^{N} d_i = (-2) + (-1) + (-4) + \cdots + (0) + (-1) = -18 \ ,$$

the sum of the $N = 9$ squared differences is

$$\sum_{i=1}^{N} d_i^2 = (-2)^2 + (-1)^2 + (-4)^2 + \cdots + (0)^2 + (-1)^2 = 68 \ ,$$

and the total sum-of-squares is

$$SS_{\text{Total}} = \sum_{i=1}^{N} d_i^2 - \left(\sum_{i=1}^{N} d_i\right)^2 \Big/ N = 68 - (18)^2/9 = 32 \ .$$

Conversely, the observed value of Student's t test statistic with respect to the observed value of test statistic δ is

$$t = \left(\frac{2}{\delta} \sum_{i=1}^{N} d_i^2 - N + 1\right)^{1/2} = \left[\frac{2(68)}{8.00} - 9 + 1\right]^{1/2} = \pm 3.00 \ .$$

Because of the relationship between test statistic δ and Student's t, the probability values given by

$$P(\delta \le \delta_0) = \frac{\text{number of } \delta \text{ values } \le \delta_0}{M}$$

and

$$P(|t| \geq |t_o|) = \frac{\text{number of } |t| \text{ values } \geq |t_o|}{M}$$

are equivalent under the Fisher–Pitman null hypothesis, where δ_o and t_o denote the observed values of test statistics δ and t, respectively, and M is the number of possible, equally-likely arrangements of the $N = 9$ matched pairs listed in Table 7.5. There are only

$$M = 2^N = 2^9 = 512$$

possible, equally-likely arrangements in the reference set of all permutations of the matched-pairs data listed in Table 7.5, making an exact analysis possible. Under the Fisher–Pitman permutation model, the exact probability of an observed δ is the proportion of δ test statistic values calculated on all possible, equally-likely arrangements of the $N = 9$ matched pairs listed in Table 7.5 that are equal to or less than the observed value of $\delta = 8.00$. For test statistic δ there are exactly 16 δ test statistic values that are equal to or less than the observed value of $\delta = 8.00$. If all M arrangements of the $N = 18$ observations listed in Table 7.5 occur with equal chance under the Fisher–Pitman null hypothesis, the exact probability value computed on the $M = 512$ possible arrangements of the observed data with $N = 9$ subjects preserved for each arrangement is

$$P(\delta \leq \delta_o) = \frac{\text{number of } \delta \text{ values } \leq \delta_o}{M} = \frac{16}{512} = 0.0313$$

where δ_o denotes the observed value of test statistic δ and M is the number of possible, equally-likely arrangements of the $N = 9$ matched pairs listed in Table 7.5.

Alternatively, for test statistic t there are 16 $|t|$ test statistic values that are equal to or greater than the observed value of $|t| = 6.00$. Then if all M arrangements of the observed data occur with equal chance under the Fisher–Pitman null hypothesis, the exact two-tail probability value is

$$P(|t| \geq |t_o|) = \frac{\text{number of } |t| \text{ values } \geq |t_o|}{M} = \frac{16}{512} = 0.0313 \, ,$$

where t_o denotes the observed value of test statistic t.

7.5.2   Chance-Corrected Measures of Effect Size

The conventional measures of effect size for a matched-pairs t test are Cohen's $\hat{d}$ measure given by

$$\hat{d} = \frac{|\bar{d} - \mu_d|}{s_d} \, ,$$

Pearson's r^2 measure given by

$$r^2 = \frac{t^2}{t^2 + N - 1},$$

and Mielke and Berry's $\Re$ measure given by

$$\Re = 1 - \frac{\delta}{\mu_\delta},$$

where test statistic δ is defined in Eq. (7.1) on p. 211 and μ_δ is the exact expected value of test statistic δ under the Fisher–Pitman null hypothesis given by

$$\mu_\delta - \frac{1}{M} \sum_{i=1}^{M} \delta_i , \tag{7.12}$$

where for a matched-pairs test, $M = 2^N$. For calculation purposes,

$$\mu_\delta = \frac{1}{N(N-1)} \sum_{i=1}^{N-1} \sum_{j=i+1}^{N} \left(|d_i - d_j|^2 + |d_i + d_j|^2 \right). \tag{7.13}$$

For the example data listed in Table 7.5 with $N = 9$ matched pairs and null hypothesis, H_0: $\mu_d = 0$, Cohen's $\hat{d}$ measure of effect size is

$$\hat{d} = \frac{|\bar{d} - \mu_d|}{s_d} = \frac{|-2.00 - 0|}{2.00} = 1.00 ,$$

indicating a large effect size ($\hat{d} \geq 0.80$) and Pearson's r^2 measure of effect size is

$$r^2 = \frac{t^2}{t^2 + N - 1} = \frac{(-3.00)^2}{(-3.00)^2 + 9 - 1} = 0.5294 ,$$

also indicating a large effect size ($r^2 \geq 0.25$). For Mielke and Berry's $\Re$ measure of effect size, the observed value of test statistic δ is $\delta = 8.00$ and following Eq. (7.4) on p. 217 the exact expected value of test statistic δ under the Fisher–Pitman null hypothesis is

$$\mu_\delta = \frac{1}{M} \sum_{i=1}^{M} \delta_i = \frac{7736.8888}{512} = 15.1111 .$$

Alternatively, following Eq. (7.5) on p. 217,

$$\mu_\delta = \frac{1}{N(N-1)} \sum_{i=1}^{N-1} \sum_{j=i+1}^{N} \left(|d_i - d_j|^2 + |d_i + d_j|^2 \right)$$

$$= \frac{1088}{9(9-1)} = 15.1111 .$$

Then the observed chance-corrected measure of effect size is

$$\Re = 1 - \frac{\delta}{\mu_\delta} = 1 - \frac{8.00}{15.1111} = +0.4707 ,$$

indicating approximately 47% agreement above what is expected by chance.

7.5.3 An Exact Analysis with $v = 1$

Consider an analysis of the example data listed in Table 7.5 on p. 223 under the Fisher–Pitman permutation model with $v = 1$, employing ordinary Euclidean scaling. For the $N = 9$ matched pairs listed in Table 7.5 with $v = 1$, the observed value of test statistic δ is

$$\delta = \binom{N}{2}^{-1} \sum_{i=1}^{N-1} \sum_{j=i+1}^{N} |d_i - d_j|^v = \binom{9}{2}^{-1} (86) = \frac{2(86)}{9(9-1)} = 2.3889 .$$

There are only

$$M = 2^N = 2^9 = 512$$

possible, equally-likely arrangements in the reference set of all permutations of the $N = 9$ matched pairs listed in Table 7.5, making an exact analysis feasible. Under the Fisher–Pitman permutation model, the exact probability of an observed δ is the proportion of δ test statistic values calculated on all possible, equally-likely arrangements of the $N = 9$ matched pairs listed in Table 7.5 that are equal to or less than the observed value of $\delta = 2.3889$. For test statistic δ there are exactly 16 δ test statistic values that are equal to or less than the observed value of $\delta = 2.3889$. If all M arrangements of the $N = 18$ observations listed in Table 7.5 occur with equal chance under the Fisher–Pitman null hypothesis, the exact probability value computed on the $M = 512$ possible arrangements of the observed data with $N = 9$ subjects preserved for each arrangement is

$$P(\delta \le \delta_0 | H_0) = \frac{\text{number of } \delta \text{ values } \le \delta_0}{M} = \frac{16}{512} = 0.0313 ,$$

where δ_o denotes the observed value of test statistic δ and M is the number of possible, equally-likely arrangements of the $N = 9$ matched pairs listed in Table 7.5. No comparison is made with Student's t test statistic for two matched samples as Student's t is undefined for ordinary Euclidean scaling.

Following Eq. (7.5) on p. 217 the exact expected value of test statistic δ under the Fisher–Pitman null hypothesis is

$$\mu_\delta = \frac{1}{M} \sum_{i=1}^{M} \delta_i = \frac{1649.7778}{512} = 3.2222$$

and the observed chance-corrected measure of effect size is

$$\Re = 1 - \frac{\delta}{\mu_\delta} = 1 - \frac{2.3889}{3.2222} = +0.2586 \, ,$$

indicating approximately 26% agreement above what is expected by chance. No comparisons are made with Cohen's $\hat{d}$ or Pearson's r^2 conventional measures of effect size for two matched samples as $\hat{d}$ and r^2 are undefined for ordinary Euclidean scaling.

7.5.4 A Comparison of $v = 2$ and $v = 1$

Unlike the tests for two independent samples discussed in Chap. 6, matched-pairs designs often exhibit very little difference under squared Euclidean scaling with $v = 2$ and ordinary Euclidean scaling with $v = 1$. To illustrate, for the example data listed in Table 7.5 on p. 223 with $N = 9$ matched pairs, $v = 2$, and $\delta = 8.00$, the exact probability value to five decimal places is $P = 0.03125$. For the same data with $v = 1$ and $\delta = 2.3889$, the exact probability value to five decimal places is also $P = 0.03125$.

Inserting an extreme value does not alter the result. Consider the example data listed in Table 7.6 which is the same data listed in Table 7.5 with one alteration: the x_1 score for Subject 9 has been increased from 8 to 18 and the associated difference score has been decreased from -4 to -14. For the example data listed in Table 7.6 with $v = 2$ and $\delta = 40.2222$, the exact probability value is unchanged at $P = 0.03125$. For the data listed in Table 7.6 with $v = 1$ and $\delta = 4.5556$, the exact probability value is unchanged at $P = 0.03125$.

For matched-pairs analyses, whenever all, or almost all, of the difference scores possess the same sign, $v = 2$ and $v = 1$ typically yield the same result, even with an included extreme score. In the case of the example data listed in Tables 7.5 and 7.6, seven of the $N = 9$ difference scores are negative, only one difference score is positive, and one is unsigned (zero).

Table 7.6 Example data for a matched-pairs test with $N = 9$ subjects, including an extreme difference score $(x_{91} = 18)$

Subject	x_1	x_2	d	d^2
1	9	7	−2	4
2	8	7	−1	1
3	7	3	−4	16
4	7	8	+1	1
5	8	6	−2	4
6	9	4	−5	25
7	7	6	−1	1
8	7	7	0	0
9	18	4	−14	196
Sum			−28	248

Table 7.7 Example data for a matched-pairs test with $N = 9$ subjects and no extreme values

Subject	x_1	x_2	d	d^2
1	7	9	+2	4
2	7	8	+1	1
3	3	7	+4	16
4	7	8	+1	1
5	8	6	−2	4
6	9	4	−5	25
7	7	6	−1	1
8	7	7	0	0
9	8	4	−4	16
Sum			−4	68

Now consider a set of data with a mix of positive and negative difference scores, such as in Table 7.7. The data listed in Table 7.7 are the same difference scores listed in Table 7.5, but some signs have been changed so that there are four positive difference scores, four negative difference scores, and one unsigned (zero) score. For the example data listed in Table 7.7 with $v = 2$ and $\delta = 13.00$, the exact probability value is $P = 0.1953$. For the data listed in Table 7.7 with $v = 1$ and $\delta = 3.0556$, the exact probability value is $P = 0.2013$ for a difference between the two probability values of only

$$\Delta_P = 0.2013 - 0.1953 = 0.0060 .$$

The analysis of the matched-pairs data listed in Table 7.7 illustrates that $v = 2$ and $v = 1$ yield similar results when the signs are mixed and there are no extreme values.

Finally, consider the example data listed in Table 7.8. The data listed in Table 7.8 are the same data listed in Table 7.7 with one alteration: the x_1 score for Subject 9 has been increased from 8 to 18 and the associated difference score has been decreased from −4 to −14. For the example data listed in Table 7.8 with $v = 2$ and $\delta = 55.5556$, the exact probability value is $P = 0.5547$. For the data listed in

Table 7.8 Example data for
a matched-pairs test with
$N = 9$ subjects, including an
extreme difference score
($x_{91} = 18$)

Subject	x_1	x_2	d	d^2
1	7	9	+2	4
2	7	8	+1	1
3	3	7	+4	16
4	7	8	+1	1
5	8	6	−2	4
6	9	4	−5	25
7	7	6	−1	1
8	7	7	0	0
9	18	4	−14	196
Sum			−14	248

Table 7.8 with $v = 1$ and $\delta = 5.6111$, the exact probability value is $P = 0.8594$, for a difference between the two probability values with $v = 2$ and $v = 1$ of

$$\Delta_P = 0.8594 - 0.5547 = 0.3047 .$$

The analysis of the matched-pairs data listed in Table 7.8 illustrates the possible differences between $v = 2$ and $v = 1$ with an extreme difference score and mixed positive and negative signs.

7.6 Example 4: Exact and Monte Carlo Analyses

For a fourth, larger example of a matched-pairs test under the Neyman–Pearson population model, consider the data on $N = 30$ matched pairs listed in Table 7.9. The data listed in Table 7.9 represent the number of correct answers on two standardized examinations with 240 multiple-choice questions each on Mathematics (x_1) and English (x_2) taken by $N = 30$ students in the 7th grade at a private charter school. For the score data listed in Table 7.9, the null hypothesis is H_0: $\mu_d = 0$, where $\mu_d = \mu_1 - \mu_2$; that is, no difference is expected between the two tests. The mean of the difference scores is $\bar{d} = +23.7667$, the standard deviation of the difference scores is $s_d = 65.8639$, the standard error of $\bar{d}$ is

$$s_{\bar{d}} = \frac{s_d}{\sqrt{N}} = \frac{65.8639}{\sqrt{30}} = 12.0250 ,$$

and the observed value of Student's t test statistic is

$$t = \frac{\bar{d} - \mu_d}{s_{\bar{d}}} = \frac{+23.7667 - 0}{12.0250} = +1.9764 .$$

Table 7.9 Examination
scores in Mathematics (x_1)
and English (x_2) for $N = 30$
students in the 7th grade at a
private charter school

Subject	x_1	x_2	d	Subject	x_1	x_2	d
1	207	118	+89	16	179	128	+51
2	200	113	+87	17	205	154	+51
3	203	116	+87	18	199	149	+50
4	198	113	+85	19	188	138	+50
5	197	112	+85	20	160	110	+50
6	193	110	+83	21	132	178	−46
7	186	109	+77	22	146	197	−51
8	185	108	+77	23	135	191	−56
9	185	109	+76	24	140	199	−59
10	181	109	+72	25	152	218	−66
11	172	104	+68	26	167	234	−67
12	184	119	+65	27	129	200	−71
13	190	130	+60	28	133	207	−74
14	186	131	+55	29	128	209	−81
15	185	133	+52	30	142	228	−86

Under the Neyman–Pearson null hypothesis, H_0: $\mu_d = 0$, test statistic t is
asymptotically distributed as Student's t with $N - 1$ degrees of freedom. With
$N - 1 = 30 - 1 = 29$ degrees of freedom, the asymptotic two-tail probability
value of $t = +1.9764$ is $P = 0.0577$, under the assumption of normality.

7.6.1   A Monte Carlo Analysis with $v = 2$

For the first analysis of the examination score data listed in Table 7.9 under the
Fisher–Pitman permutation model, employing squared Euclidean scaling with $v = 2$
for correspondence with Student's conventional matched-pairs t test, the observed
value of test statistic δ is

$$\delta = \binom{N}{2}^{-1} \sum_{i=1}^{N-1} \sum_{j=i+1}^{N} |d_i - d_j|^v = \frac{2(3,774,101)}{30(30 - 1)} = 8676.0943 .$$

Alternatively, in terms of an analysis of variance model,

$$\delta = \frac{2SS_{\text{Total}}}{N - 1} = \frac{2(125,803.3667)}{30 - 1} = 8676.0943 ,$$

where for the examination data listed in Table 7.9, the sum of the $N = 30$ differences
is

$$\sum_{i=1}^{N} d_i = (+89) + (+87) + (+87) + \cdots + (-81) + (-86) = +713 ,$$

the sum of the $N = 30$ squared differences is

$$\sum_{i=1}^{N} d_i^2 = (+89)^2 + (+87)^2 + (+87)^2 + \cdots + (-81)^2 + (-86)^2 = 142{,}749 \,,$$

and the total sum-of-squares is

$$SS_{\text{Total}} = \sum_{i=1}^{N} d_i^2 - \left(\sum_{i=1}^{N} d_i\right)^2 \bigg/ N$$

$$= 142{,}749 - (713)^2/30 = 125{,}803.3667 \,.$$

Following the expressions given in Eq. (7.2) on p. 212 for the relationships between test statistics δ and t, the observed value of test statistic δ with respect to the observed value of Student's t test statistic is

$$\delta = \frac{2\sum_{i=1}^{N} d_i^2}{t^2 + N - 1} = \frac{2(142{,}749)}{(+1.9764)^2 + 30 - 1} = 8676.0943$$

and the observed value of Student's t test statistic with respect to the observed value of test statistic δ is

$$t = \left(\frac{2}{\delta}\sum_{i=1}^{N} d_i^2 - N + 1\right)^{1/2} = \left[\frac{2(142{,}749)}{8676.0943} - 30 + 1\right]^{1/2} = \pm1.9764 \,.$$

Because of the functional relationship between test statistic δ and Student's t, the probability values given by

$$P(\delta \leq \delta_o) = \frac{\text{number of } \delta \text{ values } \leq \delta_o}{M}$$

and

$$P(|t| \geq |t_o|) = \frac{\text{number of } |t| \text{ values } \geq |t_o|}{M}$$

are equivalent under the Fisher–Pitman null hypothesis, where δ_o and t_o denote the observed values of δ and t, respectively, and M is the number of possible, equally-likely arrangements of the $N = 30$ matched-pairs examination scores listed in Table 7.9.

There are

$$M = 2^N = 2^{30} = 1{,}073{,}741{,}824$$

possible, equally-likely arrangements in the reference set of all permutations of the $N = 30$ matched-pairs examination scores listed in Table 7.9, making an exact permutation analysis impractical. When the number of possible arrangements is very large, Monte Carlo permutation methods are more practical than exact permutation methods. Monte Carlo permutation methods generate and evaluate a large random sample of all possible arrangements of the observed data. Under the Fisher–Pitman permutation model, the Monte Carlo probability value is the proportion of δ test statistic values computed on the randomly-selected arrangements of the observed data that are equal to or less than the observed test statistic value. In general, a random sample of $L = 1{,}000{,}000$ is sufficient to ensure three decimal places of accuracy [5].

For the examination score data listed in Table 7.9 a sample of $L = 1{,}000{,}000$ random arrangements of the observed data yields exactly 53,342 δ test statistic values that are equal to or less than the observed value of $\delta = 8676.0943$. If all M arrangements of the $N = 30$ observations listed in Table 7.9 occur with equal chance under the Fisher–Pitman null hypothesis, the Monte Carlo probability value of $\delta = 8676.0943$ is

$$P(\delta \leq \delta_o) = \frac{\text{number of } \delta \text{ values } \leq \delta_o}{L} = \frac{53{,}342}{1{,}000{,}000} = 0.0533 \;,$$

where δ_o denotes the observed value of δ and L is the number of randomly-selected, equally-likely arrangements of the $N = 30$ matched-pairs examination scores listed in Table 7.9. For the examination score data listed in Table 7.9, the exact expected value of test statistic δ under the Fisher–Pitman null hypothesis is

$$\mu_\delta = \frac{1}{M} \sum_{i=1}^{M} \delta_i = \frac{10{,}218{,}371{,}442{,}278.40}{1{,}073{,}741{,}824} = 9516.60$$

and the observed chance-corrected measure of effect size is

$$\Re = 1 - \frac{\delta}{\mu_\delta} = 1 - \frac{8676.0943}{9516.60} = +0.0883 \;,$$

indicating approximately 9% agreement among the $N = 30$ scores above what is expected by chance. For comparison, Cohen's measure of effect size is

$$\hat{d} = \frac{|\bar{d} - \mu_d|}{s_d} = \frac{23.7667 - 0}{65.8639} = 0.3608 \;,$$

indicating a medium effect size $(0.20 < \hat{d} < 0.80)$, and Pearson's measure of effect size is

$$r^2 = \frac{t^2}{t^2 + N - 1} = \frac{(+1.9764)^2}{(+1.9764)^2 + 30 - 1} = 0.1187 \,,$$

also indicating a medium effect size $(0.09 < r^2 < 0.25)$.

7.6.2   An Exact Analysis with $v = 2$

Although an exact permutation analysis is not practical for the score data listed in Table 7.9, it is not impossible. For an exact permutation analysis with $v = 2$, the observed value of δ is $\delta = 8676.0943$, the exact expected value of test statistic δ under the Fisher–Pitman null hypothesis is $\mu_\delta = 9516.60$, and there are exactly 56,876,624 δ test statistic values that are equal to or less than the observed value of $\delta = 8676.0943$. If all M arrangements of the $N = 30$ observations listed in Table 7.9 occur with equal chance under the Fisher–Pitman null hypothesis, the exact probability value computed on the $M = 1,073,741,824$ possible arrangements of the observed data with $N = 30$ examination scores preserved for each arrangement is

$$P(\delta \leq \delta_o | H_0) = \frac{\text{number of } \delta \text{ values} \leq \delta_o}{M} = \frac{56,876,624}{1,073,741,824} = 0.0530 \,.$$

Note that the Monte Carlo probability value of $P = 0.0533$ based on $L = 1,000,000$ randomly-selected arrangements of the observed data compares favorably with the exact probability value of $P = 0.0530$ based on all $M = 1,073,741,824$ arrangements of the observed data. The difference between the two probability values is only

$$\Delta_P = 0.0533 - 0.0530 = 0.0003 \,.$$

In general, a random sample of $L = 1,000,000$ arrangements ensures a probability value accurate to three decimal places, provided the probability value is not too small [5]. Finally, the observed chance-corrected measure of effect size is

$$\Re = 1 - \frac{\delta}{\mu_\delta} = 1 - \frac{8676.0943}{9516.60} = +0.0883 \,,$$

indicating approximately 9% agreement among the $N = 30$ scores above what is expected by chance. Alternatively, in terms of Student's t test statistic

$$\Re = \frac{t^2 - 1}{t^2 + N - 1} = \frac{(+1.9764)^2 - 1}{(+1.9764)^2 + 30 - 1} = +0.0883 \,.$$

7.6.3   A Monte Carlo Analysis with $v = 1$

For a second analysis of the data listed in Table 7.9 under the Fisher–Pitman permutation model, employing ordinary Euclidean scaling with $v = 1$, the observed value of test statistic δ is $\delta = 70.6391$, the exact expected value of test statistic δ under the Fisher–Pitman null hypothesis is

$$\mu_\delta = \frac{1}{M} \sum_{i=1}^{M} \delta_i = \frac{81{,}377{,}282{,}228.2240}{1{,}073{,}741{,}824} = 75.7885 ,$$

and the Monte Carlo probability value based on a sample of $L = 1{,}000{,}000$ random arrangements of the observed data with $N = 30$ examination scores preserved for each arrangement is

$$P(\delta \le \delta_0) = \frac{\text{number of } \delta \text{ values } \le \delta_0}{L} = \frac{50{,}302}{1{,}000{,}000} = 0.0503 ,$$

where δ_0 denotes the observed value of δ and L is the number of randomly-selected, equally-likely arrangements of the $N = 30$ matched-pairs examination scores listed in Table 7.9. No comparison is made with Student's t test statistic for two matched samples as Student's t is undefined for ordinary Euclidean scaling.

For $v = 1$, the observed chance-corrected measure of effect size is

$$\Re = 1 - \frac{\delta}{\mu_\delta} = 1 - \frac{70.6391}{75.7885} = +0.0679 ,$$

indicating approximately 7% agreement among the $N = 30$ scores above what is expected by chance. No comparisons are made with Cohen's $\hat{d}$ or Pearson's r^2 measures of effect size for matched pairs as $\hat{d}$ and r^2 are undefined for ordinary Euclidean scaling.

7.6.4   An Exact Analysis with $v = 1$

For an exact permutation analysis of the data listed in Table 7.9 with $v = 1$, the observed value of test statistic δ is $\delta = 70.6391$, the exact expected value of test statistic δ under the Fisher–Pitman null hypothesis is $\mu_\delta = 75.7885$, the exact probability value based on the $M = 1{,}073{,}741{,}824$ possible arrangements of the observed data with $N = 30$ subjects preserved for each arrangement is

$$P(\delta \le \delta_0) = \frac{\text{number of } \delta \text{ values } \le \delta_0}{M} = \frac{63{,}555{,}742}{1{,}073{,}741{,}824} = 0.0592 ,$$

and the observed chance-corrected measure of effect size is

$$\Re = 1 - \frac{\delta}{\mu_\delta} = 1 - \frac{70.6391}{75.7885} = +0.0679 \, ,$$

indicating approximately 7% agreement among the $N = 30$ scores above what is expected by chance.

7.7   Example 5: Rank-Score Permutation Analyses

Occasionally it becomes necessary for researchers to analyze rank-score data. Rank scores customarily arise under one of three scenarios. First, data may be gathered as ranks such as when respondents are asked to rank objects in order of preference. For example, frequent travelers may be asked to rank their favorite brands of hotels in which to stay or their preferred airlines on which to fly. Second, rank scores are commonly gathered and reported in the popular press. For example, each year the Social Security Administration provides a list of the most popular female and male baby names for the previous year. Third, raw interval-level data may not meet the assumptions of tests such as t or F tests and are, therefore, converted to rank scores where the nonparametric statistical tests designed for rank scores are free of many of the assumptions associated with conventional parametric statistical tests.

7.7.1   The Wilcoxon Signed-Ranks Test

The conventional approach to rank-score data under the Neyman–Pearson population model is Wilcoxon's signed-ranks test [8]. Consider a matched-pairs test for N univariate rank scores. Wilcoxon's signed-ranks test statistic is simply the smaller of the sums of the like-signed ranks. An example set of $N = 8$ rank scores is listed in Table 7.10, where eight sets of identical twins serve as subjects. At random, one twin from each pair is assigned to attend nursery school for a term. At the end of the term, the 16 children are each given a test of social perceptiveness.

Table 7.10 Perception scores of nursery- and home-schooled children with differences (d) and signed ranks

Pair	Nursery	Home	d	rank
1	82	63	+19	+7
2	69	42	+27	+8
3	73	74	−1	−1
4	43	37	+6	+4
5	58	51	+7	+5
6	56	43	+13	+6
7	76	80	−4	−3
8	85	82	+3	+2

The sums of the $(+)$ and $(-)$ signed ranks in Table 7.10 are

$$\sum(+) = 7 + 8 + 4 + 5 + 6 + 2 = 32$$

and

$$\sum(-) = 1 + 3 = 4 ,$$

respectively. Then Wilcoxon's test statistic is $T = \sum(-) = 4$.

Test statistic T is asymptotically distributed $N(0, 1)$ under the Neyman–Pearson null hypothesis as $N \to \infty$. For the $N = 8$ rank scores listed in Table 7.10, the mean value of Wilcoxon's T test statistic is

$$\mu_T = \frac{N(N+1)}{4} = \frac{8(8+1)}{4} = 18 ,$$

the standard deviation of Wilcoxon's T is

$$\sigma_T = \left[\frac{N(N+1)(2N+1)}{24} \right]^{1/2} = \left\{ \frac{8(8+1)[2(8)+1]}{24} \right\}^{1/2} = 7.1414 ,$$

and the standard score of $T = 4$ is

$$z = \frac{T - \mu_T}{\sigma_T} = \frac{4 - 18}{7.1414} = -1.9604 ,$$

yielding an asymptotic $N(0, 1)$ two-tail probability value of $P = 0.0499$, under the assumption of normality. If a correction for continuity is applied,

$$z = \frac{T + 0.50 - \mu_T}{\sigma_T} = \frac{4 + 0.50 - 18}{7.1414} = -1.8904$$

and the two-tail probability value of Wilcoxon's T is increased to $P = 0.0587$.

7.7.2 An Exact Analysis with $v = 2$

For an analysis of the rank-score data listed in Table 7.10 under the Fisher–Pitman permutation model let $v = 2$, employing squared Euclidean differences between the rank scores for correspondence with Wilcoxon's signed-ranks test, and let x_i denote the observed rank-score values for $i = 1, \ldots, N$. Then the permutation test statistic is given by

$$\delta = \binom{N}{2}^{-1} \sum_{i=1}^{N-1} \sum_{j=i+1}^{N} |x_i - x_j|^v . \tag{7.14}$$

Following Eq. (7.14) for the rank-score data listed in Table 7.10 with $N = 8$ and $v = 2$, the observed value of the permutation test statistic is

$$\delta = \frac{2}{(8)(8-1)}\Big[\big|(+7)-(+8)\big|^2 + \big|(+7)-(-1)\big|^2$$

$$+ \cdots + \big|(-3)-(+2)\big|^2\Big] = 30.2857 \;.$$

Because there are only

$$M = 2^N = 2^8 = 256$$

possible, equally-likely arrangements in the reference set of all permutations of the perceptiveness-score data listed in Table 7.10, an exact permutation analysis is feasible. Under the Fisher–Pitman permutation model, the exact probability of an observed δ is the proportion of δ test statistic values calculated on all possible, equally-likely arrangements of the $N = 8$ perceptiveness scores listed in Table 7.10 that are equal to or less than the observed value of $\delta = 30.2857$.

There are exactly 14 δ test statistic values that are equal to or less than the observed value of $\delta = 30.2857$. If all M arrangements of the $N = 8$ rank scores listed in Table 7.10 occur with equal chance under the Fisher–Pitman null hypothesis, the exact probability value of $\delta = 30.2857$ computed on the $M = 256$ possible arrangements of the observed data with $N = 8$ observations preserved for each arrangement is

$$P(\delta \le \delta_0 | H_0) = \frac{\text{number of } \delta \text{ values } \le \delta_0}{M} = \frac{14}{256} = 0.0547 \;,$$

where δ_0 denotes the observed value of test statistic δ and M is the number of possible, equally-likely arrangements of the $N = 8$ matched-pairs perceptiveness scores listed in Table 7.10.

7.7.3 The Relationship Between Statistics T and δ

The functional relationships between test statistics T and δ are given by

$$\delta = \frac{N(N+1)(2N+1)}{3(N-1)} - \frac{\big[4T - N(N+1)\big]^2}{2N(N-1)} \tag{7.15}$$

and

$$T = \frac{N(N+1)}{4} - \left\{ \frac{N\big[N(N+1)(2N+1) - 3(N-1)\delta\big]}{24} \right\}^{1/2} \;. \tag{7.16}$$

Following Eq. (7.15), the observed value of test statistic δ with respect to the observed value of Wilcoxon's T test statistic for the rank-score data listed in Table 7.10 is

$$\delta = \frac{8(8+1)[2(8)+1]}{3(8-1)} - \frac{[4(4) - 8(8+1)]^2}{2(8)(8-1)}$$

$$= 58.2857 - 28.00 = 30.2857$$

and following Eq. (7.16), the observed value of Wilcoxon's T test statistic with respect to the observed value of test statistic δ is

$$T = \frac{8(8+1)}{4}$$

$$- \left(\frac{8\{8(8+1)[2(8)+1] - 3(8-1)(30.2857)\}}{24} \right)^{1/2}$$

$$= 18.00 - 14.00 = 4.00 \ .$$

Because test statistics δ and T are equivalent under the Fisher–Pitman null hypothesis, the exact probability value of Wilcoxon's $T = 4$ is identical to the exact probability value of $\delta = 30.2557$; that is,

$$P(\delta \leq \delta_o) = \frac{\text{number of } \delta \text{ values } \leq \delta_o}{M} = \frac{14}{256} = 0.0547$$

and

$$P(T \geq T_o) = \frac{\text{number of } T \text{ values } \geq T_o}{M} = \frac{14}{256} = 0.0547 \ ,$$

where δ_o and T_o denote the observed values of test statistics δ and T, respectively, and M is the number of possible, equally-likely arrangements of the observed data listed in Table 7.10.

Following Eq. (7.4) on p. 217, the exact expected value of the $M = 256$ δ test statistic values under the Fisher–Pitman null hypothesis is

$$\mu_\delta = \frac{1}{M} \sum_{i=1}^{M} \delta_i = \frac{10,404.5722}{256} = 40.6429$$

and following Eq. (7.4) on p. 217, the observed chance-corrected measure of effect size is

$$\Re = 1 - \frac{\delta}{\mu_\delta} = 1 - \frac{30.2857}{40.6429} = +0.2548 \ ,$$

indicating approximately 25% within-group agreement above what is expected by chance. No comparisons are made with Cohen's $\hat{d}$ or Pearson's r^2 measures of effect size for matched pairs as $\hat{d}$ and r^2 are undefined for rank-score data.

7.7.4 An Exact Analysis with $v = 1$

For an analysis of the rank-score data listed in Table 7.10 on p. 236 under the Fisher–Pitman permutation model let $v = 1$, employing ordinary Euclidean differences between the rank scores. Then the observed value of the permutation test statistic is

$$\delta = \binom{N}{2}^{-1} \sum_{i=1}^{N-1} \sum_{j=i+1}^{N} |x_i - x_j|^v$$

$$= \frac{2}{(8)(8-1)} \Big[|(+7) - (+8)|^1 + |(+7) - (-1)|^1$$

$$+ \cdots + |(-3) - (+2)|^1 \Big] = 4.6429 \ .$$

There are only

$$M = 2^N = 2^8 = 256$$

possible, equally-likely arrangements in the reference set of all permutations of the perceptiveness-score data listed in Table 7.10, making an exact permutation analysis possible. Under the Fisher–Pitman permutation model, the exact probability of an observed δ is the proportion of δ test statistic values calculated on all possible, equally-likely arrangements of the $N = 8$ perceptiveness scores listed in Table 7.10 that are equal to or less than the observed value of $\delta = 4.6429$. There are exactly four δ test statistic values that are equal to or less than the observed value of $\delta = 4.6429$. If all M arrangements of the $N = 8$ rank scores listed in Table 7.10 occur with equal chance under the Fisher–Pitman null hypothesis, the exact probability value of $\delta = 4.6429$ computed on the $M = 256$ possible arrangements of the observed data with $N = 8$ observations preserved for each arrangement is

$$P(\delta \leq \delta_0 | H_0) = \frac{\text{number of } \delta \text{ values} \leq \delta_0}{M} = \frac{4}{256} = 0.0156 \ ,$$

where δ_0 denotes the observed value of test statistic δ and M is the number of possible, equally-likely arrangements of the $N = 8$ matched-pairs perceptiveness scores listed in Table 7.10.

Following Eq. (7.4) on p. 217, the exact expected value of the $M = 256\ \delta$ test statistic values under the Fisher–Pitman null hypothesis is

$$\mu_\delta = \frac{1}{M} \sum_{i=1}^{M} \delta_i = \frac{1746.2784}{256} = 6.8214$$

and following Eq. (7.3) on p. 217, the observed chance-corrected measure of effect size is

$$\Re = 1 - \frac{\delta}{\mu_\delta} = 1 - \frac{4.6429}{6.8214} = +0.3194\ ,$$

indicating approximately 32% within-group agreement above what is expected by chance. No comparisons are made with Cohen's $\hat{d}$ or Pearson's r^2 measures of effect size for matched pairs as $\hat{d}$ and r^2 are undefined for rank-score data.

7.7.5 The Sign Test

The sign test is the most elementary of all tests of differences. Although the sign test is a very simple test, it is also very useful in a variety of research settings. The sign test is so named because the test statistic is computed from data that consist of, or have been reduced to, simple plus (+) and minus (−) signs, representing positive and negative differences between values, respectively. The test statistic, denoted by S, is the smaller of the number of (+) or (−) signs. Because there are only two values, the sign test follows the discrete binomial probability distribution.

To illustrate the sign test, consider the signed-ranks data listed in Table 7.10 on p. 236, replicated in Table 7.11 with the ranks removed. For the sign data listed in Table 7.11, there are six (+) signs and two (−) signs; thus, $S = 2$. Under the Neyman–Pearson null hypothesis that the measurement of perceptiveness is equally likely for the nursery school and home children, the sign test provides the exact probability of an arrangement with $S = 2$ minus signs and $N - S = 6$ plus signs, or an arrangement more extreme.

Table 7.11 Perception scores of nursery- and home-schooled children with differences (d) and signs

Pair	Nursery	Home	d	Sign
1	82	63	+19	+
2	69	42	+27	+
3	73	74	−1	−
4	43	37	+6	+
5	58	51	+7	+
6	56	43	+13	+
7	76	80	−4	−
8	85	82	+3	+

Let p denote the probability of success on a single trial. The signs are asymptotically distributed $N(0, 1)$ under the Neyman–Pearson null hypothesis, H_0: $p = 0.50$, as $N \rightarrow \infty$. For the sign data listed in Table 7.11, the mean of the binomial probability distribution with $N = 8$ and $p = 0.50$ is

$$\mu_b = Np = (8)(0.50) = 4.00 ,$$

the standard deviation of the binomial probability distribution is

$$\sigma_b = \sqrt{Np(1 - p)} = \sqrt{(8)(0.50)(1.00 - 0.50)} = 1.4142 ,$$

and the standard score of $S = 2$ is

$$z = \frac{S - \mu_b}{\sigma_b} = \frac{2 - 4}{1.4142} = -1.4142 ,$$

yielding an asymptotic $N(0, 1)$ two-tail probability value of $P = 0.1573$ under the assumption of normality. Since $N = 8$ is a very small sample size, a correction for continuity is essential. Thus,

$$z = \frac{S + 0.50 - \mu_b}{\sigma_b} = \frac{2 + 0.50 - 4}{1.4142} = -1.0607 ,$$

yielding an asymptotic $N(0, 1)$ two-tail probability value of $P = 0.2888$, under the assumption of normality.

For comparison, the exact cumulative binomial probability value for any S is given by

$$P(S|N) = \sum_{i=0}^{S} \binom{N}{i} p^i (1 - p)^{N-i} , \qquad (7.17)$$

where p is the probability of success on a single trial. Since the null hypothesis for the sign test is simply that there is no difference expected between the number of $(+)$ and $(-)$ signs; that is H_0: $p = 0.50$, Eq. (7.17) reduces to

$$P(S|N) = \sum_{i=0}^{S} \binom{N}{i} (0.50)^N .$$

For the sign data listed in Table 7.11 with $i = 0, 1, 2$,

$$p(0|8) = \binom{8}{0}(0.50)^8 = \frac{8!}{0!\,8!}(0.50)^8 = \frac{1}{256} = 0.0039 ,$$

$$p(1|8) = \binom{8}{1}(0.50)^8 = \frac{8!}{1!\,7!}(0.50)^8 = \frac{8}{256} = 0.0312 ,$$

and

$$p(2|8) = \binom{8}{2}(0.50)^8 = \frac{8!}{2!\,6!}(0.50)^8 = \frac{28}{256} = 0.1094 \ .$$

Because the probability of success is $p = 0.50$, the binomial probability distribution is symmetrical and the exact two-tail binomial probability value is

$$P = 2(0.0039 + 0.0312 + 0.1094) = 0.2891 \ .$$

7.7.6 An Exact Analysis with $v = 2$

For an analysis of the sign data listed in Table 7.11 under the Fisher–Pitman permutation model let $v = 2$, employing squared Euclidean differences between the pairs of signs for correspondence with the sign test and let $x_i = \pm 1$ denote the observed signs for $i = 1, \ldots, N$. Then the permutation test statistic is given by

$$\delta = \binom{N}{2}^{-1} \sum_{i=1}^{N-1} \sum_{j=i+1}^{N} |x_i - x_j|^v \ . \tag{7.18}$$

Following Eq. (7.18) for the sign data listed in Table 7.11 with $N = 8$ and $v = 2$, the observed value of the permutation test statistic is

$$\delta = \frac{2}{(8)(8-1)} \Big[\big|(+1) - (+1)\big|^2 + \big|(+1) - (-1)\big|^2$$
$$+ \cdots + \big|(-1) - (+1)\big|^2 \Big] = 1.7143 \ .$$

Because there are only

$$M = 2^N = 2^8 = 256$$

possible, equally-likely arrangements in the reference set of all permutations of the sign data listed in Table 7.11, an exact permutation analysis is possible. Under the Fisher–Pitman permutation model, the exact probability of an observed δ is the proportion of δ test statistic values calculated on all possible, equally-likely arrangements of the $N = 8(+)$ and $(-)$ signs listed in Table 7.11 that are equal to or less than the observed value of $\delta = 1.7143$. There are exactly 74 δ test statistic values that are equal to or less than the observed value of $\delta = 1.7143$. If all M arrangements of the $N = 8$ signs listed in Table 7.11 occur with equal chance under the Fisher–Pitman null hypothesis, the exact probability value of $\delta = 1.7143$ computed on the $M = 256$ possible arrangements of the observed signs with $N = 8$

observations preserved for each arrangement is

$$P(\delta \leq \delta_0|H_0) = \frac{\text{number of } \delta \text{ values } \leq \delta_0}{M} = \frac{74}{256} = 0.2891 \ ,$$

which is the same probability value as the binomial probability value.

7.7.7   The Relationship Between Statistics S and δ

Under the Neyman–Pearson null hypothesis, H_0: $p = 0.50$, the functional relationships between test statistics δ and S are given by

$$\delta = \frac{2S(N-S)}{N(N-1)p^2} = \frac{8S(N-S)}{N(N-1)} \ , \tag{7.19}$$

where $p = 0.50$ and

$$S = \frac{N}{2} \pm \frac{\sqrt{4N^2 - 2\delta N(N-1)}}{4} \ . \tag{7.20}$$

Following Eq. (7.19), the observed value of test statistic δ with respect to the observed value of test statistic S for the sign data listed in Table 7.11 is

$$\delta = \frac{(8)(2)(8-2)}{(8)(8-1)} = \frac{96}{56} = 1.7143$$

and following Eq. (7.20), the observed value of test statistic S with respect to the observed value of test statistic δ is

$$S = \frac{8}{2} \pm \frac{\sqrt{4(8)^2 - 2(1.7143)(8)(8-1)}}{4} = \frac{8}{2} \pm \frac{\sqrt{64}}{4} = 4 \pm 2 \ ,$$

where the two roots of the quadratic equation yield $4 + 2 = 6$ and $4 - 2 = 2$, which are the values for $N - S = 8 - 2 = 6$ (+) signs and $S = 2$ (−) signs, respectively.

Because statistics δ and S are equivalent under the Fisher–Pitman null hypothesis, the exact probability value of $S = 2$ is identical to the exact probability value of $\delta = 1.7143$; that is,

$$P(\delta \leq \delta_0) = \frac{\text{number of } \delta \text{ values } \leq \delta_0}{M} = \frac{74}{256} = 0.2891$$

and

$$P(S \geq S_0) = \frac{\text{number of } S \text{ values } \geq S_0}{M} = \frac{74}{256} = 0.2891 \ ,$$

where δ_o and S_o denote the observed values of δ and S, respectively, and M is the number of possible, equally-likely arrangements of the sign data listed in Table 7.11.

Following Eq. (7.4) on p. 217, the exact expected value of the $M = 256$ δ test statistic values under the Fisher–Pitman null hypothesis is

$$\mu_\delta = \frac{1}{M} \sum_{i=1}^{M} \delta_i = \frac{512}{256} = 2.00$$

and following Eq. (7.3) on p. 217, the observed chance-corrected measure of effect size is

$$\Re = 1 - \frac{\delta}{\mu_\delta} = 1 - \frac{1.7143}{2.00} = +0.1429 \, ,$$

indicating approximately 14% within-group agreement above what is expected by chance. No comparisons are made with Cohen's $\hat{d}$ or Pearson's r^2 measures of effect size for matched pairs as $\hat{d}$ and r^2 are undefined for simple sign data.

7.7.8 An Exact Analysis with $v = 1$

For an analysis of the sign data listed in Table 7.11 under the Fisher–Pitman permutation model with $v = 1$, employing ordinary Euclidean differences between the pairs of signs, the observed value of the permutation test statistic is

$$\begin{aligned}
\delta = \binom{N}{2}^{-1} \sum_{i=1}^{N-1} \sum_{j=i+1}^{N} |x_i - x_j|^v \\
= \frac{2}{(8)(8-1)} \Big[\big|(+1) - (+1)\big|^1 + \big|(+1) - (-1)\big|^1 \\
+ \cdots + \big|(-1) - (+1)\big|^1 \Big] = 0.8571 \, .
\end{aligned}$$

There are only

$$M = 2^N = 2^8 = 256$$

possible, equally-likely arrangements in the reference set of all permutations of the sign data listed in Table 7.11. Under the Fisher–Pitman permutation model, the exact probability of an observed δ is the proportion of δ test statistic values calculated on all possible, equally-likely arrangements of the $N = 8$ (+) and (−) signs listed in Table 7.11 that are equal to or less than the observed value of $\delta = 0.8571$. There are exactly 74 δ test statistic values that are equal to or less than the observed value of $\delta = 0.8571$. If all arrangements of the $N = 8$ (+) and ($-$) signs listed in Table 7.11 occur with equal chance under the Fisher–Pitman null hypothesis, the exact probability value of $\delta = 0.8571$ computed on the $M = 256$ possible arrangements of the observed data with $N = 8$ observations preserved for each arrangement is

$$P(\delta \leq \delta_0 | H_0) = \frac{\text{number of } \delta \text{ values } \leq \delta_0}{M} = \frac{74}{256} = 0.2891 \ ,$$

where δ_0 denotes the observed value of test statistic δ and M is the number of possible, equally-likely arrangements of the sign data listed in Table 7.11. No comparison is made with the conventional sign test as S is undefined for ordinary Euclidean scaling.

Following Eq. (7.4) on p. 217, the exact expected value of the $M = 256$ δ test statistic values under the Fisher–Pitman null hypothesis is

$$\mu_\delta = \frac{1}{M} \sum_{i=1}^{M} \delta_i = \frac{256}{256} = 1.00$$

and following Eq. (7.3) on p. 217, the observed chance-corrected measure of effect size is

$$\Re = 1 - \frac{\delta}{\mu_{\delta_0}} = 1 - \frac{0.8571}{1.00} = +0.1429 \ ,$$

indicating approximately 14% within-group agreement above what is expected by chance. No comparisons are made with Cohen's $\hat{d}$ or Pearson's r^2 measures of effect size for matched pairs as $\hat{d}$ and r^2 are undefined for simple sign data.

Because all values for the sign test are either $+1$ or -1, the probability values for $v = 2$ and $v = 1$ are identical; that is, $P = 0.2891$. Also, the permutation test statistic value for $v = 2$ ($\delta = 1.7143$) is exactly twice the value for $v = 1$ ($\delta = 0.8571$) and the exact expected value of δ for $v = 2$ ($\mu_\delta = 2.00$) is exactly twice the expected value of δ for $v = 1$ ($\mu_\delta = 1.00$). Consequently, the chance-corrected value for the measure of effect size with $v = 2$ ($\Re = +0.1429$) is identical to the value for the measure of effect size with $v = 1$ ($\Re = +0.1429$).

7.8 Example 6: Multivariate Permutation Analyses

Oftentimes a research design calls for a test of difference between $g = 2$ matched treatment groups when multivariate ($r \geq 2$) measurements have been obtained for each of $N \geq 2$ subjects. The conventional approach to such a research design under the Neyman–Pearson population model is Hotelling's multivariate T^2 test for two matched samples [3].

Suppose that $r \geq 2$ measurements and $N \geq 2$ subjects are associated with a multivariate pre-treatment and post-treatment matched-pairs permutation test and let

$$(w_{11j}, \ldots, w_{r1j}) \quad \text{and} \quad (w_{12j}, \ldots, w_{r2j})$$

denote r-dimensional row vectors with elements comprised of the r measurements on the jth subject from the pre- and post-treatments, respectively, where $j = 1, \ldots, N$. Let

$$x_{1j} = \begin{bmatrix} x_{11j} \\ \vdots \\ x_{r1j} \end{bmatrix},$$

where $x_{k1j} = w_{k1j} - w_{k2j}$ for $k = 1, \ldots, r$, be the r dimensional column vector of differences between pre-treatment and post-treatment measurement scores for the jth subject, and let $x_{2j} = -x_{1j}$ be the r-dimensional origin reflection of x_{1j} for $j = 1, \ldots, N$. The probability under the null hypothesis is $P(x_{1j}) = P(x_{2j}) = 0.50$ for $j = 1, \ldots, N$. For the multivariate matched-pairs research design, test statistic δ is given by

$$\delta = \binom{N}{2}^{-1} \sum_{m=1}^{N-1} \sum_{n=m+1}^{N} \Delta(x_{1m}, x_{1n}), \tag{7.21}$$

where

$$\Delta(x_{1m}, x_{1n}) = \left[(x_{1m}, x_{1n})'(x_{1m}, x_{1n}) \right]^{v/2} \tag{7.22}$$

is the r-dimensional Euclidean difference between the mth and nth subjects' differences. When $v = 1$ in Eq. (7.22), $\Delta(x_{1m}, x_{1n})$ is an ordinary Euclidean scaling metric and when $v = 2$ in Eq. (7.22), $\Delta(x_{1m}, x_{1n})$ is a squared Euclidean scaling function and is not a metric function since the triangle inequality is not satisfied; that is, $\Delta(x, y) \leq \Delta(x, z) + \Delta(y, z)$.

Hotelling's multivariate matched-pairs T^2 test statistic is given by

$$T^2 = N\bar{x}_1' S^{-1} \bar{x}_1,$$

where $\mathbf{S}$ is an $r \times r$ variance-covariance matrix given by

$$
\begin{bmatrix}
\dfrac{1}{N-1} \displaystyle\sum_{I=1}^{N} (x_{1I} - \bar{x}_1)^2 & \cdots & \dfrac{1}{N-1} \displaystyle\sum_{I=1}^{N} (x_{1I} - \bar{x}_1)(x_{rI} - \bar{x}_r) \\
\vdots & & \vdots \\
\dfrac{1}{N-1} \displaystyle\sum_{I=1}^{N} (x_{rI} - \bar{x}_r)(x_{1I} - \bar{x}_1) & \cdots & \dfrac{1}{N-1} \displaystyle\sum_{I=1}^{N} (x_{rI} - \bar{x}_r)^2
\end{bmatrix}
$$

and

$$
\bar{x}_1 = \frac{1}{N} \sum_{j=1}^{N} x_{1j} .
$$

While the permutation test is applicable to all combinations of r and N, any application of Hotelling's T^2 test statistic under the Neyman–Pearson null hypothesis with the assumption of multivariate normality requires that $\min(r, N - r) \geq 1$ since the distribution of the adjusted T^2 test statistic given by

$$
F = \frac{(N-r)T^2}{(N-1)r}
$$

is asymptotically distributed as Snedecor's F with $v_1 = r$ and $v_2 = N - r$ degrees of freedom. When $v = 2$ and squared Euclidean scaling is employed, the functional relationships between Hotelling's T^2 and test statistic δ are given by

$$
T^2 = \frac{r(N-1)^2 \left[2SS_{\text{Total}} - g(N-1)\delta \right]}{g(N-r)(N-1)\delta - 2SS_{\text{Between}}} \tag{7.23}
$$

and

$$
\delta = \frac{2 \left[r(N-1)^2 SS_{\text{Total}} + T^2 SS_{\text{Between}} \right]}{g(N-1) \left[T^2(N-r) + r(N-1)^2 \right]} , \tag{7.24}
$$

respectively, where g denotes the number of treatments and SS_{Between} and SS_{Total} are defined as usual; that is, the sum-of-squares between treatments is given by

$$
SS_{\text{Between}} = N \sum_{i=1}^{g} \left(\bar{x}_{i.} - \bar{x}_{..} \right)^2 ,
$$

the sum-of-squares total is given by

$$
SS_{\text{Total}} = \sum_{i=1}^{g} \sum_{j=1}^{N} \left(x_{ij} - \bar{x}_{..} \right)^2 ,
$$

the mean of the ith of g treatments is given by

$$\bar{x}_{i.} = \frac{1}{N} \sum_{j=1}^{N} x_{ij}, \qquad i = 1, \ldots, g,$$

the grand mean over all g treatments is given by

$$\bar{x}_{..} = \frac{1}{Ng} \sum_{i=1}^{g} \sum_{j=1}^{N} x_{ij},$$

and x_{ij} is the univariate measurement score of the ith of g treatments for the jth of N judges.

If the observed values of δ and T^2 are denoted by δ_o and T_o^2, respectively, then the exact probability value of δ_o and T_o^2 is given by

$$P(T^2 \geq T_o^2 | H_0) = P(\delta \leq \delta_o | H_0) = \frac{\text{number of } \delta \text{ values } \leq \delta_o}{M},$$

where $M = (g!)^N$ in this application. When M is large a Monte Carlo method to approximate the probability value is essential. A Monte Carlo permutation procedure provides an approximate probability value for δ and is given by

$$P(\delta \leq \delta_o | H_0) = \frac{\text{number of } \delta \text{ values } \leq \delta_o}{L},$$

where L is a random sample of all possible, equally-likely arrangements of the $2Nr$ measurements.

7.8.1 The Hotelling's Matched-Pairs T^2 Test

Consider the following scenario: paired, but randomly arranged, pre-training and post-training writing samples of $r = 11$ students were blindly presented to $N = 13$ experienced teachers of language arts for grading. Each of the $N = 13$ judges scored each of the 22 writing samples on a scale from 0 to 10. The pre- and post-training writing assessment scores are listed in Tables 7.12 and 7.13, respectively.

The example analysis blocks on the $N = 13$ judges and compares the pre-training and post-training scores of the $r = 11$ students. The analysis evaluates the following question: Did the course work result in significant pre- and post-training writing differences among the students? A conventional Hotelling's matched-pairs T^2 test on the measurement scores listed in Tables 7.12 and 7.13 yields an observed T^2

Table 7.12 Pre-training writing assessment scores assigned by $N = 13$ judges to writing samples of $r = 11$ students

Judge	Student										
	1	2	3	4	5	6	7	8	9	10	11
1	1	6	1	1	8	1	5	8	6	3	1
2	3	4	6	2	8	3	6	9	9	7	3
3	1	6	2	3	7	3	3	5	5	2	4
4	2	5	5	1	8	2	4	7	8	6	4
5	3	6	5	2	8	2	3	5	9	4	2
6	0	4	3	0	8	0	3	9	7	3	0
7	1	5	0	1	7	0	1	2	8	5	1
8	5	8	4	0	2	0	2	10	2	2	0
9	1	7	2	5	9	2	6	6	9	6	3
10	2	3	2	0	6	1	5	7	5	3	3
11	1	5	2	1	7	1	2	8	8	7	4
12	0	4	1	0	9	0	2	5	3	2	1
13	4	9	2	2	5	3	3	9	8	4	3

Table 7.13 Post-training writing assessment scores assigned by $N = 13$ judges to writing samples of $r = 11$ students

Judge	Student										
	1	2	3	4	5	6	7	8	9	10	11
1	9	5	3	1	8	1	7	6	6	4	5
2	8	5	5	2	9	2	6	6	7	5	5
3	5	6	2	3	3	3	6	8	7	5	8
4	7	6	3	2	9	4	5	6	6	4	7
5	8	7	4	2	8	4	7	8	6	3	5
6	6	7	2	0	6	0	5	7	6	5	4
7	5	5	2	1	5	3	5	5	4	0	7
8	4	9	6	0	3	3	10	8	5	3	5
9	9	5	5	7	8	3	8	8	8	7	8
10	4	4	1	0	4	3	4	5	6	6	6
11	6	3	3	2	9	2	9	7	7	5	9
12	6	2	3	1	5	1	6	9	6	5	6
13	9	6	4	4	7	6	9	7	6	7	5

value of $T^2 = 766.0821$ and the observed F test statistic value is

$$F = \frac{(N - r)T^2}{(N - 1)r} = \frac{(13 - 11)(766.0821)}{(13 - 1)(11)} = 11.6073 \ .$$

Assuming independence, multivariate normality, homogeneity of variance, and homogeneity of covariance, test statistic F is asymptotically distributed as Snedecor's F under the Neyman–Pearson null hypothesis with $v_1 = r = 11$ and $v_2 = N - r = 13 - 11 = 2$ degrees of freedom. Under the Neyman–Pearson null hypothesis the observed value of $F = 11.673$ yields an asymptotic probability value of $P = 0.0819$, under the assumptions of normality and homogeneity.

7.8.2   *An Exact Analysis with v = 2*

There are only

$$M = (g!)^N = (2!)^{13} = 8192$$

possible, equally-likely arrangements in the reference set of all permutations of the scores of the $N = 13$ judges listed in Tables 7.12 and 7.13, making an exact permutation analysis possible. For this permutation analysis where $r = 11$, $g = 2$, and $N = 13$, let $v = 2$ in Eq. (7.22) on p. 247, employing squared Euclidean differences between measurement scores for correspondence with Hotelling's matched-pairs T^2 test. Following Eq. (7.21) on p. 247, the observed value of δ with $v = 2$ is $\delta = 65.9872$.

The functional relationships between test statistics T^2 and δ given in Eqs. (7.23) and (7.24), respectively, can be confirmed with the data listed in Tables 7.12 and 7.13. For the data listed in Tables 7.12 and 7.13 the sum-of-squares between treatments is

$$SS_{\text{Between}} = N \sum_{i=1}^{g} (\bar{x}_{i.} - \bar{x}_{..})^2 = 9.7346$$

and the sum-of-squares total is

$$SS_{\text{Total}} = \sum_{i=1}^{g} \sum_{j=1}^{N} (x_{ij} - \bar{x}_{..})^2 = 1553.0719 \ .$$

Then, following Eq. (7.24) on p. 248, the observed value of test statistic δ with respect to the observed value of Hotelling's T^2 test statistic for the pre- and post-training scores listed in Tables 7.12 and 7.13 is

$$
\begin{aligned}
\delta &= \frac{2\left[r(N-1)^2 SS_{\text{Total}} + T^2 SS_{\text{Between}}\right]}{g(N-1)\left[T^2(N-r) + r(N-1)^2\right]} \\[2mm]
&= \frac{2\left[11(13-1)^2(1553.0719) + (766.0821)(9.7346)\right]}{2(13-1)\left[(766.0821)(13-11) + 11(13-1)^2\right]} \\[2mm]
&= \frac{4{,}935{,}046.8072}{74{,}787.9408} = 65.9872
\end{aligned}
$$

and, following Eq. (7.23) on p. 248, the observed value of Hotelling's T^2 test statistic with respect to the observed value of test statistic δ is

$$
T^2 = \frac{r(N-1)^2\left[2SS_{\text{Total}} - g(N-1)\delta\right]}{g(N-r)(N-1)\delta - 2SS_{\text{Between}}}
$$

$$
= \frac{11(13-1)^2\left[2(1553.0719) - 2(13-1)(65.9872)\right]}{2(13-11)(13-1)(65.9872) - 2(9.7264)}
$$

$$
= \frac{2,411,562.4063}{3147.9164} = 766.0821 .
$$

If all M arrangements of the observed writing assessment scores listed in Tables 7.12 and 7.13 occur with equal chance under the Fisher–Pitman null hypothesis, the exact probability value of $\delta = 65.9872$ computed on the $M = 8192$ possible arrangements of the observed data with $N = 13$ judges preserved for each arrangement is

$$
P(\delta \leq \delta_0 | H_0) = \frac{\text{number of } \delta \text{ values } \leq \delta_0}{M} = \frac{2}{8192} = 0.2441 \times 10^{-3} ,
$$

where δ_0 denotes the observed value of test statistic δ and M is the number of possible, equally-likely arrangements of the pre- and post-training writing assessment scores listed in Tables 7.12 and 7.13.

There is a considerable difference between the Hotelling's T^2 probability value of $P = 0.0819$ and the exact probability value of $P = 0.2441 \times 10^{-3}$. The difference is quite possibly due to the violation of the assumptions of multivariate normality, homogeneity of variance, and homogeneity of covariance required by Hotelling's T^2, but not required by the permutation test.

The exact expected value of the $M = 8192$ δ test statistic values under the Fisher–Pitman null hypothesis is $\mu_\delta = 90.1731$ and the observed chance-corrected measure of effect size is

$$
\Re = 1 - \frac{\delta}{\mu_\delta} = 1 - \frac{65.9872}{90.1731} = +0.2682 ,
$$

indicating approximately 27% within-judges agreement above what is expected by chance. No comparisons are made with Cohen's $\hat{d}$ or Pearson's r^2 measures of effect size for matched pairs as $\hat{d}$ and r^2 are undefined for multivariate data.

7.8.3 An Exact Analysis with $v = 1$

For a comparison analysis of the multivariate data listed in Tables 7.12 and 7.13 under the Fisher–Pitman permutation model, let $v = 1$ instead of $v = 2$ in Eq. (7.22) on p. 247, thereby employing ordinary Euclidean differences between measurement scores. For the pre- and post-training writing assessment scores listed in Tables 7.12 and 7.13, the number of possible, equally-likely arrangements in the reference set of all permutations of the $N = 13$ judges listed in Tables 7.12 and 7.13 is still only

$$M = (g!)^N = (2!)^{13} = 8192 .$$

The observed value of test statistic δ with $v = 1$ is $\delta = 0.0928$. If all M arrangements of the $N = 13$ writing assessment scores listed in Tables 7.12 and 7.13 occur with equal chance under the Fisher–Pitman null hypothesis, the exact probability value of $\delta = 0.0928$ computed on the $M = 8192$ possible arrangements of the observed writing assessment scores with $N = 13$ judges preserved for each arrangement is

$$P(\delta \leq \delta_0 | H_0) = \frac{\text{number of } \delta \text{ values } \leq \delta_0}{M} = \frac{634}{8192} = 0.0774 ,$$

where δ_0 denotes the observed value of test statistic δ and M is the number of possible, equally-likely arrangements of the writing assessment scores listed in Tables 7.12 and 7.13.

In this example analysis there is considerable difference in probability values, where with $v = 2$, the exact probability value is $P = 0.2441 \times 10^{-3}$, and with $v = 1$, the exact probability value is $P = 0.0774$. The substantial difference in probability values is possibly due to large differences between pre-test and post-test writing assessment scores that are amplified by squaring the differences with $v = 2$; for example, Student 1 and Judge 1 with pre- and post-test scores of 1 and 9, respectively; Student 1 and Judge 9 with pre- and post-test scores of 1 and 9, respectively; Student 7 and Judge 8 with pre- and post-test scores of 2 and 10, respectively; and others in Tables 7.12 and 7.13. No comparison is made with Hotelling's T^2 test as T^2 is undefined for ordinary Euclidean scaling.

The exact expected value of the $M = 8192$ δ test statistic values under the Fisher–Pitman null hypothesis is

$$\mu_\delta = \frac{1}{M} \sum_{i=1}^{M} \delta_i = \frac{922}{8192} = 0.1125$$

and the observed chance-corrected measure of effect size is

$$\Re = 1 - \frac{\delta}{\mu_\delta} = 1 - \frac{0.0928}{0.1125} = +0.1755 ,$$

indicating approximately 18% within-judges agreement above what is expected by chance. No comparisons are made with Cohen's $\hat{d}$ or Pearson's r^2 measures of effect size for matched pairs as $\hat{d}$ and r^2 are undefined for multivariate data.

7.9 Summary

This chapter examined matched-pairs tests where the null hypothesis under the Neyman–Pearson population model typically posits no difference between two population means. The conventional matched-pairs test and two measures of effect size under the Neyman–Pearson population model of inference were described and illustrated: Student's matched-pairs t test, and Cohen's $\hat{d}$ and Pearson's r^2 measures of effect size, respectively.

Under the Fisher–Pitman permutation model of inference, test statistic δ and associated measure of effect size, $\mathfrak{R}$, were introduced and illustrated for two matched samples. For tests of two matched samples, test statistic δ was demonstrated to be flexible enough to incorporate both ordinary and squared Euclidean scaling functions with $v = 1$ and $v = 2$, respectively. Effect size measure, $\mathfrak{R}$, was shown to be applicable to either $v = 1$ or $v = 2$ without modification and to have a clear and meaningful chance-corrected interpretation in both cases.

Six examples illustrated permutation-based test statistics δ and $\mathfrak{R}$. In the first example, a small sample of $N = 5$ matched subjects was utilized to describe and illustrate the calculation of test statistics δ and $\mathfrak{R}$ for two matched samples. The second example demonstrated the permutation-based, chance-corrected measure of effect size, $\mathfrak{R}$, and related $\mathfrak{R}$ to the conventional measures of effect size for two matched samples: Cohen's $\hat{d}$ and Pearson's r^2. The third example with $N = 9$ observations illustrated the effects of extreme values on various combinations of plus-and-minus values with both $v = 2$ and $v = 1$. The fourth example with $N = 30$ observations compared exact and Monte Carlo permutation methods, illustrating the accuracy and efficiency of Monte Carlo analyses. The fifth example with $N = 8$ rank scores illustrated an application of permutation statistical methods to univariate rank-score data, including Wilcoxon's conventional signed-ranks test and the sign test. Finally, in the sixth example, both statistic δ and effect-size measure $\mathfrak{R}$ were extended to multivariate data with $N = 13$ subjects and $r = 11$ variates and compared with Hotelling's conventional T^2 test for two matched samples.

Chapter 8 continues the presentation of permutation statistical methods for independent samples initiated in Chap. 6, but extends the permutation methods to examine research designs in which more than $g = 2$ samples are considered. Research designs incorporating multiple treatments are prevalent in many fields of research. When the Neyman–Pearson null hypothesis posits no difference among the $g \geq 3$ population means, the designs are commonly known as fully- or completely-randomized analysis of variance designs.

References

1. Berry, K.J.: Algorithm 179: enumeration of all permutations of multi-sets with fixed repetition numbers. J. R. Stat. Soc. C Appl. **31**, 169–173 (1982)
2. Feinstein, A.R.: Clinical biostatistics XXIII: the role of randomization in sampling, testing, allocation, and credulous idolatry (Part 2). Clin. Pharmacol. Ther. **14**, 898–915 (1973)

3. Hotelling, H.: The generalization of Student's ratio. Ann. Math. Stat. **2**, 360–378 (1931)
4. Hotelling, H., Pabst, M.R.: Rank correlation and tests of significance involving no assumption of normality. Ann. Math. Stat. **7**, 29–43 (1936)
5. Johnston, J.E., Berry, K.J., Mielke, P.W.: Permutation tests: precision in estimating probability values. Percept. Motor Skill. **105**, 915–920 (2007)
6. Satterthwaite, F.E.: An approximate distribution of estimates of variance components. Biometrics Bull. **2**, 110–114 (1946)
7. Welch, B.L.: On the comparison of several mean values: an alternative approach. Biometrika **38**, 330–336 (1951)
8. Wilcoxon, F.: Individual comparisons by ranking methods. Biometrics Bull. **1**, 80–83 (1945)

Chapter 8
Completely-Randomized Designs

Abstract This chapter introduces permutation methods for multiple independent variables; that is, completely-randomized designs. Included in this chapter are six example analyses illustrating computation of exact permutation probability values for multi-sample tests, calculation of measures of effect size for multi-sample tests, the effect of extreme values on conventional and permutation multi-sample tests, exact and Monte Carlo permutation procedures for multi-sample tests, application of permutation methods to multi-sample rank-score data, and analysis of multi-sample multivariate data. Included in this chapter are permutation versions of Fisher's F test for one-way, completely-randomized analysis of variance, the Kruskal–Wallis one-way analysis of variance for ranks, the Bartlett–Nanda–Pillai trace test for multivariate analysis of variance, and a permutation-based alternative for the four conventional measures of effect size for multi-sample tests: Cohen's $\hat{d}$, Pearson's η^2, Kelley's $\hat{\eta}^2$, and Hays' $\hat{\omega}^2$.

This chapter presents exact and Monte Carlo permutation statistical methods for multi-sample tests. Multi-sample tests are of two types: tests for experimental differences among three or more independent samples (completely-randomized designs) and tests for experimental differences among three or more dependent samples (randomized-blocks designs).[1] Permutation statistical methods for multiple dependent samples are presented in Chap. 9. Permutation statistical methods for multiple independent samples are presented in this chapter. In addition there are mixed models with one or more independent samples and one or more dependent samples, but these models are beyond the scope of this introductory book on permutation statistical methods. Interested readers can consult a 2016 book on *Permutation Statistical Methods: An Integrated Approach* by the authors [2].

Multi-sample tests for independent samples constitute a large family of tests in conventional statistical methods. Included in this family are one-way analysis of variance with univariate responses (ANOVA), one-way analysis of variance with

---

[1]In some disciplines tests on multiple independent samples are known as between-subjects tests and tests for multiple dependent or related samples are known as within-subjects tests.

© Springer Nature Switzerland AG 2019

K. J. Berry et al., *A Primer of Permutation Statistical Methods*,
https://doi.org/10.1007/978-3-030-20933-9_8

multivariate responses (MANOVA), one-way analysis of variance with one or more covariates and univariate responses (ANCOVA), one-way analysis of variance with one or more covariates and multivariate responses (MANCOVA), and a variety of factorial designs that may be two-way, three-way, four-way, nested, balanced, unbalanced, fixed, random, or mixed.

In this chapter, permutation statistical methods for multiple independent samples are illustrated with six example analyses. The first example utilizes a small set of data to illustrate the computation of exact permutation methods for multiple independent samples, wherein the permutation test statistic, δ, is developed and compared with Fisher's conventional F-ratio test statistic. The second example develops a permutation-based measure of effect size as a chance-corrected alternative to the five conventional measures of effect size for multi-sample tests: Cohen's $\hat{d}$, Pearson's η^2, Kelley's $\hat{\eta}^2$, Hays' $\hat{\omega}_F^2$ for fixed models, and Hays' $\hat{\omega}_R^2$ for random models. The third example compares permutation statistical methods based on ordinary and squared Euclidean scaling functions, with an emphasis on the analysis of data sets containing extreme values. The fourth example utilizes a larger data set to provide a comparison of exact permutation methods and Monte Carlo permutation methods, demonstrating the efficiency and accuracy of Monte Carlo statistical methods for multi-sample tests. The fifth example illustrates the application of permutation statistical methods to univariate rank-score data, comparing permutation statistical methods to the conventional Kruskal–Wallis one-way analysis of variance for ranks test. The sixth example illustrates the application of permutation statistical methods to multivariate data, comparing permutation statistical methods with the conventional Bartlett–Nanda–Pillai trace test for multivariate data.

8.1 Introduction

The most popular univariate test for $g \geq 3$ independent samples under the Neyman–Pearson population model of statistical inference is Fisher's one-way analysis of variance wherein the null hypothesis (H_0) posits no mean differences among the g populations from which the samples are presumed to have been randomly drawn; that is, H_0: $\mu_1 = \mu_2 = \cdots = \mu_g$. It should be noted that Fisher, writing in the first edition of *Statistical Methods for Research Workers* in 1925, named the aforementioned statistic the variance-ratio test, symbolized it as z, and defined it as

$$z = \frac{1}{2} \log_e \left(\frac{\nu_1}{\nu_0} \right) ,$$

where $\nu_1 = MS_{\text{Between}}$ and $\nu_0 = MS_{\text{Within}}$ in modern notation. In 1934, in an effort to eliminate the calculation of the natural logarithm required for calculating Fisher's z test, George Snedecor at Iowa State University published tabled values in a small monograph for Fisher's variance-ratio z statistic and renamed the test statistic F, presumably in honor of Fisher [22]. It has often been reported that Fisher was displeased when the variance-ratio z test statistic was renamed F by Snedecor [4, 8].

Fisher's F-ratio test for a completely-randomized design does not determine whether or not the null hypothesis is true, but only provides the probability that, if the null hypothesis is true, the samples have been drawn from populations with identical mean values, assuming normality and homogeneity of variance.

Consider a conventional multi-sample F test with samples of independent and identically distributed univariate random variables of sizes $n_1, \ldots, n_g$, viz.,

$$\{x_{11}, \ldots, x_{n_1 1}\}, \ldots, \{x_{1g}, \ldots, x_{n_g g}\},$$

drawn from g specified populations with cumulative distribution functions $F_1(x), \ldots, F_g(x)$, respectively. For simplicity, suppose that population i is normal with mean μ_i and variance σ^2 for $i = 1, \ldots, g$. This is the standard one-way classification model with g treatment groups. Under the Neyman–Pearson population model of statistical inference, the null hypothesis of no differences among the population means tests

$$H_0\text{: } \mu_1 = \mu_2 = \cdots = \mu_g \quad \text{versus} \quad H_1\text{: } \mu_i \neq \mu_j \quad \text{for some } i \neq j$$

for g treatment groups. The permissible probability of a type I error is denoted by α and if the observed value of Fisher's F-ratio test statistic is equal to or greater than the critical value of F that defines α, the null hypothesis is rejected with a probability of type I error equal to or less than α, under the assumptions of normality and homogeneity.

For multi-sample tests with g treatment groups and N observations, Fisher's F-ratio test statistic is given by

$$F = \frac{MS_{\text{Between}}}{MS_{\text{Within}}},$$

where the mean-square between treatments is given by[2]

$$MS_{\text{Between}} = \frac{SS_{\text{Between}}}{g - 1},$$

the sum-of-squares between treatments is given by

$$SS_{\text{Between}} = \sum_{i=1}^{g} n_i \left(\bar{x}_i - \bar{\bar{x}}\right)^2,$$

---

[2]The terms MS_{Between} and MS_{Within} are only one set of descriptive labels for the numerator and denominator of the F-ratio test statistic. MS_{Between} is often replaced by either $MS_{\text{Treatment}}$ or MS_{Factor} and MS_{Within} is often replaced by MS_{Error}.

the mean-square within treatments is given by

$$MS_{\text{Within}} = \frac{SS_{\text{Within}}}{N - g} ,$$

the sum-of-squares within treatments is given by

$$SS_{\text{Within}} = \sum_{i=1}^{g} \sum_{j=1}^{n_i} \left(x_{ij} - \bar{x}_i \right)^2 ,$$

the sum-of-squares total is given by

$$SS_{\text{Total}} = SS_{\text{Between}} + SS_{\text{Within}} = \sum_{i=1}^{g} \sum_{j=1}^{n_i} \left(x_{ij} - \bar{\bar{x}} \right)^2 ,$$

the mean value for the ith of g treatment groups is given by

$$\bar{x}_i = \frac{1}{n_i} \sum_{j=1}^{n_i} x_{ij} ,$$

the grand mean for all g treatment groups combined is given by

$$\bar{\bar{x}} = \frac{1}{N} \sum_{i=1}^{g} \sum_{j=1}^{n_i} x_{ij} ,$$

and the total number of observations is

$$N = \sum_{i=1}^{g} n_i .$$

Under the Neyman–Pearson null hypothesis, H_0: $\mu_1 = \mu_2 = \cdots = \mu_g$, test statistic F is asymptotically distributed as Snedecor's F distribution with $v_1 = g - 1$ degrees of freedom in the numerator and $v_2 = N - g$ degrees of freedom in the denominator. However, if any of the g populations is not normally distributed, then the distribution of test statistic F no longer follows Snedecor's F distribution with $v_1 = g - 1$ and $v_2 = N - g$ degrees of freedom.

The assumptions underlying Fisher's F-ratio test for multiple independent samples are (1) the observations are independent, (2) the data are random samples from well-defined, normally-distributed populations, and (3) homogeneity of variance; that is, $\sigma_1^2 = \sigma_2^2 = \cdots = \sigma_g^2$.

8.2 A Permutation Approach

Now consider a test for multiple independent samples under the Fisher–Pitman permutation model of statistical inference. Under the Fisher–Pitman permutation model there is no null hypothesis specifying population parameters. Instead the null hypothesis simply states that all possible arrangements of the observations occur with equal chance [10]. Also, there is no alternative hypothesis under the permutation model and no specified α level. Moreover, there is no requirement of random sampling, no degrees of freedom, no assumption of normality, and no assumption of homogeneity of variance.

A permutation alternative to the conventional F test for multiple independent samples is easily defined. The permutation test statistic for $g \geq 3$ independent samples is given by

$$\delta = \sum_{i=1}^{g} C_i \xi_i , \tag{8.1}$$

where $C_i > 0$ is a positive treatment-group weight for $i = 1, \ldots, g$,

$$\xi_i = \binom{n_i}{2}^{-1} \sum_{j=1}^{N-1} \sum_{k=j+1}^{N} \Delta(j,k) \Psi_i(\omega_j) \Psi_i(\omega_k) \tag{8.2}$$

is the average distance-function value for all distinct pairs of objects in sample S_i for $i = 1, \ldots, g$,

$$\Delta(j,k) = |x_j - x_k|^v$$

denotes a symmetric distance-function value for a single pair of objects,

$$N = \sum_{i=1}^{g} n_i ,$$

and $\Psi(\cdot)$ is an indicator function given by

$$\Psi_i(\omega_j) = \begin{cases} 1 & \text{if } \omega_j \in S_i , \\ 0 & \text{otherwise} . \end{cases}$$

Under the Fisher–Pitman permutation model, the null hypothesis simply states that equal probabilities are assigned to each of the

$$M = \frac{N!}{\displaystyle\prod_{i=1}^{g} n_i!} \tag{8.3}$$

possible, equally-likely allocations of the N objects to the g samples [10]. The probability value associated with an observed value of δ, say δ_0, is the probability under the null hypothesis of observing a value of δ as extreme or more extreme than δ_0. Thus, an exact probability value for δ_0 may be expressed as

$$P(\delta \le \delta_0 | H_0) = \frac{\text{number of } \delta \text{ values } \le \delta_0}{M} . \tag{8.4}$$

When M is large, an approximate probability value for δ may be obtained from a Monte Carlo permutation procedure, where

$$P(\delta \le \delta_0 | H_0) = \frac{\text{number of } \delta \text{ values } \le \delta_0}{L}$$

and L denotes the number of randomly-sampled test statistic values. Typically, L is set to a large number to ensure accuracy; for example, $L = 1{,}000{,}000$ [11].

8.3 The Relationship Between Statistics F and δ

When the null hypothesis under the Neyman–Pearson population model states $H_0\colon \mu_1 = \mu_2 = \cdots = \mu_g$, $v = 2$, and the treatment-group weights are given by

$$C_i = \frac{n_i - 1}{N - g}, \qquad i = 1, \ldots, g,$$

the functional relationships between test statistic δ and Fisher's F-ratio test statistic are given by

$$\delta = \frac{2SS_{\text{Total}}}{N - g + (g - 1)F} \quad \text{and} \quad F = \frac{2SS_{\text{Total}}}{(g - 1)\delta} - \frac{N - g}{g - 1}, \tag{8.5}$$

where

$$SS_{\text{Total}} = \sum_{i=1}^{N} x_i^2 - \left(\sum_{i=1}^{N} x_i \right)^2 \Big/ N ,$$

and x_i is a univariate measurement score for the ith of N objects. The permutation analogue of the F test is generally known as the Fisher–Pitman permutation test [3].

Because of the relationship between test statistics δ and F, the exact probability values given by

$$P(\delta \le \delta_0 | H_0) = \frac{\text{number of } \delta \text{ values } \le \delta_0}{M}$$

and

$$P\left(F \geq F_o | H_0\right) = \frac{\text{number of } F \text{ values } \geq F_o}{M}$$

are equivalent under the Fisher–Pitman null hypothesis, where δ_o and F_o denote the observed values of δ and F, respectively, and M is the number of possible, equally-likely arrangements of the observed data.

A chance-corrected measure of agreement among the N measurement scores is given by

$$\Re = 1 - \frac{\delta}{\mu_\delta} , \tag{8.6}$$

where μ_δ is the arithmetic average of the M δ test statistic values calculated on all possible arrangements of the observed measurements; that is,

$$\mu_\delta = \frac{1}{M} \sum_{i=1}^{M} \delta_i . \tag{8.7}$$

Alternatively, in terms of a one-way analysis of variance model, the exact expected value of test statistic δ is a simple function of the total sum-of-squares; that is,

$$\mu_\delta = \frac{2SS_{\text{Total}}}{N - 1} .$$

8.4 Example 1: Test Statistics F and δ

A small example will serve to illustrate the relationship between test statistics F and δ. Consider the example data listed in Table 8.1 with $g = 3$ treatment groups, sample sizes of $n_1 = n_2 = 3$, $n_3 = 4$, and $N = n_1 + n_2 + n_3 = 3 + 3 + 4 = 10$ total observations. Under the Neyman–Pearson population model with sample sizes $n_1 = n_2 = 3$, and $n_3 = 4$, treatment-group means $\bar{x}_1 = 3$, $\bar{x}_2 = 4$, and $\bar{x}_3 = 8$, grand mean $\bar{\bar{x}} = 5.30$, estimated population variances $s_1^2 = s_2^2 = 1.00$ and

Table 8.1 Example data for a test of $g = 3$ independent samples with $N = 10$ observations

Treatment group		
1	2	3
2	3	7
3	4	8
4	5	8
		9

$s_3^2 = 0.6667$, the sum-of-squares between treatments is

$$SS_{\text{Between}} = \sum_{i=1}^{g} n_i (\bar{x}_i - \bar{\bar{x}})^2 = 50.10 ,$$

the sum-of-squares within treatments is

$$SS_{\text{Within}} = \sum_{i=1}^{g} \sum_{j=1}^{n_i} (x_{ij} - \bar{x}_i)^2 = 6.00 ,$$

the sum-of-squares total is

$$SS_{\text{Total}} = SS_{\text{Between}} + SS_{\text{Within}} = 50.10 + 6.00 = 56.10 ,$$

the mean-square between treatments is

$$MS_{\text{Between}} = \frac{SS_{\text{Between}}}{g - 1} = \frac{50.10}{3 - 1} = 25.05 ,$$

the mean-square within treatments is

$$MS_{\text{Within}} = \frac{SS_{\text{Within}}}{N - g} = \frac{6.00}{10 - 3} = 0.8571 ,$$

and the observed value of Fisher's F-ratio test statistic is

$$F = \frac{MS_{\text{Between}}}{MS_{\text{Within}}} = \frac{25.05}{0.8571} = 29.2250 .$$

The essential factors, sums of squares (SS), degrees of freedom (df), mean squares (MS), and variance-ratio test statistic (F) are summarized in Table 8.2.

Under the Neyman–Pearson null hypothesis, H_0: $\mu_1 = \mu_2 = \mu_3$, Fisher's F-ratio test statistic is asymptotically distributed as Snedecor's F with $v_1 = g - 1$ and $v_2 = N - g$ degrees of freedom. With $v_1 = g - 1 = 3 - 1 = 2$ and $v_2 = N - g = 10 - 3 = 7$ degrees of freedom, the asymptotic probability value of $F = 29.2250$ is $P = 0.4001 \times 10^{-3}$, under the assumptions of normality and homogeneity.

Table 8.2 Source table for the example data listed in Table 8.1

Factor	SS	df	MS	F
Between	50.10	2	25.0500	29.2250
Within	6.00	7	0.8571	
Total	56.10			

8.4.1   An Exact Analysis with $v = 2$

For the first permutation analysis of the example data listed in Table 8.1 let $v = 2$, employing squared Euclidean scaling, and let the treatment-group weights be given by

$$C_i = \frac{n_i - 1}{N - g}, \qquad i = 1, \ldots, g,$$

for correspondence with Fisher's F-ratio test statistic.

Because there are only

$$M = \frac{N!}{\displaystyle\prod_{i=1}^{g} n_i!} = \frac{10!}{3! \, 3! \, 4!} = 4200$$

possible, equally-likely arrangements in the reference set of all permutations of the $N = 10$ observations listed in Table 8.1, an exact permutation analysis is feasible. While $M = 4200$ arrangements are too many to list, Table 8.3 illustrates the calculation of the ξ, δ, and F values for a small sample of the M possible arrangements of the $N = 10$ observations listed in Table 8.1.

Following Eq. (8.1) on p. 261, the $N = 10$ observations yield $g = 3$ average distance-function values of

$$\xi_i = \xi_2 = 2.00 \quad \text{and} \quad \xi_3 = 1.3333.$$

Alternatively, in terms of a one-way analysis of variance model the average distance-function values are $\xi_1 = 2s_1^2 = 2(1.00) = 2.00$, $\xi_2 = 2s_2^2 = 2(1.00) = 2.00$, and $\xi_3 = 2s_3^2 = 2(0.6667) = 1.3333$.

Following Eq. (8.1) on p. 260, the observed value of the permutation test statistic based on $v = 2$ and treatment-group weights

$$C_i = \frac{n_i - 1}{N - g}, \qquad i = 1, 2, 3,$$

is

$$\delta = \sum_{i=1}^{g} C_i \xi_i = \frac{1}{10 - 3} \big[(3 - 1)(2.00) + (3 - 1)(2.00)$$

$$+ (4 - 1)(1.3333) \big] = 1.7143.$$

Table 8.3 Sample arrangements of the example data listed in Table 8.1 with associated ξ_1, ξ_2, δ, and F values

Number	Arrangement	ξ_1	ξ_2	ξ_3	δ	F
1	234 345 7889	2.0000	2.0000	1.3333	1.7143	29.2250
2	234 347 5889	2.0000	8.6667	6.0000	5.6190	6.4839
3	234 347 4889	2.0000	8.6667	9.8333	7.2619	4.4318
4	234 457 3889	2.0000	4.6667	14.6667	8.1905	3.3494
5	234 348 5789	2.0000	14.0000	5.8333	7.0714	4.4333
6	234 358 4789	2.0000	12.6667	9.3333	8.1905	3.3494
7	234 458 3789	2.0000	8.6667	13.8333	8.9762	2.7499
8	234 378 4589	2.0000	14.0000	11.3333	9.4286	2.4500
9	234 478 3589	2.0000	8.6667	15.1667	9.5476	2.3758
10	234 578 3489	2.0000	4.6667	17.3333	9.3333	2.5107
11	234 348 5789	2.0000	14.0000	5.8333	7.0714	4.4333
12	234 358 4789	2.0000	12.6667	9.3333	8.1905	3.3494
13	234 458 3789	2.0000	8.6667	13.8333	8.9762	2.7499
14	234 378 4589	2.0000	14.0000	11.3333	9.4286	2.4500
15	234 478 3589	2.0000	8.6667	15.1667	9.5476	2.3758
16	234 578 3489	2.0000	4.6667	17.3333	9.3333	2.5107
17	234 488 4579	2.0000	10.6667	9.8333	7.8333	3.1894
18	234 488 3579	2.0000	10.6667	13.3333	9.3333	2.5107
19	234 588 3479	2.0000	6.0000	15.1667	8.7857	2.8854
20	234 788 3459	2.0000	0.6667	13.8333	6.6905	4.8851
⋮	⋮ ⋮ ⋮	⋮	⋮	⋮	⋮	⋮
4199	889 357 2344	0.6667	8.0000	1.8333	3.2619	13.6985
4200	889 457 2343	0.6667	4.6667	1.3333	2.0952	23.2750

Alternatively, in terms of a one-way analysis of variance model the permutation test statistic is

$$\delta = 2MS_{\text{Within}} = 2(0.8571) = 1.7143 .$$

For the example data listed in Table 8.1, the sum of the $N = 10$ observations is

$$\sum_{i=1}^{N} x_i = 2 + 3 + 4 + 3 + 4 + 5 + 7 + 8 + 8 + 9 = 53 ,$$

the sum of the $N = 10$ squared observations is

$$\sum_{i=1}^{N} x_i^2 = 2^2 + 3^2 + 4^2 + 3^2 + 4^2 + 5^2 + 7^2 + 8^2 + 8^2 + 9^2 = 337 ,$$

and the total sum-of-squares is

$$SS_{\text{Total}} = \sum_{i=1}^{N} \left(x_i - \bar{\bar{x}}\right)^2 = \sum_{i=1}^{N} x_i^2 - \left(\sum_{i=1}^{N} x_i\right)^2 \bigg/ N$$

$$= 337 - (53)^2/10 = 56.10 ,$$

where $\bar{\bar{x}}$ denotes the grand mean of all $N = 10$ observations. Then following the expressions given in Eq. (8.5) on p. 262 for test statistics δ and F, the observed value of test statistic δ with respect to test statistic F is

$$\delta = \frac{2SS_{\text{Total}}}{N - g + (g-1)F} = \frac{2(56.10)}{10 - 3 + (3-1)(29.2250)} = 1.7143$$

and the observed value of test statistic F with respect to test statistic δ is

$$F = \frac{2SS_{\text{Total}}}{(g-1)\delta} - \frac{N-g}{g-1} = \frac{2(56.10)}{(3-1)(1.7143)} - \frac{10-3}{3-1} = 29.2250 .$$

Under the Fisher–Pitman permutation model, the exact probability of an observed δ is the proportion of δ test statistic values computed on all possible, equally-likely arrangements of the $N = 10$ observations listed in Table 8.1 that are equal to or less than the observed value of $\delta = 1.7143$. There are exactly 10 δ test statistic values that are equal to or less than the observed value of $\delta = 1.7143$. If all M arrangements of the $N = 10$ observations listed in Table 8.1 occur with equal chance under the Fisher–Pitman null hypothesis, the exact probability value of $\delta = 1.7143$ computed on all $M = 4200$ arrangements of the observed data with $n_1 = n_2 = 3$ and $n_3 = 4$ preserved for each arrangement is

$$P\left(\delta \leq \delta_0 | H_0\right) = \frac{\text{number of } \delta \text{ values } \leq \delta_0}{M} = \frac{10}{4200} = 0.2381 \times 10^{-2} ,$$

where δ_0 denotes the observed value of test statistic δ and M is the number of possible, equally-likely arrangements of the $N = 10$ observations listed in Table 8.1.

Alternatively, there are only 10 F values that are larger than the observed value of $F = 29.2250$. Thus, if all arrangements of the observed data occur with equal chance, the exact probability value of $F = 29.2250$ under the Fisher–Pitman null hypothesis is

$$P\left(F \geq F_0 | H_0\right) = \frac{\text{number of } F \text{ values } \geq F_0}{M} = \frac{10}{4200} = 0.2381 \times 10^{-2} ,$$

where F_0 denotes the observed value of test statistic F.

Following Eq. (8.7) on p. 263, the exact expected value of the $M = 4200\,\delta$ test statistic values under the Fisher–Pitman null hypothesis is

$$\mu_\delta = \frac{1}{M}\sum_{i=1}^{M}\delta_i = \frac{52{,}360}{4200} = 12.4667 \ .$$

Alternatively, in terms of a one-way analysis of variance model the exact expected value of test statistic δ is

$$\mu_\delta = \frac{2SS_{\text{Total}}}{N-1} = \frac{2(56.10)}{10-1} = 12.4667 \ .$$

Following Eq. (8.6) on p. 263, the observed chance-corrected measure of effect size is

$$\Re = 1 - \frac{\delta}{\mu_\delta} = 1 - \frac{1.7143}{12.4667} = +0.8625 \ ,$$

indicating approximately 86% within-group agreement above what is expected by chance. Alternatively, in terms of a one-way analysis of variance model the chance-corrected measure of effect size is

$$\Re = 1 - \frac{\delta}{\mu_\delta} = 1 - \frac{2MS_{\text{Within}}}{\dfrac{2SS_{\text{Total}}}{N-1}} = 1 - \frac{(N-1)(MS_{\text{Within}})}{SS_{\text{Total}}}$$

$$= 1 - \frac{(10-1)(0.8571)}{56.10} = +0.8625 \ .$$

8.5   Example 2: Measures of Effect Size

Measures of effect size express the practical or clinical significance of differences among multiple independent sample means, as contrasted with the statistical significance of differences. Five measures of effect size are commonly used for determining the magnitude of treatment effects for multiple independent samples: Cohen's $\hat{d}$, Pearson's η^2, Kelley's $\hat{\eta}^2$, Hays' $\hat{\omega}_F^2$ for fixed models, and Hays' $\hat{\omega}_R^2$, for random models. Cohen's $\hat{d}$ measure of effect size is given by

$$\hat{d} = \left[\frac{1}{g-1}\left(\frac{SS_{\text{Between}}}{nMS_{\text{Within}}}\right)\right]^{1/2} = \left[\frac{F}{n}\right]^{1/2} \ ,$$

where n denotes the common size of each treatment group. Pearson's η^2 measure of effect size is given by

$$\eta^2 = \frac{SS_{\text{Between}}}{SS_{\text{Total}}} = 1 - \frac{N - g}{F(g - 1) + N - g} \ ,$$

which is equivalent to Pearson's r^2 for a one-way analysis of variance design. Kelley's "unbiased" correlation ratio is given by[3]

$$\hat{\eta}^2 = \frac{SS_{\text{Total}} - (N - 1)MS_{\text{Within}}}{SS_{\text{Total}}} = 1 - \frac{N - 1}{F(g - 1) + N - g} \ ,$$

which is equivalent to an adjusted or "shrunken" squared multiple correlation coefficient reported by most computer statistical packages and given by

$$\hat{\eta}^2 = R_{\text{adj}}^2 = 1 - \frac{(1 - R^2)(N - 1)}{N - p - 1} \ ,$$

where R^2 is the squared product-moment multiple correlation coefficient and p is the number of predictors. Hays' $\hat{\omega}_F^2$ measure of effect size for a fixed-effects analysis of variance model is given by

$$\hat{\omega}_F^2 = \frac{SS_{\text{Between}} - (g - 1)MS_{\text{Within}}}{SS_{\text{Total}} + MS_{\text{Within}}} = 1 - \frac{N}{(F - 1)(g - 1) + N} \ .$$

Hays' $\hat{\omega}_R^2$ measure of effect size for a random-effects analysis of variance model is given by

$$\hat{\omega}_R^2 = \frac{MS_{\text{Between}} - MS_{\text{Within}}}{MS_{\text{Between}} + (n - 1)MS_{\text{Within}}} = 1 - \frac{n}{F + n - 1} \ ,$$

where n denotes the common size of each treatment group. Mielke and Berry's $\mathfrak{R}$ chance-corrected measure of effect size is given by

$$\mathfrak{R} = 1 - \frac{\delta}{\mu_\delta} \ ,$$

where δ is defined in Eq. (8.1) on p. 261 and μ_δ is the exact expected value of δ under the Fisher–Pitman null hypothesis given by

$$\mu_\delta = \frac{1}{M} \sum_{i=1}^{M} \delta_i \ ,$$

---

[3]It is well known that Kelley's correlation ratio is not unbiased, but since the title of Truman Kelley's 1935 article was "An unbiased correlation ratio measure," the label has persisted.

where, for a test of $g \geq 3$ independent samples, the number of possible, equally-likely arrangements of the observed data is given by

$$M = \frac{N!}{\displaystyle\prod_{i=1}^{g} n_i!} \; .$$

For the example data listed in Table 8.1 on p. 263 for $N = 10$ observations, Cohen's $\hat{d}$ measure of effect size is[4]

$$\hat{d} = \left[\frac{1}{g-1} \left(\frac{SS_{\text{Between}}}{\bar{n} MS_{\text{Within}}} \right) \right]^{1/2} = \left[\frac{F}{\bar{n}} \right]^{1/2} = \left[\frac{29.2250}{3.3333} \right]^{1/2} = \pm 2.9610 \; .$$

Pearson's r^2 measure of effect size is usually labeled as η^2 when reported with an analysis of variance. For the example data listed in Table 8.1, η^2 is

$$\eta^2 = \frac{SS_{\text{Between}}}{SS_{\text{Total}}} = 1 - \frac{N-g}{F(g-1)+N-g}$$

$$= 1 - \frac{10-3}{(29.2250)(3-1)+10-3} = 0.8930 \; ,$$

Kelley's $\hat{\eta}^2$ measure of effect size is

$$\hat{\eta}^2 = \frac{SS_{\text{Total}} - (N-1)MS_{\text{Within}}}{SS_{\text{Total}}} = 1 - \frac{N-1}{F(g-1)+N-g}$$

$$= 1 - \frac{10-1}{(29.2250)(3-1)+10-3} = 0.8625 \; ,$$

Hays' $\hat{\omega}_F^2$ measure of effect size for a fixed-effects analysis of variance model is

$$\hat{\omega}_F^2 = \frac{SS_{\text{Between}} - (g-1)MS_{\text{Within}}}{SS_{\text{Total}} + MS_{\text{Within}}} = 1 - \frac{N}{(F-1)(g-1)+N}$$

$$= 1 - \frac{10}{(29.2250-1)(3-1)+10} = 0.8495 \; ,$$

----

[4]Since the sizes of the treatment groups are not equal, the average value of $\bar{n} = 3.3333$ is used for both Cohen's $\hat{d}$ measure of effect size and Hays' $\hat{\omega}_R^2$ measure of effect size for a random-effects model. In cases where the treatment-group sizes differ greatly, a weighted average recommended by Haggard is often adopted [6].

Hays' $\hat{\omega}_R^2$ measure of effect size for a random-effects analysis of variance model is[5]

$$\hat{\omega}_R^2 = \frac{MS_{\text{Between}} - MS_{\text{Within}}}{MS_{\text{Between}} + (\bar{n} - 1)MS_{\text{Within}}} = 1 - \frac{\bar{n}}{F + \bar{n} - 1}$$

$$= 1 - \frac{3.3333}{29.2250 + 3.3333 - 1} = 0.8944 ,$$

and Mielke and Berry's $\mathfrak{R}$ chance-corrected measure of effect size is

$$\mathfrak{R} = 1 - \frac{\delta}{\mu_\delta} = 1 - \frac{1.7143}{12.4667} = +0.8625 ,$$

where the exact expected value of test statistic δ under the Fisher–Pitman null hypothesis is

$$\mu_\delta = \frac{1}{M} \sum_{i=1}^{M} \delta_i = \frac{52,360}{4200} = 12.4667 .$$

It can easily be shown that Mielke and Berry's $\mathfrak{R}$ chance-corrected measure of effect size is identical to Kelley's $\hat{\eta}^2$ measure of effect size for a one-way, completely-randomized analysis of variance design, under the Neyman–Pearson population model.

8.5.1 Comparisons of Effect Size Measures

In this section the various measures of effect size are compared and contrasted. Because Pearson's r^2 and η^2 are equivalent and Kelley's $\hat{\eta}^2$ and Mielke and Berry's $\mathfrak{R}$ are equivalent for multi-sample designs, only η^2 and $\mathfrak{R}$ are utilized for the comparisons. The functional relationships between Cohen's $\hat{d}$ measure of effect size and Pearson's η^2 (r^2) measure of effect size for $g \geq 3$ independent samples are given by

$$\hat{d} = \left[\frac{\eta^2(N - g)}{n(g - 1)(1 - \eta^2)} \right]^{1/2} \quad \text{and} \quad \eta^2 = 1 - \frac{N - g}{n\hat{d}^2(g - 1) + N - g} , \tag{8.8}$$

where n denotes the common treatment-group size. The relationships between Cohen's $\hat{d}$ measure of effect size and Mielke and Berry's $\mathfrak{R}$ $(\hat{\eta}^2)$ chance-corrected

---

[5]For a one-way completely-randomized analysis of variance, a fixed-effects model and a random-effects model yield the same F-ratio, but measures of effect size can differ under the two models.

measure of effect size are given by

$$\hat{d} = \left[\frac{\Re(N - g) + g - 1}{n(g - 1)(1 - \Re)} \right]^{1/2} \quad \text{and} \quad \Re = 1 - \frac{N - 1}{n\hat{d}^2(g - 1) + N - g} \,. \tag{8.9}$$

The relationships between Cohen's $\hat{d}$ measure of effect size and Hays' $\hat{\omega}_F^2$ measure of effect size for a fixed-effects model are given by

$$\hat{d} = \left[\frac{(N - g + 1)\hat{\omega}_F^2 + g - 1}{n(g - 1)(1 - \hat{\omega}_F^2)} \right]^{1/2} \tag{8.10}$$

and

$$\hat{\omega}_F^2 = 1 - \frac{N}{(n\hat{d}^2 - 1)(g - 1) + N} \,. \tag{8.11}$$

The relationships between Cohen's $\hat{d}$ measure of effect size and Hays' $\hat{\omega}_R^2$ measure of effect size for a random-effects model are given by

$$\hat{d} = \left[\frac{\hat{\omega}_R^2(n - 1) + 1}{n(1 - \hat{\omega}_R^2)} \right]^{1/2} \quad \text{and} \quad \hat{\omega}_R^2 = 1 - \frac{n}{n(\hat{d}^2 + 1) - 1} \,. \tag{8.12}$$

The relationships between Pearson's η^2 (r^2) measure of effect size and Mielke and Berry's $\Re$ ($\hat{\eta}^2$) measure of effect size are given by

$$\eta^2 = 1 - \frac{(N - g)(1 - \Re)}{N - 1} \quad \text{and} \quad \Re = 1 - \frac{(N - 1)(1 - \eta^2)}{N - g} \,. \tag{8.13}$$

The relationships between Pearson's η^2 (r^2) measure of effect size and Hays' $\hat{\omega}_F^2$ measure of effect size for a fixed-effects model are given by

$$\eta^2 = \frac{(N - g + 1)\hat{\omega}_F^2 + g - 1}{N + \hat{\omega}_F^2 - 1} \tag{8.14}$$

and

$$\hat{\omega}_F^2 = \frac{\eta^2(N - 1) - g + 1}{N - \eta^2 - g + 1} \,. \tag{8.15}$$

The relationships between Pearson's η^2 (r^2) measure of effect size and Hays' $\hat{\omega}_R^2$ measure of effect size for a random-effects model are given by

$$\eta^2 = 1 - \frac{(N - g)(1 - \hat{\omega}_R^2)}{(g - 1)[\hat{\omega}_R^2(n - 1) + 1] + (N - g)(1 - \hat{\omega}_R^2)} \tag{8.16}$$

and

$$\hat{\omega}_R^2 = \frac{\eta^2(N - 1) - g + 1}{(N - g)\eta^2 + (g - 1)(1 - \eta^2)(n - 1)} . \tag{8.17}$$

The relationships between Mielke and Berry's $\mathfrak{R}$ ($\hat{\eta}^2$) measure of effect size and Hays' $\hat{\omega}_F^2$ measure of effect size for a fixed-effects model are given by

$$\mathfrak{R} = \frac{N\hat{\omega}_F^2}{N + \hat{\omega}_F^2 - 1} \quad \text{and} \quad \hat{\omega}_F^2 = \frac{\mathfrak{R}(N - 1)}{N - \mathfrak{R}} . \tag{8.18}$$

The relationships between Mielke and Berry's $\mathfrak{R}$ ($\hat{\eta}^2$) measure of effect size and Hays' $\hat{\omega}_R^2$ measure of effect size for a random-effects model are given by

$$\mathfrak{R} = 1 - \frac{(N - 1)(1 - \hat{\omega}_R^2)}{n\hat{\omega}_R^2(g - 1) + (N - 1))(1 - \hat{\omega}_R^2)} \tag{8.19}$$

and

$$\hat{\omega}_R^2 = \frac{\hat{\eta}^2(N - 1)}{N\mathfrak{R} - 1 + (1 - \mathfrak{R})[n(g - 1) + 1]} . \tag{8.20}$$

And the relationships between Hays' $\hat{\omega}_F^2$ measure of effect size for a fixed-effects model and Hays' $\hat{\omega}_R^2$ measure of effect size for a random-effects model are given by

$$\hat{\omega}_F^2 = \frac{n\hat{\omega}_R^2(g - 1)}{n\hat{\omega}_R^2 + N(1 - \hat{\omega}_R^2)} \quad \text{and} \quad \hat{\omega}_R^2 = \frac{N\hat{\omega}_F^2}{N\hat{\omega}_F^2 - n(g - 1)(1 - \hat{\omega}_F^2)} . \tag{8.21}$$

8.5.2 Example Comparisons of Effect Size Measures

In this section comparisons of Cohen's $\hat{d}$, Pearson's η^2, Mielke and Berry's $\mathfrak{R}$, Hays' $\hat{\omega}_F^2$, and Hays' $\hat{\omega}_R^2$ measures of effect size are illustrated with the example data listed in Table 8.1 on p. 263 with $n_1 = n_2 = 3$, $n_3 = 4$, and $N = n_1 + n_2 + n_3 = 3 + 3 + 4 = 10$ observations. Because the treatment-group sizes are unequal, the

ns in the equations for Cohen's $\hat{d}$ and Hays' $\hat{\omega}_R^2$ are replaced with a simple average; that is, $\bar{n} = (3 + 3 + 4)/3 = 3.3333$.

Given the example data listed in Table 8.1 and following the expressions given in Eq. (8.8) for Cohen's $\hat{d}$ measure of effect size and Pearson's η^2 (r^2) measure of effect size, the observed value for Cohen's $\hat{d}$ measure of effect size with respect to the observed value of Pearson's η^2 (r^2) measure of effect size is

$$\hat{d} = \left[\frac{\eta^2(N - g)}{\bar{n}(g - 1)(1 - \eta^2)} \right]^{1/2} = \left[\frac{(0.8930)(10 - 3)}{(3.3333)(3 - 1)(1 - 0.8930)} \right]^{1/2} = \pm 2.9610$$

and the observed value for Pearson's η^2 (r^2) measure of effect size with respect to the observed value of Cohen's $\hat{d}$ measure of effect size is

$$\eta^2 = 1 - \frac{N - g}{\bar{n}\hat{d}^2(g - 1) + N - g}$$

$$= 1 - \frac{10 - 3}{(3.3333)(2.9610)^2(3 - 1) + 10 - 3} = 0.8930 .$$

Following the expressions given in Eq. (8.9) for Cohen's $\hat{d}$ measure of effect size and Mielke and Berry's $\Re$ ($\hat{\eta}^2$) measure of effect size, the observed value for Cohen's $\hat{d}$ measure of effect size with respect to the observed value of Mielke and Berry's $\Re$ ($\hat{\eta}^2$) measure of effect size is

$$\hat{d} = \left[\frac{\Re(N - g) + g - 1}{\bar{n}(g - 1)(1 - \Re)} \right]^{1/2}$$

$$= \left[\frac{0.8625(10 - 3) + 3 - 1}{(3.3333)(3 - 1)(1 - 0.8625)} \right]^{1/2} = \pm 2.9610$$

and the observed value for Mielke and Berry's $\Re$ ($\hat{\eta}^2$) measure of effect size with respect to the observed value of Cohen's $\hat{d}$ measure of effect size is

$$\Re = 1 - \frac{N - 1}{\bar{n}\hat{d}^2(g - 1) + N - g}$$

$$= 1 - \frac{10 - 1}{(3.3333)(2.9610)^2(3 - 1) + 10 - 3} = +0.8625 .$$

Following the expressions given in Eqs. (8.10) and (8.11) for Cohen's $\hat{d}$ measure of effect size and Hays' $\hat{\omega}_F^2$ measure of effect size for a fixed-effects model, the observed value for Cohen's $\hat{d}$ measure of effect size with respect to the observed value of Hays' $\hat{\omega}_F^2$ measure of effect size is

$$\hat{d} = \left[\frac{(N - g + 1)\hat{\omega}_F^2 + g - 1}{\bar{n}(g - 1)(1 - \hat{\omega}_F^2)} \right]^{1/2}$$

$$= \left[\frac{(10 - 3 + 1)(0.8495) + 3 - 1}{(3.3333)(3 - 1)(1 - 0.8495)} \right]^{1/2} = \pm 2.9610$$

and the observed value for Hays' $\hat{\omega}_F^2$ measure of effect size with respect to the observed value of Cohen's $\hat{d}$ measure of effect size is

$$\hat{\omega}_F^2 = 1 - \frac{N}{(\bar{n}\hat{d}^2 - 1)(g - 1) + N}$$

$$= 1 - \frac{10}{[(3.3333)(2.9610)^2 - 1](3 - 1) + 10} = 0.8495 .$$

Following the expressions given in Eq. (8.12) for Cohen's $\hat{d}$ measure of effect size and Hays' $\hat{\omega}_R^2$ measure of effect size for a random-effects model, the observed value for Cohen's $\hat{d}$ measure of effect size with respect to the observed value of Hays' $\hat{\omega}_R^2$ measure of effect size is

$$\hat{d} = \left[\frac{\hat{\omega}_R^2(\bar{n} - 1) + 1}{\bar{n}(1 - \hat{\omega}_R^2)} \right]^{1/2} = \left[\frac{(0.8944)(3.3333 - 1) + 1}{(3.3333)(1 - 0.8944)} \right]^{1/2} = \pm 2.9610$$

and the observed value of Hays' $\hat{\omega}_R^2$ measure of effect size with respect to the observed value of Cohen's $\hat{d}$ measure of effect size is

$$\hat{\omega}_R^2 = 1 - \frac{\bar{n}}{\bar{n}(\hat{d}^2 + 1) - 1} = 1 - \frac{3.3333}{(3.3333)[(2.9610)^2 + 1] - 1} = 0.8944 .$$

Following the expressions given in Eq. (8.13) for Pearson's η^2 (r^2) measure of effect size and Mielke and Berry's $\Re$ $(\hat{\eta}^2)$ measure of effect size, the observed value for Pearson's η^2 (r^2) measure of effect size with respect to the observed value of Mielke and Berry's $\Re$ $(\hat{\eta}^2)$ measure of effect size is

$$\eta^2 = 1 - \frac{(N - g)(1 - \Re)}{N - 1} = 1 - \frac{(10 - 3)(1 - 0.8625)}{10 - 1} = 0.8930$$

and the observed value for Mielke and Berry's $\Re$ $(\hat{\eta}^2)$ measure of effect size with respect to the observed value of Pearson's η^2 (r^2) measure of effect size is

$$\Re = 1 - \frac{(N - 1)(1 - \eta^2)}{N - g} = 1 - \frac{(10 - 1)(1 - 0.8930)}{10 - 3} = +0.8625 .$$

Following the expressions given in Eqs. (8.14) and (8.15) for Pearson's η^2 (r^2) measure of effect size and Hays' $\hat{\omega}_F^2$ measure of effect size for a fixed-effects model, the observed value for Pearson's η^2 (r^2) measure of effect size with respect to the observed value of Hays' $\hat{\omega}_F^2$ measure of effect size is

$$\eta^2 = \frac{(N - g + 1)\hat{\omega}_F^2 + g - 1}{N + \hat{\omega}_F^2 - 1} = \frac{(10 - 3 + 1)(0.8495) + 3 - 1}{10 + 0.8495 - 1} = 0.8930$$

and the observed value for Hays' $\hat{\omega}_F^2$ measure of effect size with respect to the observed value of Pearson's η^2 (r^2) measure of effect size is

$$\hat{\omega}_F^2 = \frac{\eta^2(N - 1) - g + 1}{N - \eta^2 - g + 1} = \frac{(0.8930)(10 - 1) - 3 + 1}{10 - 0.8930 - 3 + 1} = 0.8495 \ .$$

Following the expressions given in Eqs. (8.16) and (8.17) for Pearson's η^2 (r^2) measure of effect size and Hays' $\hat{\omega}_R^2$ measure of effect size for a random-effects model, the observed value for Pearson's η^2 (r^2) measure of effect size with respect to the observed value of Hays' $\hat{\omega}_R^2$ measure of effect size is

$$
\begin{aligned}
\eta^2 &= 1 - \frac{(N - g)(1 - \hat{\omega}_R^2)}{(g - 1)[\hat{\omega}_R^2(\bar{n} - 1) + 1] + (N - g)(1 - \hat{\omega}_R^2)} \\
&= 1 - \frac{(10 - 3)(1 - 0.8944)}{(3 - 1)[(0.8944)(3.3333 - 1) + 1] + (10 - 3)(1 - 0.8944)} \\
&= 0.8930
\end{aligned}
$$

and the observed value for Hays' $\hat{\omega}_R^2$ measure of effect size with respect to the observed value of Pearson's η^2 (r^2) measure of effect size is

$$
\begin{aligned}
\hat{\omega}_R^2 &= \frac{\eta^2(N - 1) - g + 1}{(N - g)\eta^2 + (g - 1)(1 - \eta^2)(\bar{n} - 1)} \\
&= \frac{0.8930(10 - 1) - 3 + 1}{(10 - 3)(0.8930) + (3 - 1)(1 - 0.8930)(3.3333 - 1)} = 0.8944 \ .
\end{aligned}
$$

Following the expressions given in Eq. (8.18) for Mielke and Berry's $\mathfrak{R}$ ($\hat{\eta}^2$) measure of effect size and Hays' $\hat{\omega}_F^2$ measure of effect size for a fixed-effects model, the observed value for Mielke and Berry's $\mathfrak{R}$ ($\hat{\eta}^2$) measure of effect size with respect to the observed value of Hays' $\hat{\omega}_F^2$ measure of effect size is

$$\mathfrak{R} = \frac{N\hat{\omega}_F^2}{N + \hat{\omega}_F^2 - 1} = \frac{(10)(0.8495)}{10 + 0.8495 - 1} = +0.8625$$

and the observed value for Hays' $\hat{\omega}_F^2$ measure of effect size with respect to the observed value of Mielke and Berry's $\Re$ ($\hat{\eta}^2$) measure of effect size is

$$\hat{\omega}_F^2 = \frac{\Re(N-1)}{N-\Re} = \frac{(0.8625)(10-1)}{10-0.8625} = 0.8495 \ .$$

Following the expressions given in Eqs. (8.19) and (8.20) for Mielke and Berry's $\Re$ ($\hat{\eta}^2$) measure of effect size and Hays' $\hat{\omega}_R^2$ measure of effect size for a random-effects model, the observed value for Mielke and Berry's $\Re$ ($\hat{\eta}^2$) measure of effect size with respect to the observed value of Hays' $\hat{\omega}_R^2$ measure of effect size is

$$\Re = 1 - \frac{(N-1)(1-\hat{\omega}_R^2)}{\bar{n}\hat{\omega}_R^2(g-1)+(N-1)(1-\hat{\omega}_R^2)}$$

$$= 1 - \frac{(10-1)(1-0.8944)}{(3.3333)(0.8944)(3-1)+(10-1)(1-0.8944)} = +0.8625$$

and the observed value for Hays' $\hat{\omega}_R^2$ measure of effect size with respect to the observed value for Mielke and Berry's $\Re$ ($\hat{\eta}^2$) measure of effect size is

$$\hat{\omega}_R^2 = \frac{\hat{\eta}^2(N-1)}{N\Re - 1 + (1-\Re)[\bar{n}(g-1)+1]}$$

$$= \frac{(0.8625)(10-1)}{(10)(0.8625)-1+(1-0.8625)[(3.3333)(3-1)+1]} = 0.8944 \ .$$

Following the expressions given in Eq. (8.21) for Hays' $\hat{\omega}_F^2$ measure of effect size for a fixed-effects model and Hays' $\hat{\omega}_R^2$ measure of effect size for a random-effects model, the observed value for Hays' $\hat{\omega}_F^2$ measure of effect size with respect to the observed value of Hays' $\hat{\omega}_R^2$ measure of effect size is

$$\hat{\omega}_F^2 = \frac{\bar{n}\hat{\omega}_R^2(g-1)}{\bar{n}\hat{\omega}_R^2(g-1)+N(1-\hat{\omega}_R^2)}$$

$$= \frac{(3.3333)(0.8944)(3-1)}{(3.3333)(0.8944)(3-1)+(10)(1-0.8944)} = 0.8495$$

and the observed value for Hays' $\hat{\omega}_R^2$ measure of effect size with respect to the observed value of Hays' $\hat{\omega}_F^2$ measure of effect size is

$$\hat{\omega}_R^2 = \frac{N\hat{\omega}_F^2}{N\hat{\omega}_F^2 + \bar{n}(g-1)(1-\hat{\omega}_F^2)}$$

$$= \frac{(10)(0.8495)}{(10)(0.8495)+(3.3333)(3-1)(1-0.8495)} = 0.8944 \ .$$

8.6   Example 3: Analyses with $v = 2$ and $v = 1$

For a third example of tests of differences among $g \geq 3$ independent samples, consider the example data set given in Table 8.4 with $g = 4$ treatment groups, sample sizes of $n_1 = n_2 = n_3 = n_4 = 7$, and $N = 28$ total observations. Under the Neyman–Pearson population model with sample sizes $n_1 = n_2 = n_3 = n_4 = 7$, treatment-group means $\bar{x}_1 = 20.4286$, $\bar{x}_2 = 20.8571$, $\bar{x}_3 = 9.1429$, and $\bar{x}_4 = 14.1429$, grand mean $\bar{\bar{x}} = 16.1429$, estimated population variances $s_1^2 = 27.9524$, $s_2^2 = 35.4762$, and $s_3^2 = s_4^2 = 8.8095$, the sum-of-squares between treatments is

$$SS_{\text{Between}} = \sum_{i=1}^{g} n_i \left(\bar{x}_i - \bar{\bar{x}} \right)^2 = 655.1429 \, ,$$

the sum-of-squares within treatments is

$$SS_{\text{Within}} = \sum_{i=1}^{g} \sum_{j=1}^{n_i} \left(x_{ij} - \bar{x}_i \right)^2 = 486.2857 \, ,$$

the sum-of-squares total is

$$SS_{\text{Total}} = SS_{\text{Between}} + SS_{\text{Within}} = 655.1429 + 486.2857 = 1141.4286 \, ,$$

the mean-square between treatments is

$$MS_{\text{Between}} = \frac{SS_{\text{Between}}}{g - 1} = \frac{655.1429}{4 - 1} = 218.3810 \, ,$$

the mean-square within treatments is

$$MS_{\text{Within}} = \frac{SS_{\text{Within}}}{N - g} = \frac{486.28571}{28 - 4} = 20.2619 \, ,$$

Table 8.4 Example data for a test of $g = 4$ independent samples with $N = 28$ observations

Treatment group			
1	2	3	4
15	24	10	15
23	14	5	13
18	15	8	10
16	19	13	17
25	30	6	18
29	26	10	11
17	18	12	15

Table 8.5 Source table for
the data listed in Table 8.4

Factor	SS	df	MS	F
Between	655.1429	3	218.3810	10.7779
Within	486.1429	24	20.2619	
Total	1141.4286			

and the observed value of Fisher's F-ratio test statistic is

$$F = \frac{MS_{\text{Between}}}{MS_{\text{Within}}} = \frac{218.3810}{20.2619} = 10.7779 \ .$$

The essential factors, sums of squares (SS), degrees of freedom (df), mean squares (MS), and variance-ratio test statistic (F) are summarized in Table 8.5.

Under the Neyman–Pearson null hypothesis, H_0: $\mu_1 = \mu_2 = \mu_3 = \mu_4$, Fisher's F-ratio test statistic is asymptotically distributed as Snedecor's F with $v_1 = g - 1$ and $v_2 = N - g$ degrees of freedom. With $v_1 = g - 1 = 4 - 1 = 3$ and $v_2 = N - g = 28 - 4 = 24$ degrees of freedom, the asymptotic probability value of $F = 10.7778$ is $P = 0.1122 \times 10^{-3}$, under the assumptions of normality and homogeneity.

8.6.1   A Monte Carlo Analysis with $v = 2$

For the first analysis of the example data listed in Table 8.4 on p. 278 under the Fisher–Pitman permutation model let $v = 2$, employing squared Euclidean scaling, and let the treatment-group weights be given by

$$C_i = \frac{n_i - 1}{N - g} \ , \qquad i = 1, \ldots, g \ ,$$

for correspondence with Fisher's F-ratio test statistic.

Because there are

$$M = \frac{N!}{\prod\limits_{i=1}^{g} n_i!} = \frac{28!}{7! \, 7! \, 7! \, 7!} = 472{,}518{,}347{,}558{,}400$$

possible, equally-likely arrangements in the reference set of all permutations of the $N = 28$ observations listed in Table 8.4, an exact permutation analysis is not possible and a Monte Carlo analysis is required.

Following Eq. (8.2) on p. 261, the $N = 28$ observations yield $g = 4$ average distance-function values of

$$\xi_i = 55.9048 \ , \quad \xi_2 = 70.9524 \ , \quad \text{and} \quad \xi_3 = \xi_4 = 17.6190 \ .$$

Alternatively, in terms of a one-way analysis of variance model the average distance-function values are $\xi_1 = 2s_1^2 = 2(27.9524) = 55.9048$, $\xi_2 = 2s_2^2 = 2(34.4762) = 70.9524$, $\xi_3 = 2s_3^2 = 2(8.8095) = 2(8.8095) = 17.6190$, and $\xi_4 = 2s_4^2 = 2(8.8095) = 17.6190$.

Following Eq. (8.1) on p. 261, the observed value of the permutation test statistic based on $v = 2$ and treatment-group weights

$$C_i = \frac{n_i - 1}{N - g} , \qquad i = 1, \ldots, 4 ,$$

is

$$\delta = \sum_{i=1}^{g} C_i \xi_i = \frac{7 - 1}{28 - 4}(55.9048 + 70.9524$$

$$+ 17.6190 + 17.6190) = 40.5238 .$$

Alternatively, in terms of a one-way analysis of variance model the permutation test statistic is

$$\delta = 2MS_{\text{Within}} = 2(20.2619) = 40.5238 .$$

For the example data listed in Table 8.4, the sum of the $N = 28$ observations is

$$\sum_{i=1}^{N} x_i = 15 + 23 + 18 + \cdots + 11 + 15 = 452 ,$$

the sum of the $N = 28$ squared observations is

$$\sum_{i=1}^{N} x_i^2 = 15^2 + 23^2 + 18^2 + \cdots + 11^2 + 15^2 = 8438 ,$$

and the total sum-of-squares is

$$SS_{\text{Total}} = \sum_{i=1}^{N} (x_i - \bar{\bar{x}})^2 = \sum_{i=1}^{N} x_i^2 - \left(\sum_{i=1}^{N} x_i\right)^2 \Big/ N$$

$$= 8438 - (452)^2/28 = 1141.4286 ,$$

where $\bar{\bar{x}}$ denotes the grand mean of all $N = 28$ observations.

Then following the expressions given in Eq. (8.5) on p. 262 for test statistics δ and F, the observed value for test statistic δ with respect to the observed value of test statistic F is

$$\delta = \frac{2SS_{\text{Total}}}{N - g + (g - 1)F} = \frac{2(1141.4286)}{28 - 4 + (4 - 1)(10.7779)} = 40.5238$$

and the observed value of test statistic F with respect to the observed value of test statistic δ is

$$F = \frac{2SS_{\text{Total}}}{(g - 1)\delta} - \frac{N - g}{g - 1} = \frac{2(1141.4286)}{(4 - 1)(40.5238)} - \frac{28 - 4}{4 - 1} = 10.7779 \;.$$

Under the Fisher–Pitman permutation model, the Monte Carlo probability of an observed δ is the proportion of δ test statistic values computed on the randomly-selected, equally-likely arrangements of the $N = 28$ observations listed in Table 8.4 that are equal to or less than the observed value of $\delta = 40.5238$. There are exactly 138 δ test statistic values that are equal to or less than the observed value of $\delta = 40.5238$. If all M arrangements of the $N = 28$ observations listed in Table 8.4 occur with equal chance under the Fisher–Pitman null hypothesis, the Monte Carlo probability value of $\delta = 40.5238$ computed on $L = 1,000,000$ random arrangements of the observed data with $n_1 = n_2 = n_3 = n_4 = 7$ preserved for each arrangement is

$$P(\delta \leq \delta_o) = \frac{\text{number of } \delta \text{ values} \leq \delta_o}{L} = \frac{138}{1,000,000} = 0.1380 \times 10^{-3} \;,$$

where δ_o denotes the observed value of test statistic δ and L is the number of randomly-selected, equally-likely arrangements of the $N = 28$ observations listed in Table 8.4.

In terms of a one-way analysis of variance model, there are only 138 F values that are larger than the observed value of $F = 10.7779$. Thus, if all arrangements of the observed data occur with equal chance, the exact probability value of $F = 10.7779$ under the Fisher–Pitman null hypothesis is

$$P(F \geq F_o) = \frac{\text{number of } F \text{ values} \geq F_o}{L} = \frac{138}{1,000,000} = 0.1380 \times 10^{-3} \;,$$

where F_o denotes the observed value of test statistic F and L is the number of random, equally-likely arrangements of the example data listed in Table 8.4.

Following Eq. (8.7) on p. 263, the exact expected value of the $M = 4200$ δ test statistic values under the Fisher–Pitman null hypothesis is

$$\mu_\delta = \frac{1}{M} \sum_{i=1}^{M} \delta_i = \frac{39,951,568,041,566,987}{472,518,347,558,400} = 84.5503 \;.$$

Alternatively, in terms of a one-way analysis of variance model the exact expected value of test statistic δ under the Fisher–Pitman null hypothesis is

$$\mu_\delta = \frac{2SS_{Total}}{N-1} = \frac{2(1141.4286)}{28-1} = 84.5503 \; .$$

Following Eq. (8.6) on p. 263, the observed chance-corrected measure of effect size is

$$\Re = 1 - \frac{\delta}{\mu_\delta} = 1 - \frac{40.5238}{84.5503} = +0.5207 \; ,$$

indicating approximately 52% within-group agreement above what is expected by chance. Alternatively, in terms of a one-way analysis of variance model, the observed chance-corrected measure of effect size is

$$\Re = 1 - \frac{(N-1)(MS_{Within})}{SS_{Total}} = 1 - \frac{(28-1)(20.2619)}{1141.4286} = +0.5207 \; .$$

Alternatively, in terms of Fisher's F-ratio test statistic the chance-corrected measure of effect size is

$$\Re = 1 - \frac{N-1}{F(g-1)+N-g} = 1 - \frac{28-1}{10.7779(4-1)+28-4} = +0.5207 \; .$$

8.6.2   Measures of Effect Size

For the example data listed in Table 8.4, Cohen's $\hat{d}$ measure of effect size is

$$\hat{d} = \left[\frac{1}{g-1} \left(\frac{SS_{Between}}{nMS_{Within}} \right) \right]^{1/2} = \left[\frac{1}{4-1} \left(\frac{655.1429}{(7)(20.2619)} \right) \right]^{1/2} = \pm 1.2408 \; ,$$

Pearson's η^2 (r^2) measure of effect size is

$$\eta^2 = \frac{SS_{Between}}{SS_{Total}} = \frac{655.1429}{1141.4286} = 0.5740 \; ,$$

Kelley's $\hat{\eta}^2$ measure of effect size is

$$\hat{\eta}^2 = \frac{SS_{Total} - (N-1)MS_{Within}}{SS_{Total}}$$

$$= \frac{1141.4286 - (28-1)(20.2619)}{1141.4286} = 0.5207 \; ,$$

Hays' $\hat{\omega}_F^2$ measure of effect size for a fixed-effects model is

$$\hat{\omega}_F^2 = \frac{SS_{\text{Between}} - (g - 1)MS_{\text{Within}}}{SS_{\text{Total}} + MS_{\text{Within}}}$$

$$= \frac{655.1429 - (4 - 1)(20.2619)}{1141.4286 + 20.2619} = 0.5116 ,$$

Hays' $\hat{\omega}_R^2$ measure of effect size for a random-effects model is

$$\hat{\omega}_R^2 = \frac{MS_{\text{Between}} - MS_{\text{Within}}}{MS_{\text{Between}} + (n - 1)MS_{\text{Within}}}$$

$$= \frac{655.1429 - 20.2619}{655.1429 + (7 - 1)(20.2619)} = 0.8174 ,$$

and the observed chance-corrected measure of effect size is

$$\Re = 1 - \frac{\delta}{\mu_\delta} = 1 - \frac{40.5238}{84.5503} = +0.5207 ,$$

indicating approximately 52% within-group agreement above what is expected by chance.

8.6.3 A Monte Carlo Analysis with $v = 1$

Consider a second analysis of the example data listed in Table 8.4 on p. 278 under the Fisher–Pitman permutation model with $v = 1$ and treatment-group weights

$$C_i = \frac{n_i - 1}{N - g} , \qquad i = 1, \ldots, g .$$

For $v = 1$, the average distance-function values for the $g = 4$ treatment groups are

$$\xi_1 = 6.2857 , \quad \xi_2 = 7.2381 , \quad \text{and} \quad \xi_3 = \xi_4 = 3.6190 ,$$

respectively, and the observed permutation test statistic is

$$\delta = \sum_{i=1}^{g} C_i \xi_i$$

$$= \left(\frac{7 - 1}{28 - 4} \right) (6.2857 + 7.2381 + 3.6190 + 3.6190) = 5.1905 .$$

Because there are

$$M = \frac{N!}{\displaystyle\prod_{i=1}^{g} n_i!} = \frac{28!}{7!\,7!\,7!\,7!} = 472{,}518{,}347{,}558{,}400$$

possible, equally-likely arrangements in the reference set of all permutations of the $N = 28$ observations listed in Table 8.4, an exact permutation analysis is impossible and a Monte Carlo permutation analysis is required. Under the Fisher–Pitman permutation model, the Monte Carlo probability of an observed δ is the proportion of δ test statistic values computed on the randomly-selected, equally-likely arrangements of the $N = 28$ observations listed in Table 8.4 that are equal to or less than the observed value of $\delta = 5.1905$. There are exactly 204 δ test statistic values that are equal to or less than the observed value of $\delta = 5.1905$. If all M arrangements of the $N = 28$ observations listed in Table 8.4 occur with equal chance under the Fisher–Pitman null hypothesis, the Monte Carlo probability value of $\delta = 5.1905$ computed on $L = 1{,}000{,}000$ random arrangements of the observed data with $n_1 = n_2 = n_3 = n_4 = 7$ preserved for each arrangement is

$$P\big(\delta \le \delta_0 | H_0\big) = \frac{\text{number of } \delta \text{ values } \le \delta_0}{L} = \frac{204}{1{,}000{,}000} = 0.2040 \times 10^{-3}\,,$$

where δ_0 denotes the observed value of test statistic δ and L is the number of randomly-selected, equally-likely arrangements of the $N = 28$ observations listed in Table 8.4. No comparison is made with Fisher's F-ratio test statistic as F is undefined for ordinary Euclidean scaling.

For the example data listed in Table 8.4, the exact expected value of test statistic δ under the Fisher–Pitman null hypothesis is

$$\mu_\delta = \frac{1}{M} \sum_{i=1}^{M} \delta_i = \frac{3{,}497{,}628{,}060{,}462{,}033}{472{,}518{,}347{,}558{,}400} = 7.4021 \tag{8.22}$$

and the observed chance-corrected measure of effect size is

$$\Re = 1 - \frac{\delta}{\mu_\delta} = 1 - \frac{5.1905}{7.4021} = +0.2988\,,$$

indicating approximately 30% within-group agreement above what is expected by chance. No comparisons are made with Cohen's $\hat{d}$, Pearson's η^2 (r^2), Kelley's $\hat{\eta}^2$, Hays' $\hat{\omega}_F^2$, or Hays' $\hat{\omega}_R^2$ conventional measures of effect size as $\hat{d}$, η^2, $\hat{\eta}^2$, $\hat{\omega}_F^2$, and $\hat{\omega}_R^2$ are undefined for ordinary Euclidean scaling.

8.6.4 The Effects of Extreme Values

To illustrate the robustness to the inclusion of extreme values of ordinary Euclidean scaling with $v = 1$, consider the example data listed in Table 8.4 on p. 278 with one alteration. The seventh (last) observation in Group 4 in Table 8.4 has been increased from $x_{7,4} = 15$ to $x_{7,4} = 75$, as shown in Table 8.6. Under the Neyman–Pearson population model with sample sizes $n_1 = n_2 = n_3 = n_4 = 7$, treatment-group means $\bar{x}_1 = 20.4286$, $\bar{x}_2 = 20.8571$, $\bar{x}_3 = 9.1429$, and $\bar{x}_4 = 22.7143$, grand mean $\bar{\bar{x}} = 18.2857$, estimated population variances $s_1^2 = 27.9524$, $s_2^2 = 35.4762$, $s_3^2 = 8.8095$, and $s_4^2 = 540.2381$, the sum-of-squares between treatments is

$$SS_{\text{Between}} = \sum_{i=1}^{g} n_i \left(\bar{x}_i - \bar{\bar{x}} \right)^2 = 800.8571 \; ,$$

the sum-of-squares within treatments is

$$SS_{\text{Within}} = \sum_{i=1}^{g} \sum_{j=1}^{n_i} \left(x_{ij} - \bar{x}_i \right)^2 = 3674.8571,$$

the sum-of-squares total is

$$SS_{\text{Total}} = SS_{\text{Between}} + SS_{\text{Within}} = 800.8571 + 3674.8571 = 4475.7142 \; ,$$

the mean-square between treatments is

$$MS_{\text{Between}} = \frac{SS_{\text{Between}}}{g - 1} = \frac{655.1429}{4 - 1} = 266.9524 \; ,$$

the mean-square within treatments is

$$MS_{\text{Within}} = \frac{SS_{\text{Within}}}{N - g} = \frac{486.28571}{28 - 4} = 153.1190 \; ,$$

Table 8.6 Example data for a test of $g = 4$ independent samples with $N = 28$ observations and one extreme value, $x_{7,4} = 75$

Treatment group			
1	2	3	4
15	24	10	15
23	14	5	13
18	15	8	10
16	19	13	17
25	30	6	18
29	26	10	11
17	18	12	75

Table 8.7 Source table for
the data listed in Table 8.6

Factor	SS	df	MS	F
Between	800.8571	3	266.9524	1.7434
Within	3674.8571	24	153.1190	
Total	4475.7142			

and the observed value of Fisher's F-ratio test statistic is

$$F = \frac{MS_{\text{Between}}}{MS_{\text{Within}}} = \frac{266.9524}{153.1190} = 1.7434 .$$

The essential factors, sums of squares (SS), degrees of freedom (df), mean squares
(MS), and variance-ratio test statistic (F) are summarized in Table 8.7.

Under the Neyman–Pearson null hypothesis, H_0: $\mu_1 = \mu_2 = \mu_3 = \mu_4$, Fisher's
F-ratio test statistic is asymptotically distributed as Snedecor's F with $v_1 = g - 1$
and $v_2 = N - g$ degrees of freedom. With $v_1 = g - 1 = 4 - 1 = 3$ and $v_2 = N - g =$
$28 - 4 = 24$ degrees of freedom, the asymptotic probability value of $F = 1.7434$
is $P = 0.1849$, under the assumptions of normality and homogeneity. The original
F-ratio test statistic value with observation $x_{7,4} = 15$ was $F = 10.7779$ with an
asymptotic probability value of $P = 0.1122 \times 10^{-3}$, yielding a difference between
the two probability values of

$$\Delta_P = 0.1849 - 0.1122 \times 10^{-3} = 0.1848 .$$

8.6.5 A Monte Carlo Analysis with $v = 2$

For the first analysis of the example data listed in Table 8.6 on p. 285 under the
Fisher–Pitman permutation model let $v = 2$, employing squared Euclidean scaling,
and let the treatment-group weights be given by

$$C_i = \frac{n_i - 1}{N - g} , \qquad i = 1, \ldots, g ,$$

for correspondence with Fisher's F-ratio test statistic.

Because there are

$$M = \frac{N!}{\prod\limits_{i=1}^{g} n_i!} = \frac{28!}{7! \, 7! \, 7! \, 7!} = 472{,}518{,}347{,}558{,}400$$

possible, equally-likely arrangements in the reference set of all permutations of
the $N = 28$ observations listed in Table 8.6, an exact permutation analysis is not
possible and a Monte Carlo analysis is required.

Following Eq. (8.2) on p. 261, the $N = 28$ observations yield $g = 4$ average distance-function values of

$$\xi_i = 55.9048, \quad \xi_2 = 70.9524, \quad \xi_3 = 17.6190, \quad \text{and} \quad \xi_4 = 1080.4762.$$

Alternatively, under an analysis of variance model, $\xi_1 = 2s_1^2 = 2(27.9524) = 55.9048$, $\xi_2 = 2s_2^2 = 2(35.4762) = 70.9524$, $\xi_3 = 2s_3^2 = 2(8.8095) = 17.6190$, and $\xi_4 = 2s_4^2 = 2(540.2381) = 1080.4762$.

Following Eq. (8.1) on p. 261, the observed value of the permutation test statistic based on $v = 2$ and treatment-group weights

$$C_i = \frac{n_i - 1}{N - g}, \quad i = 1, \ldots, 4,$$

is

$$\delta = \sum_{i=1}^{g} C_i \xi_i = \frac{7 - 1}{28 - 4} (55.9048 + 70.9524$$

$$+ 17.6190 + 1080.4762) = 306.2381.$$

Under the Fisher–Pitman permutation model, the Monte Carlo probability of an observed δ is the proportion of δ test statistic values computed on the randomly-selected, equally-likely arrangements of the $N = 28$ observations listed in Table 8.6 that are equal to or less than the observed value of $\delta = 306.2381$. There are exactly 128,239 δ test statistic values that are equal to or less than the observed value of $\delta = 306.2381$. If all M arrangements of the $N = 28$ observations listed in Table 8.6 occur with equal chance under the Fisher–Pitman null hypothesis, the Monte Carlo probability value of $\delta = 306.2381$ computed on $L = 1{,}000{,}000$ random arrangements of the observed data with $n_1 = n_2 = n_3 = n_4 = 7$ preserved for each arrangement is

$$P\left(\delta \leq \delta_0 | H_0\right) = \frac{\text{number of } \delta \text{ values} \leq \delta_0}{L} = \frac{128{,}239}{1{,}000{,}000} = 0.1282,$$

where δ_0 denotes the observed value of test statistic δ and L is the number of randomly-selected, equally-likely arrangements of the $N = 28$ observations listed in Table 8.6. For comparison, the original value of test statistic δ based on $v = 2$ with observation $x_{7,4} = 15$ was $\delta = 40.5238$ with a Monte Carlo probability value of $P = 0.1380 \times 10^{-3}$, yielding a difference between the two probability values of

$$\Delta_P = 0.1282 - 0.1380 \times 10^{-3} = 0.1281.$$

8.6.6 A Monte Carlo Analysis with $v = 1$

For the second analysis of the example data listed in Table 8.6 on p. 285 under the Fisher–Pitman permutation model let $v = 1$, employing ordinary Euclidean scaling, and let the treatment-group weights be given by

$$C_i = \frac{n_i - 1}{N - g}, \qquad i = 1, \ldots, g .$$

Setting $v = 1$ can be expected to reduce the outsized effect of extreme value $x_{7,4} = 75$.

Because there are

$$M = \frac{N!}{\prod\limits_{i=1}^{g} n_i!} = \frac{28!}{7! \, 7! \, 7! \, 7!} = 472{,}518{,}347{,}558{,}400$$

possible, equally-likely arrangements in the reference set of all permutations of the $N = 28$ observations listed in Table 8.6, an exact permutation analysis is not possible and a Monte Carlo analysis is required.

Following Eq. (8.2) on p. 261, the $N = 28$ observations yield $g = 4$ average distance-function values of

$$\xi_i = 6.2857 , \quad \xi_2 = 7.2381 , \quad \xi_3 = 3.6190 , \quad \text{and} \quad \xi_4 = 20.2857 .$$

Following Eq. (8.1) on p. 261, the observed value of the permutation test statistic based on $v = 1$ and treatment-group weights

$$C_i = \frac{n_i - 1}{N - g}, \qquad i = 1, \ldots, 4 ,$$

is

$$\delta = \sum_{i=1}^{g} C_i \xi_i = \frac{7 - 1}{28 - 4} \left(6.2857 + 7.2381 + 3.6190 + 20.2857 \right) = 9.3571 .$$

Under the Fisher–Pitman permutation model, the exact probability of an observed δ is the proportion of δ test statistic values computed on the randomly-selected, equally-likely arrangements of the $N = 28$ observations listed in Table 8.6 that are equal to or less than the observed value of $\delta = 9.3571$. There are exactly 1960 δ test statistic values that are equal to or less than the observed value of $\delta = 9.3571$. If all M arrangements of the $N = 28$ observations listed in Table 8.6 occur with equal chance, the Monte Carlo probability value of $\delta = 9.3571$

computed on $L = 1,000,000$ random arrangements of the observed data with $n_1 = n_2 = n_3 = n_4 = 7$ preserved for each arrangement is

$$P(\delta \leq \delta_0 | H_0) = \frac{\text{number of } \delta \text{ values } \leq \delta_0}{L} = \frac{1960}{1,000,000} = 0.1960 \times 10^{-2} ,$$

where δ_0 denotes the observed value of δ and L is the number of randomly-selected, equally-likely arrangements of the $N = 28$ observations listed in Table 8.6.

The original value of test statistic δ based on $v = 1$ with observation $x_{7,4} = 15$ was $\delta = 5.1905$ with a Monte Carlo probability value of $P = 0.2040 \times 10^{-3}$, yielding a difference between the two probability values of only

$$\Delta_P = 0.1960 \times 10^{-2} - 0.2040 \times 10^{-3} = 0.1756 \times 10^{-2} .$$

Multi-sample permutation tests based on ordinary Euclidean scaling with $v = 1$ tend to be relatively robust with respect to extreme values when compared with permutation tests based on squared Euclidean scaling with $v = 2$.

8.7   Example 4: Exact and Monte Carlo Analyses

For a fourth, larger example of tests for differences among $g \geq 3$ independent samples, consider the example data given in Table 8.8 with $g = 4$ treatment groups, sample sizes of $n_1 = n_2 = 3$, $n_3 = 4$, $n_4 = 5$, and $N = n_1 + n_2 + n_3 + n_4 = 3 + 3 + 4 + 5 = 15$ total observations. Under the Neyman–Pearson population model with sample sizes $n_1 = n_2 = 3$, $n_3 = 4$, and $n_4 = 5$, treatment-group means $\bar{x}_1 = 11.00$, $\bar{x}_2 = 12.00$, $\bar{x}_3 = 13.50$, and $\bar{x}_4 = 19.00$, grand mean $\bar{\bar{x}} = 14.5333$, estimated population variances $s_1^2 = s_2^2 = 1.00$, $s_3^2 = 1.6667$, and $s_4^2 = 62.50$, the sum-of-squares between treatments is

$$SS_{\text{Between}} = \sum_{i=1}^{g} n_i (\bar{x}_i - \bar{\bar{x}})^2 = 160.7333 ,$$

Table 8.8 Example data for a test of $g = 4$ independent samples with $N = 15$ observations

Treatment group			
1	2	3	4
10	11	12	14
11	12	13	15
12	13	14	16
		15	17
			33

Table 8.9 Source table for
the data listed in Table 8.8

Factor	SS	df	MS	F
Between	160.7333	3	53.5778	2.2755
Within	259.0000	11	23.5455	
Total	419.7333			

the sum-of-squares within treatments is

$$
SS_{\text{Within}} = \sum_{i=1}^{g} \sum_{j=1}^{n_i} \left(x_{ij} - \bar{x}_i \right)^2 = 259.00 \, ,
$$

the sum-of-squares total is

$$
SS_{\text{Total}} = SS_{\text{Between}} + SS_{\text{Within}} = 160.7333 + 259.00 = 419.7333 \, ,
$$

the mean-square between treatments is

$$
MS_{\text{Between}} = \frac{SS_{\text{Between}}}{g - 1} = \frac{160.7333}{4 - 1} = 53.5778 \, ,
$$

the mean-square within treatments is

$$
MS_{\text{Within}} = \frac{SS_{\text{Within}}}{N - g} = \frac{259.00}{15 - 4} = 23.5455 \, ,
$$

and the observed value of Fisher's F-ratio test statistic is

$$
F = \frac{MS_{\text{Between}}}{MS_{\text{Within}}} = \frac{53.5778}{23.5455} = 2.2755 \, .
$$

The essential factors, sums of squares (SS), degrees of freedom (df), mean squares (MS), and variance-ratio test statistic (F) are summarized in Table 8.9.

Under the Neyman–Pearson null hypothesis, H_0: $\mu_1 = \mu_2 = \mu_3 = \mu_4$, Fisher's F-ratio test statistic is asymptotically distributed as Snedecor's F with $\nu_1 = g - 1$ and $\nu_2 = N - g$ degrees of freedom. With $\nu_1 = g - 1 = 4 - 1 = 3$ and $\nu_2 = N - g = 15 - 4 = 11$ degrees of freedom, the asymptotic probability value of $F = 2.2755$ is $P = 0.1366$, under the assumptions of normality and homogeneity.

8.7.1 A Permutation Analysis with $v = 2$

For the first analysis of the example data listed in Table 8.8 under the Fisher–Pitman permutation model let $v = 2$, employing squared Euclidean scaling, and let the treatment-group weighting functions be given by

$$C_i = \frac{n_i - 1}{N - g} , \qquad i = 1, \ldots, g ,$$

for correspondence with Fisher's F-ratio test statistic.

Because there are

$$M = \frac{N!}{\prod\limits_{i=1}^{g} n_i!} = \frac{15!}{3!\, 3!\, 4!\, 5!} = 12{,}612{,}600$$

possible, equally-likely arrangements in the reference set of all permutations of the $N = 15$ observations listed in Table 8.8, an exact permutation analysis is not practical and a Monte Carlo analysis is utilized.

Following Eq. (8.2) on p. 261, the $N = 15$ observations yield $g = 4$ average distance-function values of

$$\xi_1 = \xi_2 = 2.00 , \quad \xi_3 = 3.3333 , \quad \text{and} \quad \xi_4 = 125.00 .$$

Alternatively, in terms of a one-way analysis of variance model the average distance-function values are $\xi_1 = 2s_1^2 = 2(1.00) = 2.00$, $\xi_2 = 2s_2^2 = 2(1.00) = 2.00$, $\xi_3 = 2s_3^2 = 2(1.667) = 3.3333$, and $\xi_4 = 2s_4^2 = 2(62.50) = 125.00$.

Following Eq. (8.1) on p. 261, the observed value of the permutation test statistic based on $v = 2$ and treatment-group weights

$$C_i = \frac{n_i - 1}{N - g} , \qquad i = 1, \ldots, 4 ,$$

is

$$\delta = \sum_{i=1}^{g} C_i \xi_i = \frac{1}{15 - 4} \big[(3 - 1)(2.00) + (3 - 1)(2.00)$$

$$+ (4 - 1)(3.3333) + (5 - 1)(125.00) \big] = 47.0909 .$$

Alternatively, in terms of a one-way analysis of variance model the permutation test statistic is

$$\delta = 2MS_{\text{Within}} = 2(23.5455) = 47.0909 .$$

For the example data listed in Table 8.8, the sum of the $N = 15$ observations is

$$\sum_{i=1}^{N} x_i = 10 + 11 + 12 + \cdots + 17 + 33 = 218 ,$$

the sum of the $N = 15$ squared observations is

$$\sum_{i=1}^{N} x_i^2 = 10^2 + 11^2 + 12^2 + \cdots + 17^2 + 33^2 = 3588 ,$$

and the total sum-of-squares is

$$SS_{\text{Total}} = \sum_{i=1}^{N} (x_i - \bar{\bar{x}})^2 = \sum_{i=1}^{N} d_i^2 - \left(\sum_{i=1}^{N} d_i \right)^2 \Big/ N$$

$$= 3588 - (218)^2/15 = 419.7333 ,$$

where $\bar{\bar{x}}$ denotes the grand mean of all $N = 15$ observations. Then following the expressions given in Eq. (8.5) on p. 262 for test statistics δ and F, the observed value for test statistic δ with respect to the observed value of test statistic F is

$$\delta = \frac{2SS_{\text{Total}}}{N - g + (g - 1)F} = \frac{2(419.7333)}{15 - 4 + (4 - 1)(2.2755)} = 47.0909$$

and the observed value for test statistic F with respect to the observed value of test statistic δ is

$$F = \frac{2SS_{\text{Total}}}{(g - 1)\delta} - \frac{N - g}{g - 1} = \frac{2(419.7333)}{(4 - 1)(47.0909)} - \frac{15 - 4}{4 - 1} = 2.2755 .$$

Under the Fisher–Pitman permutation model, the Monte Carlo probability of an observed δ is the proportion of δ test statistic values computed on the randomly-selected, equally-likely arrangements of the $N = 15$ observations listed in Table 8.8 that are equal to or less than the observed value of $\delta = 47.0909$. There are exactly 53,200 δ test statistic values that are equal to or less than the observed value of $\delta = 47.0909$. If all M arrangements of the $N = 15$ observations listed in Table 8.8 occur with equal chance under the Fisher–Pitman null hypothesis, the Monte Carlo probability value of $\delta = 47.0909$ computed on $L = 1{,}000{,}000$ randomly-selected arrangements of the observed data with $n_1 = n_2 = 3 = n_3 = 4$, and $n_4 = 5$ preserved for each arrangement is

$$P(\delta \le \delta_0 | H_0) = \frac{\text{number of } \delta \text{ values} \le \delta_0}{L} = \frac{53{,}200}{1{,}000{,}000} = 0.0532 ,$$

where δ_0 denotes the observed value of test statistic δ and L is the number of randomly-selected, equally-likely arrangements of the $N = 15$ observations listed in Table 8.8.

Alternatively, in terms of a one-way analysis of variance model, there are 53,200 F values that are equal to or greater than the observed value of $F = 2.2755$. Thus, if all arrangements of the observed data occur with equal chance, the exact probability value of $F = 2.2755$ under the Fisher–Pitman null hypothesis is

$$P\left(F \geq F_o | H_0\right) = \frac{\text{number of } F \text{ values } \geq F_o}{L} = \frac{53,200}{1,000,000} = 0.0532 ,$$

where F_o denotes the observed value of test statistic F.

Following Eq. (8.7) on p. 263, the exact expected value of the $M = 12,612,600$ δ test statistic values under the Fisher–Pitman null hypothesis is

$$\mu_\delta = \frac{1}{M} \sum_{i=1}^{M} \delta_i = \frac{756,275,456}{12,612,600} = 59.9619 .$$

In terms of a one-way analysis of variance model the exact expected value of test statistic δ is

$$\mu_\delta = \frac{2SS_{\text{Total}}}{N-1} = \frac{2(419.7333)}{15-1} = 59.9619 .$$

Following Eq. (8.6) on p. 263, the observed chance-corrected measure of effect size is

$$\Re = 1 - \frac{\delta}{\mu_\delta} = 1 - \frac{47.0909}{59.9619} = +0.2147 ,$$

indicating approximately 21% within-group agreement above what is expected by chance. Alternatively, in terms of a one-way analysis of variance model, the observed measure of effect size is

$$\Re = 1 - \frac{(N-1)(MS_{\text{Within}})}{SS_{\text{Total}}} = 1 - \frac{(15-1)(23.5455)}{419.7333} = +0.2147 .$$

8.7.2 Measures of Effect Size

For the example data listed in Table 8.8 on p. 289, the average treatment-group size is

$$\bar{n} = \frac{1}{g} \sum_{i=1}^{g} n_i = \frac{3+3+4+5}{4} = 3.75 ,$$

Cohen's $\hat{d}$ measure of effect size is

$$\hat{d} = \left[\frac{1}{g-1} \left(\frac{SS_{\text{Between}}}{\bar{n}MS_{\text{Within}}} \right) \right]^{1/2}$$

$$= \left[\frac{1}{4-1} \left(\frac{160.7333}{(3.75)(23.5455)} \right) \right]^{1/2} = \pm 0.7336 ,$$

Pearson's η^2 (r^2) measure of effect size is

$$\eta^2 = \frac{SS_{\text{Between}}}{SS_{\text{Total}}} = \frac{160.7333}{419.7333} = 0.3829 ,$$

Kelley's $\hat{\eta}^2$ measure of effect size is

$$\hat{\eta}^2 = \frac{SS_{\text{Total}} - (N-1)MS_{\text{Within}}}{SS_{\text{Total}}}$$

$$= \frac{419.7333 - (15-1)(23.5455)}{419.7333} = 0.2147 ,$$

Hays' $\hat{\omega}_{\text{F}}^2$ measure of effect size for a fixed-effects model is

$$\hat{\omega}_{\text{F}}^2 = \frac{SS_{\text{Between}} - (g-1)MS_{\text{Within}}}{SS_{\text{Total}} + MS_{\text{Within}}}$$

$$= \frac{160.7333 - (4-1)(23.5455)}{419.7333 + 23.5455} = 0.2033 ,$$

Hays' $\hat{\omega}_{\text{R}}^2$ measure of effect size for a random-effects model is

$$\hat{\omega}_{\text{R}}^2 = \frac{MS_{\text{Between}} - MS_{\text{Within}}}{MS_{\text{Between}} + (\bar{n}-1)MS_{\text{Within}}}$$

$$= \frac{53.5777 - 23.5455}{53.5777 + (3.75)(23.5455)} = 0.2117 ,$$

and Mielke and Berry's $\Re$ chance-corrected measure of effect size is

$$\Re = 1 - \frac{\delta}{\mu_\delta} = 1 - \frac{47.0909}{56.9619} = +0.2147 ,$$

indicating approximately 21% within-group agreement above what is expected by chance.

8.7.3 An Exact Analysis with $v = 2$

While an exact permutation analysis with $M = 12{,}612{,}600$ possible arrangements of the observed data may be impractical, it is not impossible. An exact analysis of the $N = 15$ observations listed in Table 8.8 on p. 289 under the Fisher–Pitman permutation model yields $g = 4$ average distance-function values of

$$\xi_1 = \xi_2 = 2.00 , \quad \xi_3 = 3.3333 , \quad \text{and} \quad \xi_4 = 125.00 .$$

The observed value of the permutation test statistic based on $v = 2$ and treatment-group weights

$$C_i = \frac{n_i - 1}{N - g} , \quad i = 1, \ldots, 4 ,$$

is

$$\delta = \sum_{i=1}^{g} C_i \xi_i = \frac{1}{15 - 4} \big[(3 - 1)(2.00) + (3 - 1)(2.00)$$

$$+ (4 - 1)(3.3333) + (5 - 1)(125.00) \big] = 47.0909 .$$

Under the Fisher–Pitman permutation model, the exact probability of an observed δ is the proportion of δ test statistic values computed on all possible, equally-likely arrangements of the $N = 15$ observations listed in Table 8.8 that are equal to or less than the observed value of $\delta = 47.0909$. There are exactly $673{,}490$ δ test statistic values that are equal to or less than the observed value of $\delta = 47.0909$. If all M arrangements of the $N = 15$ observations listed in Table 8.8 occur with equal chance under the Fisher–Pitman null hypothesis, the exact probability value of $\delta = 47.0909$ computed on the $M = 12{,}612{,}600$ possible arrangements of the observed data with $n_1 = n_2 = 3 = n_3 = 4$, and $n_4 = 5$ preserved for each arrangement is

$$P\big(\delta \le \delta_0 | H_0\big) = \frac{\text{number of } \delta \text{ values} \le \delta_0}{M} = \frac{673{,}490}{12{,}612{,}600} = 0.0534 ,$$

where δ_0 denotes the observed value of test statistic δ and M is the number of possible, equally-likely arrangements of the $N = 15$ observations listed in Table 8.8.

Carrying the Monte Carlo probability value based on $L = 1{,}000{,}000$ random arrangements and the exact probability value based on $M = 12{,}612{,}600$ possible arrangements to a few extra decimal places allows for a more direct comparison of the Monte Carlo and exact permutation approaches. The Monte Carlo approximate probability value and the corresponding exact probability value to six decimal places are

$$P = 0.053242 \quad \text{and} \quad P = 0.053398 ,$$

respectively. The difference between the two probability values is only

$$\Delta_P = 0.053398 - 0.053242 = 0.000156 \, ,$$

demonstrating the efficiency and accuracy of a Monte Carlo approach for permutation methods when L is large and the exact probability value is not too small. In general, $L = 1,000,000$ random arrangements of the observed data is sufficient to ensure three decimal places of accuracy [11].

8.7.4 A Monte Carlo Analysis with $v = 1$

Consider a second analysis of the example data listed in Table 8.8 on p. 289 under the Fisher–Pitman permutation model with $v = 1$ and treatment-group weights

$$C_i = \frac{n_i - 1}{N - g} \, , \qquad i = 1, \ldots, g \, .$$

For $v = 1$, employing ordinary Euclidean scaling between the observations, thereby reducing the effects of any extreme values, the average distance-function values for the $g = 4$ treatment groups are

$$\xi_1 = \xi_2 = 1.3333 \, , \quad \xi_3 = 1,6667 \, , \quad \text{and} \quad \xi_4 = 8.00 \, ,$$

respectively, and the observed permutation test statistic is

$$\delta = \sum_{i=1}^{g} C_i \xi_i = \left(\frac{1}{15 - 4} \right) (3 - 1)(1.3333) + (3 - 1)(1.3333)$$

$$+ (4 - 1)(1.6667) + (5 - 1)(8.00) = 3.8485 \, .$$

Because there are

$$M = \frac{N!}{\displaystyle\prod_{i=1}^{g} n_i!} = \frac{15!}{3! \, 3! \, 4! \, 5!} = 12,612,600$$

possible, equally-likely arrangements in the reference set of all permutations of the $N = 28$ observations listed in Table 8.8, a Monte Carlo permutation analysis is recommended.

Under the Fisher–Pitman permutation model, the Monte Carlo probability of an observed δ is the proportion of δ test statistic values computed on the randomly-selected, equally-likely arrangements of the $N = 15$ observations listed in Table 8.8

that are equal to or less than the observed value of $\delta = 3.8485$. There are exactly 18,000 δ test statistic values that are equal to or less than the observed value of $\delta = 3.8485$. If all M arrangements of the $N = 15$ observations listed in Table 8.8 occur with equal chance under the Fisher–Pitman null hypothesis, the Monte Carlo probability value of $\delta = 3.8485$ computed on $L = 1,000,000$ random arrangements of the observed data with $n_1 = n_2 = 3$, $n_3 = 4$, and $n_4 = 5$ preserved for each arrangement is

$$P\left(\delta \leq \delta_o | H_0\right) = \frac{\text{number of } \delta \text{ values } \leq \delta_o}{L} = \frac{18,000}{1,000,000} = 0.0180 ,$$

where δ_o denotes the observed value of test statistic δ and L is the number of randomly-selected, equally-likely arrangements of the $N = 15$ observations listed in Table 8.8.

For comparison, the approximate Monte Carlo probability value based on $v = 2$, $L = 1,000,000$, and

$$C_i = \frac{n_i - 1}{N - g} , \qquad i = 1, \ldots, g ,$$

is $P = 0.0532$. The difference between the two probability values, $P = 0.0180$ and $P = 0.0532$, is due to the single extreme value of $x_{5,4} = 33$ in the fourth treatment group. No comparison is made with Fisher's F-ratio test statistic as F is undefined for ordinary Euclidean scaling.

For the example data listed in Table 8.8 on p. 289, the exact expected value of the $M = 12,612,600$ δ test statistic values under the Fisher–Pitman null hypothesis is

$$\mu_\delta = \frac{1}{M} \sum_{i=1}^{M} \delta_i = \frac{59,579,400}{12,612,600} = 4.7238 \tag{8.23}$$

and the observed chance-corrected measure of effect size is

$$\Re = 1 - \frac{\delta}{\mu_\delta} = 1 - \frac{3.8485}{4.7238} = +0.1853 ,$$

indicating approximately 19% within-group agreement above what is expected by chance. No comparisons are made with Cohen's $\hat{d}$, Pearson's η^2 (r^2), Kelley's $\hat{\eta}^2$, Hays' $\hat{\omega}_F^2$, or Hays' $\hat{\omega}_R^2$ conventional measures of effect size as $\hat{d}$, η^2, $\hat{\eta}^2$, $\hat{\omega}_F^2$, and $\hat{\omega}_R^2$ are undefined for ordinary Euclidean scaling.

8.7.5   An Exact Analysis with $v = 1$

An exact permutation analysis of the observations listed in Table 8.8 with $v = 1$ yields $g = 4$ average distance-function values of

$$\xi_1 = \xi_2 = 1.3333 , \quad \xi_3 = 1,6667 , \quad \text{and} \quad \xi_4 = 8.00 .$$

The observed value of the permutation test statistic based on $v = 1$ and treatment-group weights

$$C_i = \frac{n_i - 1}{N - g} , \quad i = 1, \ldots, 4 ,$$

is

$$\delta = \sum_{i=1}^{g} C_i \xi_i = \frac{1}{15 - 4}[(3 - 1)(1.3333) + (3 - 1)(1.3333)$$

$$+ (4 - 1)(1.6667) + (5 - 1)(8.00)] = 3.8485 .$$

Under the Fisher–Pitman permutation model, the exact probability of an observed δ is the proportion of δ test statistic values computed on all possible, equally-likely arrangements of the $N = 15$ observations listed in Table 8.8 that are equal to or less than the observed value of $\delta = 3.8485$. There are exactly 225,720 δ test statistic values that are equal to or less than the observed value of $\delta = 3.8485$. If all M arrangements of the $N = 15$ observations listed in Table 8.8 occur with equal chance under the Fisher–Pitman null hypothesis, the exact probability value of $\delta = 3.8485$ computed on the $M = 12,612,600$ possible arrangements of the observed data with $n_1 = n_2 = 3$, $n_3 = 4$, and $n_4 = 5$ preserved for each arrangement is

$$P(\delta \leq \delta_0 | H_0) = \frac{\text{number of } \delta \text{ values} \leq \delta_0}{M} = \frac{225,720}{12,612,600} = 0.0179 ,$$

where δ_0 denotes the observed value of test statistic δ and M is the number of possible, equally-likely arrangements of the $N = 15$ observations listed in Table 8.8.

The exact expected value of the $M = 12,612,600$ δ test statistic values under the Fisher–Pitman null hypothesis is

$$\mu_\delta = \frac{1}{M} \sum_{i=1}^{M} \delta_i = \frac{59,579,400}{12,612,600} = 4.7238$$

and the observed chance-corrected measure of effect size is

$$\Re = 1 - \frac{\delta}{\mu_\delta} = 1 - \frac{3.8485}{4.7238} = +0.1853 ,$$

indicating approximately 19% within-group agreement above what is expected by chance. No comparisons are made with Cohen's $\hat{d}$, Pearson's η^2 (r^2), Kelley's $\hat{\eta}^2$, Hays' $\hat{\omega}_F^2$, or Hays' $\hat{\omega}_R^2$ conventional measures of effect size as $\hat{d}$, η^2, $\hat{\eta}^2$, $\hat{\omega}_F^2$, and $\hat{\omega}_R^2$ are undefined for ordinary Euclidean scaling.

Finally, note the effect of a single extreme value ($x_{4,5} = 33$) in Treatment 4 in the analysis based on ordinary Euclidean scaling with $v = 1$, compared with the analysis based on squared Euclidean scaling with $v = 2$. In the analysis based on $v = 2$, the value for the fourth average distance-function value was $\xi_4 = 125.00$, but in the analysis based on $v = 1$, ξ_4 was reduced to only $\xi_4 = 8.00$. Also, in the analysis based on $v = 2$ the exact probability value was $P = 0.0534$, but in the analysis based on $v = 1$ the exact probability value was only $P = 0.0179$, a reduction of approximately 66%. For comparison, the asymptotic probability value of $F = 2.2755$ with $v_1 = g - 1 = 4 - 1 = 3$ and $v_2 = N - g = 15 - 4 = 11$ degrees of freedom was $P = 0.1366$.

8.8 Example 5: Rank-Score Permutation Analyses

In many research applications it becomes necessary to analyze rank-score data, typically because the required parametric assumptions of normality and homogeneity cannot be met. Consequently, the raw scores are often converted to rank scores and analyzed under a less-restrictive model. While it is never necessary to convert raw scores to rank scores under the Fisher–Pitman permutation model, sometimes the observed data are simply collected as rank scores. Thus, this fifth example serves merely to demonstrate the relationship between a g-sample test of rank-score observations under the population model and the same test under the permutation model. The conventional approach to univariate rank-score data for multiple independent samples under the Neyman–Pearson population model is the Kruskal–Wallis g-sample rank-sum test. As Kruskal and Wallis explained, the rank-sum test stemmed from two statistical methods: rank transformations of the original raw scores and permutations of the rank-order statistics [12].

8.8.1 The Kruskal–Wallis Rank-Sum Test

Consider g random samples of possibly different sizes and denote the size of the ith sample by n_i for $i = 1, \ldots, g$. Let

$$N = \sum_{i=1}^{g} n_i$$

denote the total number of observations, assign rank 1 to the smallest of the N observations, rank 2 to the next smallest observation, continuing to the largest observation that is assigned rank N, and let R_i denote the sum of the rank scores in the ith sample, $i = 1, \ldots, g$. If there are no tied rank scores, the Kruskal–Wallis g-sample rank-sum test statistic is given by

$$H = \frac{12}{N(N+1)} \sum_{i=1}^{g} \frac{R_i}{n_i} - 3(N+1) . \tag{8.24}$$

When $g = 2$, H is equivalent to the Wilcoxon [25], Festinger [5], Mann–Whitney [15], Haldane–Smith [7], and van der Reyden [24] two-sample rank-sum tests.

For an example analysis of g-sample rank-score data, consider the rank scores listed in Table 8.10 with $g = 3$ samples, $n_1 = n_2 = n_3 = 6$, $N = 18$, and no tied rank scores.

The conventional Kruskal–Wallis g-sample rank-sum test on the $N = 18$ rank scores listed in Table 8.10 yields an observed test statistic of

$$H = \frac{12}{N(N+1)} \sum_{i=1}^{g} \frac{R_i}{n_i} - 3(N+1)$$

$$= \frac{12}{18(18+1)} \left[\frac{(63)^2}{6} + \frac{(30)^2}{6} + \frac{(78)^2}{6} \right] - 3(18+1) = 7.0526 ,$$

where test statistic H is asymptotically distributed as Pearson's chi-squared under the Neyman–Pearson null hypothesis with $g - 1$ degrees of freedom as $N \to \infty$. Under the Neyman–Pearson null hypothesis with $g - 1 = 3 - 1 = 2$ degrees of freedom, the observed value of $H = 7.0526$ yields an asymptotic probability value of $P = 0.0294$, under the assumption of normality.

Table 8.10 Ranking of $g = 3$ with $n_1 = n_2 = n_3 = 6$ and $N = 18$

	Treatment group		
	1	2	3
	4	2	17
	7	3	14
	10	11	12
	15	1	13
	9	8	16
	18	5	6
R_i	63	30	78

8.8.2   A Monte Carlo Analysis with $v = 2$

For the first analysis of the rank-score data listed in Table 8.10 under the Fisher–Pitman permutation model let $v = 2$, employing squared Euclidean scaling between the pairs of rank scores, and let the treatment-groups weights be given by

$$C_i = \frac{n_i - 1}{N - g}, \qquad i = 1, \ldots, g,$$

for correspondence with the Kruskal–Wallis g-sample rank-sum test. The average distance-function values for the $g = 3$ samples are

$$\xi_1 = 53.40, \quad \xi_2 = 29.60, \quad \text{and} \quad \xi_3 = 30.40,$$

and the observed value of the permutation test statistic based on $v = 2$ is

$$\delta = \sum_{i=1}^{g} C_i \xi_i = \frac{6 - 1}{18 - 3}(53.40 + 29.60 + 30.40) = 37.80.$$

Because there are

$$M = \frac{N!}{\displaystyle\prod_{i=1}^{g} n_i!} = \frac{18!}{6!\,6!\,6!} = 17,153,136$$

possible, equally-likely arrangements in the reference set of all permutations of the $N = 18$ rank scores listed in Table 8.10, an exact permutation analysis is not practical and a Monte Carlo permutation analysis is utilized.

Under the Fisher–Pitman permutation model, the Monte Carlo probability of an observed δ is the proportion of δ test statistic values computed on the randomly-selected, equally-likely arrangements of the $N = 18$ rank scores listed in Table 8.10 that are equal to or less than the observed value of $\delta = 37.80$. There are exactly $21,810$ δ test statistic values that are equal to or less than the observed value of $\delta = 37.80$. If all M arrangements of the $N = 18$ observations listed in Table 8.10 occur with equal chance under the Fisher–Pitman null hypothesis, the Monte Carlo probability value of $\delta = 37.80$ computed on $L = 1,000,000$ random arrangements of the observed data with $n_1 = n_2 = n_3 = 6$ preserved for each arrangement is

$$P(\delta \leq \delta_o | H_0) = \frac{\text{number of } \delta \text{ values} \leq \delta_o}{L} = \frac{21,810}{1,000,000} = 0.0218,$$

where δ_o denotes the observed value of test statistic δ and L is the number of randomly-selected, equally-likely arrangements of the $N = 18$ rank scores listed in Table 8.10. It should be noted that whereas the Kruskal–Wallis test statistic, H, as defined in Eq. (8.24) does not allow for tied rank scores, test statistic δ automatically accommodates tied rank scores.

The functional relationships between test statistics δ and H are given by

$$\delta = \frac{2\left(T - \left\{\frac{S}{6}\left[H + 3(N+1)\right]\right\}\right)}{N - g} \tag{8.25}$$

and

$$H = \frac{6}{S}\left[T - \frac{\delta}{2}(N - g)\right] - 3(N+1), \tag{8.26}$$

where, if no rank scores are tied, S and T may simply be expressed as

$$S = \sum_{i=1}^{N} i = \frac{N(N+1)}{2} \quad \text{and} \quad T = \sum_{i=1}^{N} i^2 = \frac{N(N+1)(2N+1)}{6}.$$

Note that in Eqs. (8.25) and (8.26), S, T, N, and g are invariant under permutation, along with the constants 2, 3, and 6.

The relationships between test statistics δ and H can be confirmed with the rank-score data listed in Table 8.10. For the rank scores listed in Table 8.10 with no tied values, the observed value of S is

$$S = \sum_{i=1}^{N} i = \frac{N(N+1)}{2} = \frac{18(18+1)}{2} = 171,$$

and the observed value of T is

$$T = \sum_{i=1}^{N} i^2 = \frac{N(N+1)(2N+1)}{6} = \frac{18(18+2)[(2)(18)+1]}{6} = 2109.$$

Then following Eq. (8.25), the observed value of the permutation test statistic for the $N = 18$ rank scores listed in Table 8.10 is

$$\delta = \frac{2\left(T - \left\{\frac{S}{6}\left[H + 3(N+1)\right]\right\}\right)}{N - g} = \frac{N(N+1)(N - 1 - H)}{6(N - g)}$$

$$= \frac{18(18+1)(18 - 1 - 7.0526)}{6(18 - 3)} = 37.80$$

and, following Eq. (8.26), the observed value of the Kruskal–Wallis test statistic is

$$H = \frac{6}{S}\left[T - \frac{\delta}{2}(N - g)\right] - 3(N + 1) = N - 1 - \frac{6\delta(N - g)}{N(N + 1)}$$

$$= 18 - 1 - \frac{6(37.80)(18 - 3)}{18(18 + 1)} = 7.0526 .$$

Because of the relationship between test statistics δ and H, the Monte Carlo probability value of the realized value of $H = 7.0526$ is identical to the Monte Carlo probability value of $\delta = 37.80$ under the Fisher–Pitman null hypothesis. Thus,

$$P(H \geq H_0|H_0) = \frac{\text{number of } H \text{ values} \geq H_o}{L} = \frac{21,810}{1,000,000} = 0.0218 ,$$

where H_o denotes the observed value of test statistic H.

The exact expected value of the $M = 17,153,136\ \delta$ test statistic values under the Fisher–Pitman null hypothesis is

$$\mu_\delta = \frac{1}{M}\sum_{i=1}^{M}\delta_i = \frac{977,728,752}{17,153,136} = 57.00$$

and the observed chance-corrected measure of effect size is

$$\Re = 1 - \frac{\delta}{\mu_\delta} = 1 - \frac{37.80}{57.00} = +0.3368 ,$$

indicating approximately 34% within-group agreement above what is expected by chance. No comparisons are made with Cohen's $\hat{d}$, Pearson's η^2 (r^2), Kelley's $\hat{\eta}^2$, Hays' $\hat{\omega}^2$, or Hays' $\hat{\omega}_R^2$ measures of effect size as $\hat{d}$, η^2, $\hat{\eta}^2$, $\hat{\omega}_F^2$, and $\hat{\omega}_R^2$ are undefined for rank-score data.

8.8.3 An Exact Analysis with $v = 2$

Although an exact permutation analysis with $M = 17,153,136$ possible arrangements of the observed data may be impractical, it is not impossible. An exact permutation analysis of the $N = 18$ observations listed in Table 8.10 yields $g = 3$ average distance-function values of

$$\xi_1 = 53.40 , \quad \xi_2 = 29.60 , \quad \text{and} \quad \xi_3 = 30.40 ,$$

and the observed value of the permutation test statistic based on $v = 2$ and treatment-group weights

$$C_i = \frac{N_i - 1}{N - g}, \qquad i = 1, 2, 3,$$

is

$$\delta = \sum_{i=1}^{g} C_i \xi_i = \frac{6-1}{18-3}(53.40 + 29.60 + 30.40) = 37.80.$$

There are

$$M = \frac{N!}{\prod\limits_{i=1}^{g} n_i!} = \frac{18!}{6! \, 6! \, 6!} = 17{,}153{,}136$$

possible, equally-likely arrangements in the reference set of all permutations of the $N = 18$ rank scores listed in Table 8.10, making an exact permutation analysis feasible. Under the Fisher–Pitman permutation model, the exact probability of an observed δ is the proportion of δ test statistic values computed on all possible, equally-likely arrangements of the $N = 18$ rank scores listed in Table 8.10 that are equal to or less than the observed value of $\delta = 37.80$. There are exactly 376,704 δ test statistic values that are equal to or less than the observed value of $\delta = 37.80$. If all M arrangements of the $N = 18$ rank scores listed in Table 8.10 occur with equal chance under the Fisher–Pitman null hypothesis, the exact probability value of $\delta = 37.80$ computed on the $M = 17{,}153{,}136$ possible arrangements of the observed data with $n_1 = n_2 = n_3 = 6$ preserved for each arrangement is

$$P(\delta \le \delta_0 | H_0) = \frac{\text{number of } \delta \text{ values } \le \delta_0}{M} = \frac{376{,}704}{17{,}153{,}136} = 0.0220,$$

where δ_0 denotes the observed value of test statistic δ and M is the number of possible, equally-likely arrangements of the $N = 18$ rank scores listed in Table 8.10. For comparison, the Monte Carlo probability value based on $v = 2$, $L = 1{,}000{,}000$ random arrangements of the observed data, and treatment-group weights given by

$$C_i = \frac{n_i - 1}{N - g}, \qquad i = 1, 2, 3,$$

is $P = 0.0218$ for a difference between the two probability values of only

$$\Delta_P = 0.0220 - 0.0218 = 0.0002.$$

8.8.4   An Exact Analysis with $v = 1$

For a second analysis of the rank-score data listed in Table 8.10, let the treatment-group weights be given by

$$C_i = \frac{n_i - 1}{N - g} , \qquad i = 1, \ldots, g ,$$

as in the previous example but set $v = 1$, employing ordinary Euclidean scaling between the pairs of rank scores. The $N = 18$ rank scores listed in Table 8.10 yield $g = 3$ average distance-function values of

$$\xi_1 = 6.3333 , \quad \xi_2 = 4.6667 , \quad \text{and} \quad \xi_3 = 4.5333 ,$$

and the observed value of the permutation test statistic based on $v = 1$ is

$$\delta = \sum_{i=1}^{g} C_i \xi_i = \frac{6 - 1}{18 - 3}(6.3333 + 4.6667 + 4.5333) = 5.1778 .$$

Under the Fisher–Pitman permutation model, the exact probability of an observed δ is the proportion of δ test statistic values computed on all possible, equally-likely arrangements of the $N = 18$ rank scores listed in Table 8.10 that are equal to or less than the observed value of $\delta = 5.1778$. There are exactly 547,662 δ test statistic values that are equal to or less than the observed value of $\delta = 5.1778$. If all M arrangements of the $N = 18$ rank scores listed in Table 8.10 occur with equal chance under the Fisher–Pitman null hypothesis, the exact probability value of $\delta = 5.1778$ computed on the $M = 17,153,136$ possible arrangements of the observed data with $n_1 = n_2 = n_3 = 6$ preserved for each arrangement is

$$P(\delta \leq \delta_0 | H_0) = \frac{\text{number of } \delta \text{ values} \leq \delta_0}{M} = \frac{547,662}{17,153,136} = 0.0319 ,$$

where δ_0 denotes the observed value of test statistic δ and M is the number of possible, equally-likely arrangements of the $N = 18$ rank scores listed in Table 8.10. For comparison, the exact probability value based on $v = 2$, $M = 17,153,136$, and

$$C_i = \frac{n_i - 1}{N - g} , \qquad i = 1, 2, 3 ,$$

is $P = 0.0220$. No comparison is made with the conventional Kruskal–Wallis g-sample rank-sum test as H is undefined for ordinary Euclidean scaling.

The exact expected value of the $M = 17,153,136$ δ test statistic values under the Fisher–Pitman null hypothesis is

$$
\mu_\delta = \frac{1}{M} \sum_{i=1}^M \delta_i = \frac{108,636,5232}{17,153,136} = 6.3333 \; ,
$$

and the observed chance-corrected measure of effect size is

$$
\Re = 1 - \frac{\delta}{\mu_\delta} = 1 - \frac{5.1778}{6.3333} = +0.1825 \; ,
$$

indicating approximately 18% within-group agreement above what is expected by chance. No comparisons are made with Cohen's $\hat{d}$, Pearson's r^2 (η^2), Kelley's $\hat{\eta}^2$, Hays' $\hat{\omega}_F^2$, or Hays' $\hat{\omega}_R^2$ measures of effect size as $\hat{d}, r^2, \hat{\eta}^2, \hat{\omega}_F^2$, and $\hat{\omega}_R^2$ are undefined for rank-score data.

8.9 Example 6: Multivariate Permutation Analyses

It is sometimes desirable to test for differences among $g \geq 3$ independent treatment groups where $r \geq 2$ measurement scores have been obtained from each object. The conventional approach is a one-way multivariate analysis of variance (MANOVA) for which a number of statistical tests have been proposed, including the Bartlett–Nanda–Pillai (BNP) trace test [1, 16, 19], Wilks' likelihood-ratio test [26], Roy's maximum-root test [20, 21], and the Lawley–Hotelling trace test [9, 13, 14]. The Bartlett–Nanda–Pillai trace test is considered to be the most powerful and robust of the four tests [17, 18, 23, p. 269].

8.9.1 The Bartlett–Nanda–Pillai Trace Test

To illustrate a conventional multivariate analysis of variance, consider the BNP trace test given by

$$
V^{(s)} = \text{trace}\left[\mathbf{B}(\mathbf{W} + \mathbf{B})^{-1}\right],
$$

where $\mathbf{W}$ denotes the Within matrix summarizing within-object variability, $\mathbf{B}$ denotes the hypothesized Between matrix summarizing between-object variability, and $s = \min(r, g-1)$. For a conventional test of significance, the BNP trace statistic, $V^{(s)}$, can be transformed into a conventional F test statistic by

$$
F = \frac{2u + s + 1}{2t + s + 1} \left(\frac{V^{(s)}}{s - V^{(s)}} \right) , \tag{8.27}
$$

Table 8.11 Example
multivariate response
measurement scores with
$r = 2$ measurement scores,
$g = 3$ treatment groups,
$n_1 = 5, n_2 = 4, n_3 = 3$, and
$N = 12$ observations

Treatment group		
1	2	3
(5.8, 6.0)	(4.1, 2.9)	(4.2, 7.8)
(6.2, 3.9)	(3.9, 4.1)	(5.1, 5.9)
(3.9, 4.1)	(4.9, 3.9)	(4.8, 7.2)
(5.1, 5.2)	(2.1, 5.1)	
(3.0, 2.8)		

where $s = \min(r, g - 1)$, $u = 0.50(N - g - r - 1)$, $t = 0.50(|r - q| - 1)$, and
$q = g - 1$. Assuming independence, normality, and homogeneity of variance and
covariance, test statistic F is asymptotically distributed as Snedecor's F under the
Neyman–Pearson null hypothesis with $v_1 = s(2t + s + 1)$ and $v_2 = s(2u + s + 1)$
degrees of freedom.

To illustrate the BNP trace test, consider the multivariate observations listed in
Table 8.11, where $r = 2$ measurements, $g = 3$ treatment groups, $n_1 = 5, n_2 = 4$,
and $n_3 = 3$ sample sizes, and $N = 12$ multivariate observations.

A conventional BNP analysis of the multivariate observations listed in Table 8.11
yields

$$\mathbf{W} = \begin{bmatrix} 11.71000 & 1.17000 \\ 1.17000 & 10.42667 \end{bmatrix}, \quad \mathbf{B} = \begin{bmatrix} 2.75250 & 3.19755 \\ 3.19755 & 17.30242 \end{bmatrix},$$

$$\mathbf{W} + \mathbf{B} = \begin{bmatrix} 14.46250 & 4.36755 \\ 4.36755 & 27.72909 \end{bmatrix},$$

$$(\mathbf{W} + \mathbf{B})^{-1} = \begin{bmatrix} 0.07260 & -0.01143 \\ -0.01143 & 0.03786 \end{bmatrix},$$

$$\mathbf{B}(\mathbf{W} + \mathbf{B})^{-1} = \begin{bmatrix} 0.16328 & 0.08960 \\ 0.03476 & 0.61852 \end{bmatrix},$$

and

$$V^{(2)} = \mathrm{trace}\left[\mathbf{B}(\mathbf{W} + \mathbf{B})^{-1}\right] = 0.16328 + 0.61852 = 0.7818 .$$

Then, $q = g - 1 = 3 - 1 = 2$, $s = \min(r, q) = \min(2, 3 - 1) = 2$,
$u = 0.50(N - g - r - 1) = 0.50(12 - 3 - 2 - 1) = 3$, $t = 0.50(|r - q| - 1) =$
$0.50(|2 - 2| - 1) = -0.50$, and following Eq. (8.27) on p. 306, the observed value

of Fisher's F-ratio test statistic is

$$F = \frac{2(3) + 2 + 1}{2(-0.50) + 2 + 1} \left(\frac{0.7818}{2 - 0.7818} \right) = \frac{9}{2}(0.6414) = 2.8879 .$$

Assuming independence, normality, homogeneity of variance, and homogeneity of covariance, test statistic F is asymptotically distributed as Snedecor's F with $v_1 = s(2t+s+1) = 2[(2)(-0.50)+2+1] = 4$ and $v_2 = s(2u+s+1) = 2[(2)(3)+ 2 + 1] = 18$ degrees of freedom. Under the Neyman–Pearson null hypothesis, the observed value of $F = 2.8879$ with $v_1 = 4$ and $v_2 = 18$ degrees of freedom yields an asymptotic probability value of $P = 0.0521$.

8.9.2   An Exact Analysis with $v = 2$

For the first analysis of the observed data listed in Table 8.11 under the Fisher–Pitman permutation model let $v = 2$, employing squared Euclidean scaling between the pairs of multivariate observations, and let the treatment-group weights be given by

$$C_i = \frac{n_i - 1}{N - g} , \qquad i = 1, \ldots, g ,$$

for correspondence with the BNP trace test. An exact permutation analysis is feasible for the multivariate observations listed in Table 8.11 as there are only

$$M = \frac{N!}{\displaystyle\prod_{i=1}^{g} n_i !} = \frac{12!}{5! \, 4! \, 3!} = 27,720$$

possible, equally-likely arrangements in the reference set of all permutations of the $N = 12$ multivariate scores listed in Table 8.11.

Following Eq. (8.2) on p. 261, the multivariate observations listed in Table 8.11 yield $g = 3$ average distance-function values of

$$\xi_1 = 0.3242 , \quad \xi_2 = 0.2994 , \quad \text{and} \quad \xi_3 = 0.1207 .$$

Following Eq. (8.1) on p. 261, the observed value of the permutation test statistic based on $v = 2$ and treatment-group weights

$$C_i = \frac{n_i - 1}{N - g} , \qquad i = 1, 2, 3 ,$$

is

$$\delta = \sum_{i=1}^{g} C_i \xi_i = \frac{1}{12 - 3} \big[(5 - 1)(0.3242) + (4 - 1)(0.2994)$$

$$+ (3 - 1)(0.1207) \big] = 0.2707 \ .$$

Under the Fisher–Pitman permutation model, the exact probability of an observed δ is the proportion of δ test statistic values computed on all possible, equally-likely arrangements of the $N = 12$ multivariate observations listed in Table 8.11 that are equal to or less than the observed value of $\delta = 0.2707$. There are exactly 967 δ test statistic values that are equal to or less than the observed value of $\delta = 0.2702$. If all M arrangements of the $N = 12$ multivariate scores listed in Table 8.11 occur with equal chance under the Fisher–Pitman null hypothesis, the exact probability value of $\delta = 0.2707$ computed on the $M = 27{,}720$ possible arrangements of the observed data with $n_1 = 5$, $n_2 = 4$, and $n_3 = 3$ multivariate observations preserved for each arrangement is

$$P\big(\delta \le \delta_0 | H_0\big) = \frac{\text{number of } \delta \text{ values } \le \delta_0}{M} = \frac{967}{27{,}720} = 0.0349 \ ,$$

where δ_0 denotes the observed value of test statistic δ and M is the number of possible, equally-likely arrangements of the $N = 12$ multivariate observations listed in Table 8.11.

Following Eq. (8.7) on p. 263, the exact expected value of the $M = 27{,}720$ δ test statistic values under the Fisher–Pitman null hypothesis is

$$\mu_\delta = \frac{1}{M} \sum_{i=1}^{M} \delta_i = \frac{10{,}080}{27{,}720} = 0.3636$$

and, following Eq. (8.6) on p. 263, the observed chance-corrected measure of effect size is

$$\Re = 1 - \frac{\delta}{\mu_\delta} = 1 - \frac{0.2707}{0.3636} = +0.2556 \ ,$$

indicating approximately 26% within-group agreement above what is expected by chance.

A convenient, although positively biased, measure of effect size for the BNP trace test is given by

$$\eta^2 = \frac{V^{(2)}}{S} = \frac{0.7818}{2} = 0.3909 \ ,$$

which can be compared with the unbiased chance-corrected measure of effect size, $\Re = +0.2556$. No comparisons are made with Cohen's $\hat{d}$, Kelley's $\hat{\eta}^2$, Hays' $\hat{\omega}_F^2$, or Hays' $\hat{\omega}_R^2$ measures of effect size as $\hat{d}$, $\hat{\eta}^2$, $\hat{\omega}_F^2$, and $\hat{\omega}_R^2$ are undefined for multivariate data.

The functional relationships between statistic δ and the $V^{(2)}$ BNP trace statistic are given by

$$\delta = \frac{2(r - V^{(2)})}{N - g} \quad \text{and} \quad V^{(2)} = r - \frac{\delta(N - g)}{2} . \tag{8.28}$$

Following the expressions given in Eq. (8.28) for test statistics δ and V^2, the observed value for test statistic δ with respect to the observed value of test statistic V^2 is

$$\delta = \frac{2(r - V^{(2)})}{N - g} = \frac{2(2 - 0.7818)}{12 - 3} = 0.2707$$

and the observed value for test statistic V^2 with respect to the observed value of test statistic δ is

$$V^{(2)} = r - \frac{\delta(N - g)}{2} = 2 - \frac{(0.2707)(12 - 3)}{2} = 0.7818 .$$

8.9.3 An Exact Analysis with $v = 1$

For a second analysis of the multivariate measurement scores listed in Table 8.11 on p. 307 under the Fisher–Pitman permutation model, let the treatment-group weights again be given by

$$C_i = \frac{n_i - 1}{N - g} , \quad i = 1, \ldots, g ,$$

but set $v = 1$ instead of $v = 2$, employing ordinary Euclidean scaling between the $N = 12$ multivariate scores. Following Eq. (8.2) on p. 261, the multivariate scores listed in Table 8.11 yield $g = 3$ average distance-function values of

$$\xi_1 = 2.3933 , \quad \xi_2 = 1.9326 , \quad \text{and} \quad \xi_3 = 1.4284 .$$

Following Eq. (8.1) on p. 261, the observed value of the permutation test statistic based on $v = 1$ and treatment-group weights

$$C_i = \frac{n_i - 1}{N - g} , \quad i = 1, 2, 3 ,$$

is

$$\delta = \sum_{i=1}^{g} C_i \xi_i = \frac{1}{12-3}\left[(5-1)(2.3933) + (4-1)(1.9326)\right.$$

$$\left. + (3-1)(1.4284)\right] = 2.0253 \ .$$

There are only

$$M = \frac{N!}{\prod_{i=1}^{g} n_i!} = \frac{12!}{5! \ 4! \ 3!} = 27{,}720$$

possible, equally-likely arrangements in the reference set of all permutations of the $N = 12$ multivariate observations listed in Table 8.11, making an exact permutation analysis feasible.

Under the Fisher–Pitman permutation model, the exact probability of an observed δ is the proportion of δ test statistic values computed on all possible, equally-likely arrangements of the $N = 12$ multivariate observations listed in Table 8.11 that are equal to or less than the observed value of $\delta = 2.0253$. There are exactly 618 δ test statistic values that are equal to or less than the observed value of $\delta = 2.0253$. If all M arrangements of the $N = 12$ multivariate observations listed in Table 8.11 occur with equal chance under the Fisher–Pitman null hypothesis, the exact probability value of $\delta = 2.0253$ computed on the $M = 27{,}720$ possible arrangements of the observed data with $n_1 = 5$, $n_2 = 4$, and $n_3 = 3$ multivariate observations preserved for each arrangement is

$$P\left(\delta \leq \delta_0 | H_0\right) = \frac{\text{number of } \delta \text{ values } \leq \delta_0}{M} = \frac{618}{27{,}720} = 0.0223 \ ,$$

where δ_0 denotes the observed value of test statistic δ and M is the number of possible, equally-likely arrangements of the $N = 12$ multivariate observations listed in Table 8.11. No comparison is made with the Bartlett–Nanda–Pillai trace test as the BNP test is undefined for ordinary Euclidean scaling.

Following Eq. (8.7) on p. 263, the exact expected value of the $M = 27{,}720$ δ test statistic values under the Fisher–Pitman null hypothesis is

$$\mu_\delta = \frac{1}{M} \sum_{i=1}^{M} \delta_i = \frac{69{,}854}{27{,}720} = 2.5200$$

and, following Eq. (8.6) on p. 263, the observed chance-corrected measure of effect size is

$$\Re = 1 - \frac{\delta}{\mu_\delta} = 1 - \frac{2.0253}{2.5200} = +0.1963 \ ,$$

indicating approximately 20% within-group agreement above that expected by chance. No comparison is made with the conventional measure of effect size as η^2 is undefined for ordinary Euclidean scaling.

8.10 Summary

This chapter examined statistical methods for multiple independent samples where the null hypothesis posits no differences among the $g \geq 3$ populations that the g random samples are presumed to represent. Under the Neyman–Pearson population model of statistical inference, a conventional one-way analysis of variance and five measures of effect size were described and illustrated: Fisher's F-ratio test statistic, and Cohen's $\hat{d}$, Pearson's η^2, Kelley's $\hat{\eta}^2$, Hays' $\hat{\omega}_F^2$, and Hays' $\hat{\omega}_R^2$ measures of effect size, respectively.

Under the Fisher–Pitman permutation model of statistical inference, test statistic δ and associated measure of effect size, $\Re$, were described and illustrated for multi-sample tests. For tests of $g \geq 3$ independent samples, test statistic δ was demonstrated to be flexible enough to incorporate both ordinary and squared Euclidean scaling functions with $v = 1$ and $v = 2$, respectively. Effect size measure $\Re$ was shown to be applicable to either $v = 1$ or $v = 2$ without modification and to have a clear and meaningful chance-corrected interpretation.

Six examples illustrated permutation-based statistics δ and $\Re$. In the first example, a small sample of $N = 10$ observations in $g = 3$ treatment groups was utilized to describe and illustrate the calculation of test statistics δ and $\Re$ for multiple independent samples. The second example with $N = 10$ observations in $g = 3$ treatment groups demonstrated the chance-corrected measure of effect size, $\Re$, and related $\Re$ to the five conventional measures of effect size for $g \geq 3$ independent samples: Cohen's $\hat{d}$, Pearson's η^2, Kelley's $\hat{\eta}^2$, Hays' $\hat{\omega}_F^2$, and Hays' $\hat{\omega}_R^2$. The third example with $N = 28$ observations in $g = 4$ treatment groups illustrated the effects of extreme values on analyses using $v = 1$ for ordinary Euclidean scaling and $v = 2$ for squared Euclidean scaling. The fourth example with $N = 15$ observations in $g = 4$ treatment groups compared exact and Monte Carlo permutation statistical methods, illustrating the accuracy and efficiency of Monte Carlo analyses. The fifth example with $N = 18$ rank scores in $g = 3$ treatment groups illustrated an application of permutation statistical methods to univariate rank-score data, comparing a permutation analysis of the rank-score data with the conventional Kruskal–Wallis g-sample one-way analysis of variance for ranks. In the sixth example, both test statistic δ and effect size measure $\Re$ were extended to multivariate data with $N = 12$ multivariate observations in $g = 3$ treatment groups and compared the permutation analysis of the multivariate data to the conventional Bartlett–Nanda–Pillai trace test for multivariate independent samples.

Chapter 9 continues the presentation of permutation statistical methods for $g \geq 3$ samples, but examines research designs in which the subjects in the $g \geq 3$ samples are matched on specific characteristics; that is, not independent. Research designs that posit no differences among matched treatment groups have a long history and are ubiquitous in the contemporary statistical literature and are generally known as randomized-blocks designs, of which there exist a large variety.

References

1. Bartlett, M.S.: A note on tests of significance in multivariate analysis. Proc. Camb. Philos. Soc. **34**, 33–40 (1939)
2. Berry, K.J., Mielke, P.W., Johnston, J.E.: Permutation Statistical Methods: An Integrated Approach. Springer, Cham (2016)
3. Boik, R.J.: The Fisher–Pitman permutation test: a non-robust alternative to the normal theory F test when variances are heterogeneous. Brit. J. Math. Stat. Psychol. **40**, 26–42 (1987)
4. Box, J.F.: R. A. Fisher: The Life of a Scientist. Wiley, New York (1978)
5. Festinger, L.: The significance of differences between means without reference to the frequency distribution function. Psychometrika **11**, 97–105 (1946)
6. Haggard, E.A.: Intraclass Correlation and the Analysis of Variance. Dryden, New York (1958)
7. Haldane, J.B.S., Smith, C.A.B.: A simple exact test for birth-order effect. Ann. Eugenic. **14**, 117–124 (1948)
8. Hall, N.S.: R. A. Fisher and his advocacy of randomization. J. Hist. Biol. **40**, 295–325 (2007)
9. Hotelling, H.: A generalized T test and measure of multivariate dispersion. In: Neyman, J. (ed.) Proceedings of the Second Berkeley Symposium on Mathematical Statistics and Probability, vol. II, pp. 23–41. University of California Press, Berkeley (1951)
10. Hotelling, H., Pabst, M.R.: Rank correlation and tests of significance involving no assumption of normality. Ann. Math. Stat. **7**, 29–43 (1936)
11. Johnston, J.E., Berry, K.J., Mielke, P.W.: Permutation tests: precision in estimating probability values. Percept. Motor Skill. **105**, 915–920 (2007)
12. Kruskal, W.H., Wallis, W.A.: Use of ranks in one-criterion variance analysis. J. Am. Stat. Assoc. **47**, 583–621 (1952). [Erratum: J. Am. Stat. Assoc. **48**, 907–911 (1953)]
13. Lawley, D.N.: A generalization of Fisher's z test. Biometrika **30**, 180–187 (1938)
14. Lawley, D.N.: Corrections to "A generalization of Fisher's z test". Biometrika **30**, 467–469 (1939)
15. Mann, H.B., Whitney, D.R.: On a test of whether one of two random variables is stochastically larger than the other. Ann. Math. Stat. **18**, 50–60 (1947)
16. Nanda, D.N.: Distribution of the sum of roots of a determinantal equation. Ann. Math. Stat. **21**, 432–439 (1950)
17. Olson, C.L.: On choosing a test statistic in multivariate analysis of variance. Psychol. Bull. **83**, 579–586 (1976)
18. Olson, C.L.: Practical considerations in choosing a MANOVA test statistic: a rejoinder to Stevens. Psychol. Bull. **86**, 1350–1352 (1979)
19. Pillai, K.C.S.: Some new test criteria in multivariate analysis. Ann. Math. Stat. **26**, 117–121 (1955)
20. Roy, S.N.: On a heuristic method of test construction and its use in multivariate analysis. Ann. Math. Stat. **24**, 220–238 (1953)
21. Roy, S.N.: Some Aspects of Multivariate Analysis. Wiley, New York (1957)
22. Snedecor, G.W.: Calculation and Interpretation of Analysis of Variance and Covariance. Collegiate Press, Ames (1934)
23. Tabachnick, B.G., Fidell, L.S.: Using Multivariate Statistics, 5th edn. Pearson, Boston (2007)
24. van der Reyden, D.: A simple statistical significance test. Rhod. Agric. J. **49**, 96–104 (1952)
25. Wilcoxon, F.: Individual comparisons by ranking methods. Biometrics Bull. **1**, 80–83 (1945)
26. Wilks, S.S.: Certain generalizations in the analysis of variance. Biometrika **24**, 471–494 (1932)

Chapter 9
Randomized-Blocks Designs

Abstract This chapter introduces permutation methods for multiple matched samples, i.e., randomized-blocks designs. Included in this chapter are six example analyses illustrating computation of exact permutation probability values for randomized-blocks designs, calculation of measures of effect size for randomized-blocks designs, the effect of extreme values on conventional and permutation randomized-blocks designs, exact and Monte Carlo permutation procedures for randomized-blocks designs, application of permutation methods to randomized-blocks designs with rank-score data, and analysis of randomized-blocks designs with multivariate data. Included in this chapter are permutation versions of Fisher's F test for a one-way randomized-blocks design, Friedman's two-way analysis of variance for ranks, and a permutation-based alternative for the four conventional measures of effect size for randomized-blocks designs: Hays' $\hat{\omega}^2$, Pearson's η^2, Cohen's partial η^2, and Cohen's f^2.

This chapter presents exact and Monte Carlo permutation statistical methods for tests of experimental differences among three or more matched or otherwise related samples, commonly called randomized-blocks designs under the Neyman–Pearson population model of statistical inference. As with matched-pairs tests discussed in Chap. 7, the samples may either be matched on specific criteria; for example, age, education, gender, or the same subjects may be observed at different times or under different treatments or interventions. While most randomized-blocks designs take observations at two, three, or four time periods, there have been a number of long-running studies that follow clients over many years. The best-known of these are the Fels Longitudinal Study founded in 1929 as a division of the Fels Research Institute in Yellow Springs, Ohio, the Framingham Heart Study initiated in 1948 in Framingham, Massachusetts, and the Terman Genetic Study of Genius founded at Stanford University in 1921. All three studies continue today.[1]

---

[1] Studies such as these that observe the same or matched subjects for many years are often referred to as "panel studies" and require a different statistical approach.

© Springer Nature Switzerland AG 2019
K. J. Berry et al., *A Primer of Permutation Statistical Methods*,
https://doi.org/10.1007/978-3-030-20933-9_9

As in previous chapters, six examples illustrate permutation statistical methods for randomized-blocks designs. The first example utilizes a small set of data to illustrate the computation of exact permutation methods for multiple matched samples, wherein the permutation test statistic, δ, is developed and compared with Fisher's conventional F-ratio test statistic for multiple dependent samples. The second example develops a permutation-based measure of effect size as a chance-corrected alternative to the four conventional measures of effect size for randomized-blocks designs: Hays' $\hat{\omega}^2$, Pearson's η^2, Cohen's partial η^2, and Cohen's f^2. The third example compares permutation statistical methods based on ordinary and squared Euclidean scaling functions, with an emphasis on the analysis of data sets containing extreme values. The fourth example utilizes a larger set of data to provide a comparison of exact permutation methods and Monte Carlo permutation methods, demonstrating the efficiency and accuracy of Monte Carlo permutation statistical methods for multiple matched samples. The fifth example illustrates the application of permutation statistical methods to univariate rank-score data, comparing permutation statistical methods to Friedman's conventional two-way analysis of variance for ranks. The sixth example illustrates the application of permutation statistical methods to multivariate data.

9.1 Introduction

The standard univariate test for $g \geq 3$ matched samples under the Neyman–Pearson population model of inference is Fisher's randomized-blocks analysis of variance wherein the null hypothesis (H_0) posits no mean differences among the g populations from which the samples presumably have been randomly drawn; that is, H_0: $\mu_1 = \mu_2 = \cdots = \mu_g$. Fisher's randomized-blocks analysis of variance does not determine whether or not the null hypothesis is true, but only provides the probability that, if the null hypothesis is true, the samples have been randomly drawn from populations with identical mean values, assuming normality.

Consider samples of $N = bg$ independent random variables x_{ij} with cumulative distribution functions $F_i(x + \beta_j)$ for $i = 1, \ldots, g$ and $j = 1, \ldots, b$, respectively, where g denotes the number of treatments and b denotes the number of blocks. For simplicity, assume that the x_{ij} values are randomly drawn from a normal distribution with mean $\mu_i + \beta_j$ and variance σ_x^2, $i = 1, \ldots, g$ and $j = 1, \ldots, b$. Under the Neyman–Pearson population model, the null hypothesis of no mean differences tests

$$H_0: \mu_1 = \mu_2 = \cdots = \mu_g \quad \text{versus} \quad H_1: \mu_i \neq \mu_j \quad \text{for some } i \neq j$$

for g treatment groups. The permissible probability of a type I error is denoted by α and if the observed value of Fisher's F is equal to or greater than the critical value of F that defines α, the null hypothesis is rejected with a probability of type I error equal to or less than α, under the assumption of normality.

For multi-sample tests with g treatment groups and b blocks, Fisher's F-ratio test statistic is given by

$$F = \frac{MS_{\text{Treatments}}}{MS_{\text{Error}}} ,$$

where the mean-square treatments is given by

$$MS_{\text{Treatments}} = \frac{SS_{\text{Treatments}}}{g - 1} ,$$

the sum-of-squares treatments is given by

$$SS_{\text{Treatments}} = b \sum_{i=1}^{g} \left(\bar{x}_{i.} - \bar{x}_{..} \right)^2 ,$$

the mean-square error is given by

$$MS_{\text{Error}} = \frac{SS_{\text{Error}}}{(b - 1)(g - 1)} ,$$

the sum-of-squares error is given by

$$SS_{\text{Error}} = \sum_{i=1}^{g} \sum_{j=1}^{b} \left(x_{ij} - \bar{x}_{i.} - \bar{x}_{.j} + \bar{x}_{..} \right)^2 ,$$

the sum-of-squares blocks is given by

$$SS_{\text{Blocks}} = g \sum_{j=1}^{b} \left(\bar{x}_{.j} - \bar{x}_{..} \right)^2 ,$$

the sum-of-squares total is given by

$$SS_{\text{Total}} = \sum_{i=1}^{g} \sum_{j=1}^{b} \left(x_{ij} - \bar{x}_{..} \right)^2 ,$$

the mean value for the ith of g treatments is

$$\bar{x}_{i.} = \frac{1}{b} \sum_{j=1}^{b} x_{ij} , \qquad i = 1, \ldots, g ,$$

the mean value for the jth of b blocks is

$$\bar{x}_{.j} = \frac{1}{g} \sum_{i=1}^{g} x_{ij} , \qquad j = 1, \ldots, b ,$$

the grand mean over all b blocks and g treatments is given by

$$\bar{x}_{..} = \frac{1}{gb} \sum_{i=1}^{g} \sum_{j=1}^{b} x_{ij} ,$$

and x_{ij} denotes the value of the jth block in the ith treatment for $j = 1, \ldots, b$ and $i = 1, \ldots, g$.

Under the Neyman–Pearson null hypothesis, H_0: $\mu_1 = \mu_2 = \cdots = \mu_g$, Fisher's F-ratio test statistic is asymptotically distributed as Snedecor's F with $v_1 = g - 1$ degrees of freedom (df) in the numerator and $v_2 = (b - 1)(g - 1)$ df in the denominator. If the x_{ij} values, $i = 1, \ldots, g$ and $j = 1, \ldots, b$, are not randomly sampled from a normally-distributed population, then Fisher's F-ratio test statistic no longer follows Snedecor's F distribution with $v_1 = g - 1$ and $v_2 = (b-1)(g-1)$ degrees of freedom.

The assumptions underlying Fisher's F test for multiple matched samples are (1) the observations are independent, (2) the data are random samples from well-defined, normally-distributed populations, (3) homogeneity of variance, and (4) homogeneity of covariance.

9.2   A Permutation Approach

Alternatively, consider a test for multiple matched samples under the Fisher–Pitman permutation model of statistical inference. Under the Fisher–Pitman permutation model there is no null hypothesis specifying population parameters. Instead the null hypothesis simply states that all possible arrangements of the observations occur with equal chance [4]. Moreover, there is no alternative hypothesis under the permutation model and no specified α level. Also, there is no requirement of random sampling, no degrees of freedom, no assumption of normality, no assumption of homogeneity of variance, and no assumption of homogeneity of covariance. This is not to imply that the results of permutation statistical methods are unaffected by homogeneity of variance and covariance, but homogeneity of variance and covariance are not requirements for permutation methods as they are for conventional statistical methods under the Neyman–Pearson population model.

A permutation alternative to Fisher's conventional F-ratio test for $g \geq 3$ matched samples is given by

$$\delta = \left[g \binom{b}{2} \right]^{-1} \sum_{i=1}^{g} \sum_{j=1}^{b-1} \sum_{k=j+1}^{b} \Delta \left(x_{ij}, x_{ik} \right) , \tag{9.1}$$

where the symmetric distance functions are given by

$$\Delta(x, y) = \left[(x_i - y_i)^2\right]^{v/2} \tag{9.2}$$

and $v > 0$. When $v = 1$, ordinary Euclidean scaling is employed, and when $v = 2$, squared Euclidean scaling is employed [7].

Under the Fisher–Pitman permutation model, the null hypothesis states that equal probabilities are assigned to each of the

$$M = \left(g!\right)^b$$

possible allocations of the observations to the g treatments within each of the b blocks. The probability value associated with an observed value of δ is the probability under the Fisher–Pitman null hypothesis of observing a value of δ that is equal to or less than the observed value of δ. An exact probability value for δ may be expressed as

$$P(\delta \leq \delta_0 | H_0) = \frac{\text{number of } \delta \text{ values } \leq \delta_0}{M},$$

where δ_0 denotes the observed value of test statistic δ and M is the number of possible, equally-likely arrangements of the observed data.

When M is large, an approximate probability value for test statistic δ may be obtained from a Monte Carlo procedure, where a large random sample of arrangements of the observed data is drawn. Then an approximate probability value for test statistic δ is given by

$$P(\delta \leq \delta_0 | H_0) = \frac{\text{number of } \delta \text{ values } \leq \delta_0}{L},$$

where L denotes the number of the randomly-selected, equally-likely arrangements of the observed data.

9.3   The Relationship Between Statistics F and δ

When the null hypothesis under the Neyman–Pearson population model states H_0: $\mu_1 = \mu_2 = \cdots = \mu_g$ and $v = 2$, the functional relationships between test statistic δ and Fisher's F test statistic are given by

$$F = \frac{(b - 1)[2SS_{\text{Total}} - g(b - 1)\delta]}{g(b - 1)\delta - 2SS_{\text{Blocks}}} \tag{9.3}$$

and

$$\delta = \frac{2[F\,SS_{\text{Blocks}} + (b-1)SS_{\text{Total}}]}{g(b-1)(F+b-1)} \ . \tag{9.4}$$

Because of the relationship between test statistics δ and F, the exact probability values given by

$$P(\delta \le \delta_0|H_0) = \frac{\text{number of } \delta \text{ values } \le \delta_0}{M}$$

and

$$P(F \ge F_0|H_0) = \frac{\text{number of } F \text{ values } \ge F_0}{M} \ .$$

are equivalent under the Fisher–Pitman null hypothesis, where δ_0 and F_0 denote the observed values of test statistics δ and F, respectively, and M is the number of possible, equally-likely arrangements of the observed data.

A chance-corrected measure of agreement is given by

$$\Re = 1 - \frac{\delta}{\mu_\delta} \ , \tag{9.5}$$

where μ_δ, the exact expected value of the M δ test statistic values calculated on all possible arrangements of the observed measurements, is given by

$$\mu_\delta = \frac{1}{M} \sum_{i=1}^{M} \delta_i \ . \tag{9.6}$$

9.4   Example 1: Test Statistics F and δ

A small example will serve to illustrate the relationships between test statistics F and δ. Consider the example randomized-blocks data listed in Table 9.1 with $g = 2$ treatment groups, $b = 4$ blocks, and $N = bg = (4)(2) = 8$ total observations.

Table 9.1 Example data with $g = 2$ treatments and $b = 4$ blocks

	Treatment	
Block	1	2
1	105	21
2	144	52
3	109	97
4	113	32

Under the Neyman–Pearson population model with treatment means $\bar{x}_{1.} = 117.75$ and $\bar{x}_{2.} = 50.50$, block means $\bar{x}_{.1} = 63.00$, $\bar{x}_{.2} = 98.00$, $\bar{x}_{.3} = 103.00$, and $\bar{x}_{.4} = 72.50$, grand mean $\bar{x}_{..} = 84.1250$, the sum-of-squares total is

$$SS_{Total} = \sum_{i=1}^{g} \sum_{j=1}^{b} \left(x_{ij} - \bar{x}_{..}\right)^2 = 13{,}372.8750 \, ,$$

the sum-of-squares treatments is

$$SS_{Treatments} = b \sum_{i=1}^{g} \left(\bar{x}_{i.} - \bar{x}_{..}\right)^2 = 9045.1250 \, ,$$

the mean-square treatments is

$$MS_{Treatments} = \frac{SS_{Treatments}}{g-1} = \frac{9045.1250}{2-1} = 9045.1250 \, ,$$

the sum-of-squares blocks is

$$SS_{Blocks} = g \sum_{j=1}^{b} \left(\bar{x}_{.j} - \bar{x}_{..}\right)^2 = 2260.3750 \, ,$$

the sum-of-squares error is

$$SS_{Error} = \sum_{i=1}^{g} \sum_{j=1}^{b} \left(x_{ij} - \bar{x}_{i.} - \bar{x}_{.j} + \bar{x}_{..}\right)^2 = 2067.3750 \, ,$$

the mean-square error is

$$MS_{Error} = \frac{SS_{Error}}{(b-1)(g-1)} = \frac{2067.3750}{(4-1)(2-1)} = 689.1250 \, ,$$

and the observed value of Fisher's F-ratio test statistic is

$$F = \frac{MS_{Treatments}}{MS_{Error}} = \frac{9045.1250}{689.1250} = 13.1255 \, .$$

For computational efficiency, SS_{Error} can easily be obtained by simple subtraction; for example,

$$SS_{Error} = SS_{Total} - SS_{Blocks} - SS_{Treatments}$$
$$= 13{,}372.8750 - 2260.3750 - 9045.1250 = 2067.3750 \, .$$

Table 9.2 Source table for the data listed in Table 9.1

Factor	SS	df	MS	F
Blocks	2260.3750			
Treatments	9045.1250	1	9045.1250	13.1255
Error	2067.3750	3	689.1250	
Total	13,372.8750			

The essential factors, sums of squares (SS), degrees of freedom (df), mean squares (MS), and variance-ratio test statistic (F) are summarized in Table 9.2.

Under the Neyman–Pearson null hypothesis, H_0: $\mu_1 = \mu_2 = \cdots = \mu_g$, Fisher's F-ratio test statistic is asymptotically distributed as Snedecor's F with $v_1 = g - 1$ and $v_2 = (b-1)(g-1)$ degrees of freedom. With $v_1 = g - 1 = 2 - 1 = 1$ and $v_2 = (b-1)(g-1) = (4-1)(2-1) = 3$ degrees of freedom, the asymptotic probability value of $F = 13.1255$ is $P = 0.0362$, under the assumptions of normality and homogeneity.

9.4.1 An Exact Analysis with v = 2

For an exact analysis under the Fisher–Pitman permutation model let $v = 2$, employing squared Euclidean scaling for correspondence with Fisher's F-ratio test statistic. Following Eq. (9.2) on p. 319 with $v = 2$ for Treatment 1, the six distance-function values are

$$\Delta(1, 2) = \left(\left|105 - 144\right|^2\right)^{2/2} = 1521 ,$$

$$\Delta(1, 3) = \left(\left|105 - 109\right|^2\right)^{2/2} = 16 ,$$

$$\Delta(1, 4) = \left(\left|105 - 113\right|^2\right)^{2/2} = 64 ,$$

$$\Delta(2, 3) = \left(\left|144 - 109\right|^2\right)^{2/2} = 1225 ,$$

$$\Delta(2, 4) = \left(\left|144 - 113\right|^2\right)^{2/2} = 961 ,$$

$$\Delta(3, 4) = \left(\left|109 - 113\right|^2\right)^{2/2} = 16 ,$$

and for Treatment 2, the six distance-function values are

$$\Delta(1,2) = \left(\left|21 - 52\right|^2\right)^{2/2} = 961 ,$$

$$\Delta(1,3) = \left(\left|21 - 97\right|^2\right)^{2/2} = 5776 ,$$

$$\Delta(1,4) = \left(\left|21 - 32\right|^2\right)^{2/2} = 121 ,$$

$$\Delta(2,3) = \left(\left|52 - 97\right|^2\right)^{2/2} = 2025 ,$$

$$\Delta(2,4) = \left(\left|52 - 32\right|^2\right)^{2/2} = 400 ,$$

$$\Delta(3,4) = \left(\left|97 - 32\right|^2\right)^{2/2} = 4225 .$$

Following Eq. (9.1) on p. 318, the observed value of test statistic δ is

$$\delta = \left[g\binom{b}{2}\right]^{-1} \sum_{i=1}^{g} \sum_{j=1}^{b-1} \sum_{k=j+1}^{b} \Delta\left(x_{ij}, x_{ik}\right)$$

$$= \left[2\binom{4}{2}\right]^{-1} \left[\Delta(1,2) + \Delta(1,3) + \cdots + \Delta(3,4)\right]$$

$$= \frac{1}{12}\left(1521 + 16 + 64 + \cdots + 400 + 4225\right) = 1442.5833 .$$

Alternatively, in terms of a randomized-blocks analysis of variance model the observed permutation test statistic is

$$\delta = \frac{2(SS_{\text{Total}} - SS_{\text{Treatments}})}{N - g}$$

$$= \frac{2(13{,}372.8750 - 9045.1250)}{8 - 2} = 1442.5833 .$$

Based on the expressions given in Eqs. (9.3) and (9.4) on p. 319, the observed value of test statistic F with respect to the observed value of test statistic δ is

$$F = \frac{(b-1)[2SS_{\text{Total}} - g(b-1)\delta]}{g(b-1)\delta - 2SS_{\text{Blocks}}}$$

$$= \frac{(4-1)[2(13{,}372.8750) - (2)(4-1)(1442.5833)]}{2(4-1)(1442.5833) - 2(2260.3750)} = 13.1255$$

and the observed value of test statistic δ with respect to the observed value of test statistic F is

$$
\begin{aligned}
\delta &= \frac{2[F SS_{\text{Blocks}} + (b-1)SS_{\text{Total}}]}{g(b-1)(F+b-1)} \\
&= \frac{2[(13.1255)(2260.3750) + (4-1)(13{,}372.8750)]}{2(4-1)(13.1255+4-1)} = 1442.5833 .
\end{aligned}
$$

Because there are only

$$
M = \left(g!\right)^{b} = \left(2!\right)^{4} = 16
$$

possible, equally-likely arrangements in the reference set of all permutations of the $N = 8$ observations listed in Table 9.1, an exact permutation analysis is feasible. Under the Fisher–Pitman permutation model, the exact probability of an observed δ is the proportion of δ test statistic values computed on all possible, equally-likely arrangements of the $N = 8$ observations listed in Table 9.1 that are equal to or less than the observed value of $\delta = 1442.5833$. Table 9.3 lists the $M = 16$ possible δ values, ordered from the lowest ($\delta_1 = 1442.5833$) to the highest ($\delta_{16} = 4302.5833$).

It is readily apparent from Table 9.3 that there are duplicate arrangements of the observed scores and duplicate δ values; for example, Order 1 {105, 144, 109, 113} minus Order 2 {21, 52, 97, 32} yields the same absolute difference as Order 15 {21, 52, 97, 32} minus Order 16 {105, 144, 109, 113}. It is more efficient to fix the

Table 9.3 Permutations of the observed scores listed in Table 9.1 with values for δ based on $v = 2$ ordered from lowest to highest

Order	Treatment 1	Treatment 2	δ
1	{105, 144, 109, 113}	{ 21, 52, 97, 32}	1442.5833
2	{ 21, 52, 97, 32}	{105, 144, 109, 113}	1442.5833
3	{105, 144, 97, 113}	{ 21, 52, 109, 32}	1956.5833
4	{ 21, 52, 109, 32}	{105, 144, 97, 113}	1956.5833
5	{ 21, 52, 97, 113}	{105, 144, 109, 32}	3980.5833
6	{105, 144, 109, 32}	{ 21, 52, 97, 113}	3980.5833
7	{ 21, 144, 109, 113}	{105, 52, 97, 32}	4032.5833
8	{105, 52, 97, 32}	{ 21, 144, 109, 113}	4032.5833
9	{105, 52, 109, 113}	{ 21, 144, 97, 32}	4156.5833
10	{ 21, 144, 97, 32}	{105, 52, 109, 113}	4156.5833
11	{ 21, 52, 109, 113}	{105, 144, 97, 32}	4170.5833
12	{105, 144, 97, 32}	{ 21, 52, 109, 113}	4170.5833
13	{ 21, 144, 97, 113}	{105, 52, 109, 32}	4210.5833
14	{105, 52, 109, 32}	{ 21, 144, 97, 113}	4210.5833
15	{105, 52, 97, 113}	{ 21, 144, 109, 32}	4302.5833
16	{ 21, 144, 109, 32}	{105, 52, 97, 113}	4302.5833

Table 9.4 Permutations of the observed scores listed in Table 9.1 with values for δ based on $v = 2$ ordered from lowest to highest

Order	Treatment 1	Treatment 2	δ
1	{105, 144, 109, 113}	{ 21, 52, 97, 32}	1442.5833
2	{105, 144, 97, 113}	{ 21, 52, 109, 32}	1956.5833
3	{ 21, 52, 97, 113}	{105, 144, 109, 32}	3980.5833
4	{ 21, 144, 109, 113}	{105, 52, 97, 32}	4032.5833
5	{105, 52, 109, 113}	{ 21, 144, 97, 32}	4156.5833
6	{ 21, 52, 109, 113}	{105, 144, 97, 32}	4170.5833
7	{ 21, 144, 97, 113}	{105, 52, 109, 32}	4210.5833
8	{105, 52, 97, 113}	{ 21, 144, 109, 32}	4302.5833
Total			28,252.6667

scores in one block and permute the remaining blocks. Thus,

$$M = \left(g!\right)^{b} = \left(2!\right)^{4} = 16 \quad \text{is replaced by} \quad M = \left(g!\right)^{b-1} = \left(2!\right)^{4-1} = 8$$

and the results are listed in Table 9.4. There is only one δ value in Table 9.4 that is equal to or less than the observed value of $\delta = 1442.5833$. If all M arrangements of the $N = 8$ observations listed in Table 9.4 occur with equal chance under the Fisher–Pitman null hypothesis, the exact probability value of $\delta = 1442.5833$ computed on all $M = 8$ arrangements of the observed data with $b = 4$ blocks preserved for each arrangement is

$$P(\delta \leq \delta_0 | H_0) = \frac{\text{number of } \delta \text{ values } \leq \delta_0}{M} = \frac{1}{8} = 0.1250 \,,$$

where δ_0 denotes the observed value of test statistic δ and M is the number of possible, equally-likely arrangements of the $N = 8$ observations listed in Table 9.1. Alternatively, there is only one F value that is equal to or greater than the observed value of $F = 13.1255$, as illustrated in Table 9.5. Thus if all M arrangements of the $N = 8$ observations listed in Table 9.1 occur with equal

Table 9.5 Permutations of the observed scores listed in Table 9.1 with values for Fisher's F-ratio ordered from highest to lowest

Order	Treatment 1	Treatment 2	F-ratio
1	{105, 144, 109, 113}	{ 21, 52, 97, 32}	13.1255
2	{105, 144, 97, 113}	{ 21, 52, 109, 32}	6.2364
3	{ 21, 52, 97, 113}	{105, 144, 109, 32}	0.4435
4	{ 21, 144, 109, 113}	{105, 52, 97, 32}	0.3889
5	{105, 52, 109, 113}	{ 21, 144, 97, 32}	0.2654
6	{ 21, 52, 109, 113}	{105, 144, 97, 32}	0.2520
7	{ 21, 144, 97, 113}	{105, 52, 109, 32}	0.2144
8	{105, 52, 97, 113}	{ 21, 144, 109, 32}	0.1311

chance under the Fisher–Pitman null hypothesis, the exact probability value of $F = 13.1255$ is

$$P(F \geq F_0 | H_0) = \frac{\text{number of } F \text{ values} \geq F_0}{M} = \frac{1}{8} = 0.1250 \,,$$

where F_0 denotes the observed value of test statistic F.

There is a considerable difference between the conventional asymptotic probability value for F ($P = 0.0362$) and the exact permutation probability value for δ ($P = 0.1250$). The difference between the two probability values of

$$\Delta_P = 0.1250 - 0.0362 = 0.0888$$

is most likely due to the very small number of blocks. A continuous mathematical function such as Snedecor's F cannot be expected to provide a precise fit to only $M = 8$ discrete data points.

Following Eq. (9.6) on p. 320, the exact expected value of the $M = 8$ δ test statistic values under the Fisher–Pitman null hypothesis is

$$\mu_\delta = \frac{1}{M} \sum_{i=1}^{M} \delta_i = \frac{28,252.6667}{8} = 3531.5833 \,.$$

Following Eq. (9.5) on p. 320, the observed chance-corrected measure of effect size is

$$\Re = 1 - \frac{\delta}{\mu_\delta} = 1 - \frac{1442.5833}{3531.5833} = +0.5915 \,,$$

indicating approximately 59% within-block agreement above what is expected by chance.

9.5 Example 2: Measures of Effect Size

Many researchers deplore the sole reliance on tests of statistical significance and recommend that indices of effect size—magnitude of experimental effects—accompany tests of significance. Measures of effect size express the practical or clinical significance of differences among sample means, as contrasted with the statistical significance of the differences. Consequently, the reporting of measures of effect size in addition to tests of significance has become increasingly important in the contemporary research literature. For example, a 2018 article in *The Lancet* sought to establish the risk thresholds for alcohol consumption using a meta-analysis for 83 observational studies with a total of 599,912 consumers of alcohol, concluding that no level of alcohol consumption is safe [11]. A critique of the article in the *New York Times* noted that no measure of effect size was included:

> [W]hen we compile observational study on top of observational study, we become more likely to achieve statistical significance without improving clinical significance. In other words, very small differences are real, but that doesn't mean those differences are critical [1, p. A12].

Five conventional measures of effect size for randomized-blocks analysis of variance designs are described and compared in this section: Hays' $\hat{\omega}^2$, Pearson's η^2, Cohen's partial η^2, Cohen's f^2, and Mielke and Berry's $\mathfrak{R}$.

Hays' $\hat{\omega}^2$ measure of effect size is given by

$$\hat{\omega}^2 = \frac{(g-1)(MS_{\text{Treatments}} - MS_{\text{Error}})}{SS_{\text{Total}} + MS_{\text{Within Blocks}}} \,, \tag{9.7}$$

where the mean-square within blocks is given by

$$MS_{\text{Within Blocks}} = \frac{SS_{\text{Within Blocks}}}{b(g-1)} \,,$$

b and g denote the number of blocks and treatments, respectively, and the sum-of-squares within blocks is given by

$$SS_{\text{Within Blocks}} = SS_{\text{Total}} - SS_{\text{Blocks}} \,. \tag{9.8}$$

Pearson's η^2 measure of effect size is given by[2]

$$\eta^2 = \frac{SS_{\text{Treatments}}}{SS_{\text{Total}}} \,. \tag{9.9}$$

Cohen's partial η^2 measure of effect size is given by

$$\eta^2_{\text{Partial}} = \frac{SS_{\text{Treatments}}}{SS_{\text{Total}} - SS_{\text{Error}}} \,. \tag{9.10}$$

Cohen's f^2 measure of effect size is given by

$$f^2 = \frac{SS_{\text{Treatments}}}{SS_{\text{Total}} - SS_{\text{Treatments}}} \,. \tag{9.11}$$

Mielke and Berry's chance-corrected measure of effect size is given by

$$\mathfrak{R} = 1 - \frac{\delta}{\mu_\delta} \,, \tag{9.12}$$

---

[2]Pearson's η^2 measure of effect size is often erroneously referred to as the "correlation ratio." Technically, η is the correlation ratio and η^2 is the differentiation ratio [9, p. 137].

where δ is defined in Eq. (9.1) on p. 318 and μ_δ is the exact expected value of test statistic δ under the Fisher–Pitman null hypothesis given by

$$\mu_\delta = \frac{1}{M} \sum_{i=1}^{M} \delta_i \,,$$

where for a test of $g \geq 3$ matched samples, the number of possible arrangements of the observed data is given by

$$M = (g!)^{b-1} \,, \tag{9.13}$$

where g and b denote the number of treatments and blocks, respectively.

9.5.1 An Example Analysis

To illustrate the calculation of the five measures of effect size, suppose that a fast-food chain of restaurants decides to evaluate the service at four randomly-chosen restaurants. The customer-service director for the chain hires six evaluators with varied experiences in food-service evaluations to act as raters. In this example, the $g = 4$ restaurants are the treatments and the $b = 6$ raters are the blocks. The six raters evaluate the service at each of the four restaurants in random order. A rating scale from 0 (low) to 100 (high) is used. Table 9.6 summarizes the evaluation data. Under the Neyman–Pearson population model with treatment means $\bar{x}_{1.} = 77.5000$, $\bar{x}_{2.} = 66.6667$, $\bar{x}_{3.} = 91.0000$, and $\bar{x}_{4.} = 79.3333$, block means $\bar{x}_{.1} = 71.7500$, $\bar{x}_{.2} = 79.0000$, $\bar{x}_{.3} = 78.2500$, $\bar{x}_{.4} = 78.7500$, $\bar{x}_{.5} = 81.5000$, and $\bar{x}_{.6} = 82.500$, grand mean $\bar{x}_{..} = 78.6250$, the sum-of-squares total is

$$SS_{\text{Total}} = \sum_{i=1}^{g} \sum_{j=1}^{b} \left(x_{ij} - \bar{x}_{..}\right)^2 = 2295.6250 \,,$$

Table 9.6 Example restaurant data with $g = 4$ treatments and $b = 6$ blocks

	Restaurant			
Rater	A	B	C	D
1	70	61	82	74
2	77	75	88	76
3	76	67	90	80
4	80	63	96	76
5	84	66	92	84
6	78	68	98	86

the sum-of-squares treatments is

$$SS_{\text{Treatments}} = b \sum_{i=1}^{g} \left(\bar{x}_{i.} - \bar{x}_{..}\right)^2 = 1787.4583 ,$$

the mean-square treatments is

$$MS_{\text{Treatments}} = \frac{SS_{\text{Treatments}}}{g-1} = \frac{1787.4583}{4-1} = 595.8194 ,$$

the sum-of-squares blocks is

$$SS_{\text{Blocks}} = g \sum_{j=1}^{b} \left(\bar{x}_{.j} - \bar{x}_{..}\right)^2 = 283.3750 ,$$

the sum-of-squares error is

$$SS_{\text{Error}} = SS_{\text{Total}} - SS_{\text{Blocks}} - SS_{\text{Treatments}}$$
$$= 2295.6250 - 283.3750 - 1787.4583 = 224.7917 ,$$

the mean-square error is

$$MS_{\text{Error}} = \frac{SS_{\text{Error}}}{(b-1)(g-1)} = \frac{224.7917}{(6-1)(4-1)} = 14.9861 ,$$

and the observed value of Fisher's F-ratio test statistic is

$$F = \frac{MS_{\text{Treatments}}}{MS_{\text{Error}}} = \frac{595.8194}{14.9861} = 39.7581 .$$

The essential factors, sums of squares (SS), degrees of freedom (df), mean squares (MS), and variance-ratio test statistic (F) are summarized in Table 9.7.

Table 9.7 Source table for the data listed in Table 9.6

Factor	SS	df	MS	F
Blocks	283.3750			
Treatments	1787.4583	3	595.8194	39.7581
Error	224.7917	15	14.9861	
Total	2295.6250			

Given the summary data in Table 9.7, Hays' $\hat{\omega}^2$ measure of effect size is

$$\hat{\omega}^2 = \frac{(g-1)(MS_{\text{Treatments}} - MS_{\text{Error}})}{SS_{\text{Total}} + MS_{\text{Within Blocks}}}$$

$$= \frac{(4-1)(595.8194 - 14.9861)}{2295.6250 - 111.7917} = 0.7238 ,$$

where the mean-square within blocks is

$$MS_{\text{Within Blocks}} = \frac{SS_{\text{Within Blocks}}}{b(g-1)} = \frac{2012.2500}{6(4-1)} = 111.7917 ,$$

and the sum-of-squares within blocks is

$$SS_{\text{Within Blocks}} = SS_{\text{Total}} - SS_{\text{Blocks}}$$

$$= 2295.6250 - 283.3750 = 2012.2500 .$$

Following Eq. (9.9) on p. 327, Pearson's η^2 measure of effect size is

$$\eta^2 = \frac{SS_{\text{Treatments}}}{SS_{\text{Total}}} = \frac{1787.4583}{2295.6250} = 0.7786 .$$

Following Eq. (9.10) on p. 327, Cohen's partial η^2 measure of effect size is

$$\eta^2_{\text{Partial}} = \frac{SS_{\text{Treatments}}}{SS_{\text{Total}} - SS_{\text{Error}}} = \frac{1787.4583}{2295.6250 - 224.7917} = 0.8632 .$$

Following Eq. (9.11) on p. 327, Cohen's f^2 measure of effect size is

$$f^2 = \frac{SS_{\text{Treatments}}}{SS_{\text{Total}} - SS_{\text{Treatments}}} = \frac{1787.4583}{2295.6250 - 1787.4583} = 3.5175 .$$

Cohen's f^2 measure of effect size can also be defined in terms of Pearson's η^2 measure of effect size and calculated as

$$f^2 = \frac{\eta^2}{1 - \eta^2} = \frac{0.7786}{1 - 0.7786} = 3.5175 .$$

Following Eq. (9.13) on p. 328 with $\delta = 50.8167$,

$$M = (g!)^{b-1} = (4!)^{6-1} = 7962,624 ,$$

and following Eq. (9.6) on p. 320 the exact expected value of test statistic δ under the Fisher–Pitman null hypothesis is

$$\mu_\delta = \frac{1}{M} \sum_{i=1}^{M} \delta_i = \frac{1,560,873,370}{7,962,624} = 196.0250 \, .$$

Then following Eq. (9.5) on p. 320, Mielke and Berry's chance-corrected measure of effect size is

$$\Re = 1 - \frac{\delta}{\mu_\delta} = 1 - \frac{50.8167}{196.0250} = +0.7408 \, ,$$

indicating approximately 78% within-blocks agreement above what is expected by chance.

A number of criticisms have been directed at the four conventional measures of effect size: Hays' $\hat{\omega}^2$, Pearson's η^2, Cohen's partial η^2, and Cohen's f^2. As can be seen in Eq. (9.8) on p. 327, in the unusual case when $MS_{\text{Treatments}}$ is smaller than MS_{Error}, yielding $F < 1$, Hays' $\hat{\omega}^2$ will be negative and it is difficult to interpret a squared measure of effect size that is negative. Moreover, unless a measure of effect size norms properly between the limits of 0 and 1, intermediate values are difficult to interpret.

Because Pearson's η^2 is simply the ratio of $SS_{\text{Treatments}}$ to SS_{Total}, η^2 norms properly between 0 and 1, providing an interpretation of the total variability in the dependent variable that is accounted for by variation in the independent variable. Moreover, when there is one degree of freedom in the numerator ($g = 2$ treatments), η^2 is equal to the product-moment coefficient of determination, r^2, and when there is more than one degree of freedom in the numerator ($g \geq 3$ treatments), η^2 is equal to the squared multiple product-moment correlation coefficient, R^2. Most researchers are familiar with Pearson's r^2 and R^2 correlation coefficients, making η^2 a useful index to understand the magnitude of effect sizes. Consequently, Pearson's η^2 is the most widely reported measure of effect size for randomized-blocks designs. On the other hand, η^2 is a biased estimator of effect size, systematically overestimating the size of treatment effects. Finally, as Sechrest and Yeaton concluded:

> As a general proposition it can be stated that *all measures of variance accounted for are specific to the characteristics of the experiment from which the estimates were obtained,* and therefore the ultimate interpretation of proportion of variance accounted for is a dubious prospect at best [10, p. 592].[3]

Cohen's partial η^2 is especially troublesome as reported by Kennedy [5], Levine and Hullett [6], Pedhazur [8, pp. 507–510], and Richardson [9]. In a classical one-way, completely-randomized analysis of variance design, η^2 and η^2_{Partial} yield identical results. However, η^2 and η^2_{Partial} yield different results in randomized-

---

[3] Emphasis in the original.

blocks analysis of variance designs, with η_{Partial}^2 values being equal to or greater than η^2 values. Thus if η^2 systematically overestimates effect size, η_{Partial}^2 overestimates effect size even more so. As Levine and Hullett concluded in reference to η^2:

> [B]ecause eta squared is always equal to partial eta squared or smaller, it may be seen as a more conservative estimate than partial eta squared and this may be appealing to many readers, reviewers, and editors [6, p. 620].

Since Cohen's η_{Partial}^2 is not a percentage of the total sum-of-squares, it therefore is not additive like η^2. Moreover, η^2 has the advantage of being equivalent to the familiar r^2 and R^2 Pearson product-moment correlation coefficients.

Pedhazur pointed to another limitation of both η^2 and η_{Partial}^2 as measures of effect size. While both η^2 and η_{Partial}^2 have a logical upper bound of 1, the only situation in which η^2 and η_{Partial}^2 can achieve an upper limit of 1 is when all values in each treatment are of one score, but differ among treatments. Pedhazur demonstrated that if the dependent variable is normally distributed, both η^2 and η_{Partial}^2 have an upper limit of approximately 0.64 [8, p. 507]. Finally, Levine and Hullett concluded that "[O]ur examination of the literature revealed little reason for the reporting of partial eta squared" [6, p. 620].

Cohen's f^2 measure of effect size is seldom found in the literature as it is simply a function of Pearson's η^2. Cohen's f^2 is difficult to interpret as it varies between zero and infinity; for example, anytime Pearson's $\eta^2 > 0.50$, f^2 will exceed unity. Cohen suggested that small, medium, and large effects are reflected in values of f^2 equal to 0.01, 0.0625, and 0.16, respectively. In general, researchers desire more precision than simply small, medium, and large effect sizes.

On a more positive note, $\Re$ is a measure of effect size that possesses a clear and useful chance-corrected interpretation. Positive values of $\Re$ indicate agreement greater than expected by chance, negative values of $\Re$ indicate agreement less than expected by chance, and a value of zero indicates chance agreement. Moreover, $\Re$ is a universal measure of effect size and can be used in a wide variety of statistical applications, including one-sample t tests, matched-pairs t tests, simple and multiple regression, all manner of analysis of variance designs, and numerous contingency table analyses.

9.6 Example 3: Analyses with $v = 2$ and $v = 1$

For a third example of tests of differences among $g \geq 3$ matched samples, consider the example data set given in Table 9.8 with $g = 3$ treatments, $b = 8$ blocks, and $N = bg = 24$ total observations. Under the Neyman–Pearson population model with treatment-group means $\bar{x}_{1.} = 229.25$, $\bar{x}_{2.} = 236.25$, and $\bar{x}_{3.} = 247.00$, block means $\bar{x}_{.1} = 241.00$, $\bar{x}_{.2} = 290.00$, $\bar{x}_{.3} = 118.6667$, $\bar{x}_{.4} = 246.3333$, $\bar{x}_{.5} = 122.6667$, $\bar{x}_{.6} = 336.00$, $\bar{x}_{.7} = 176.3333$, and $\bar{x}_{.8} = 369.00$, grand mean

Table 9.8 Example data for comparing analyses with $v = 2$ and $v = 1$ given $g = 3$ treatments and $b = 8$ blocks

		Treatment	
Block	1	2	3
1	221	247	255
2	283	302	285
3	103	130	123
4	254	223	262
5	115	113	140
6	322	344	342
7	161	181	187
8	375	350	382

$\bar{x}_{..} = 237.50$, the sum-of-squares total is

$$SS_{\text{Total}} = \sum_{i=1}^{g} \sum_{j=1}^{b} \left(x_{ij} - \bar{x}_{..} \right)^2 = 186{,}448.00 \, ,$$

the sum-of-squares treatments is

$$SS_{\text{Treatments}} = b \sum_{i=1}^{g} \left(\bar{x}_{i.} - \bar{x}_{..} \right)^2 = 1279.00 \, ,$$

the mean-square treatments is

$$MS_{\text{Treatments}} = \frac{SS_{\text{Treatments}}}{g - 1} = \frac{1279.00}{3 - 1} = 639.50 \, ,$$

the sum-of-squares blocks is

$$SS_{\text{Blocks}} = g \sum_{j=1}^{b} \left(\bar{x}_{.j} - \bar{x}_{..} \right)^2 = 182{,}671.3333 \, ,$$

the sum-of-squares error is

$$SS_{\text{Error}} = SS_{\text{Total}} - SS_{\text{Blocks}} - SS_{\text{Treatments}}$$

$$= 186{,}448.00 - 182{,}671.3333 - 1279.00 = 2497.6667 \, ,$$

the mean-square error is

$$MS_{\text{Error}} = \frac{SS_{\text{Error}}}{(b - 1)(g - 1)} = \frac{2497.6667}{(8 - 1)(3 - 1)} = 178.4048 \, ,$$

Table 9.9 Source table for
the data listed in Table 9.8

Factor	SS	df	MS	F
Blocks	182,671.3333			
Treatments	1279.0000	2	639.5000	3.5845
Error	2497.6667	14	178.4048	
Total	186,448.0000			

and the observed value of Fisher's F-ratio test statistic is

$$F = \frac{MS_{\text{Treatments}}}{MS_{\text{Error}}} = \frac{639.50}{178.4048} = 3.5845 \;.$$

The essential factors, sums of squares (SS), degrees of freedom (df), mean squares (MS), and variance-ratio test statistic (F) are summarized in Table 9.9.

Under the Neyman–Pearson null hypothesis, $H_0: \mu_1 = \mu_2 = \cdots = \mu_g$, Fisher's F-ratio test statistic is asymptotically distributed as Snedecor's F with $\nu_1 = g - 1$ and $\nu_2 = (b - 1)(g - 1)$ degrees of freedom. With $\nu_1 = g - 1 = 3 - 1 = 2$ and $\nu_2 = (b - 1)(g - 1) = (8 - 1)(3 - 1) = 14$ degrees of freedom, the asymptotic probability of $F = 3.5845$ is $P = 0.0553$, under the assumptions of normality and homogeneity.

9.6.1   An Exact Analysis with $v = 2$

For the example data listed in Table 9.8 with $g = 3$ treatments, $b = 8$ blocks, and $N = bg = 24$ observations, the observed value of the permutation test statistic with $v = 2$ is

$$\delta = \frac{2[F\,SS_{\text{Blocks}} + (b - 1)SS_{\text{Total}}]}{g(b - 1)(F + b - 1)}$$

$$= \frac{2[(3.5845)(182,671.3333) + (8 - 1)(186,448.00)]}{3(8 - 1)(3.5845 + 8 - 1)} = 17,635.1430 \;.$$

Alternatively, in terms of a randomized-blocks analysis of variance model the observed permutation test statistic is

$$\delta = \frac{2(SS_{\text{Total}} - SS_{\text{Treatments}})}{N - g}$$

$$= \frac{2(186,448.00 - 1279.00)}{24 - 3} = 17,635.1430 \;.$$

Because there are only

$$M = (g!)^{b-1} = (3!)^{8-1} = 279{,}936$$

possible, equally-likely arrangements in the reference set of all permutations of the observations listed in Table 9.8, an exact permutation analysis is feasible. Under the Fisher–Pitman permutation model, the exact probability of an observed δ is the proportion of δ test statistic values computed on all possible, equally-likely arrangements of the $N = 24$ observations listed in Table 9.8 that are equal to or less than the observed value of $\delta = 17{,}635.1430$. There are exactly $15{,}840$ δ test statistic values that are equal to or less than the observed value of $\delta = 17{,}635.1430$. If all M arrangements of the $N = 24$ observations listed in Table 9.8 occur with equal chance under the Fisher–Pitman null hypothesis, the exact probability value computed on the $M = 279{,}936$ possible arrangements of the observed data with $b = 8$ blocks preserved for each arrangement is

$$P(\delta \le \delta_0 | H_0) = \frac{\text{number of } \delta \text{ values } \le \delta_0}{M} = \frac{15{,}840}{279{,}936} = 0.0566 \, ,$$

where δ_0 denotes the observed value of test statistic δ and M is the number of possible, equally-likely arrangements of the $N = 24$ observations listed in Table 9.8.

There are exactly $15{,}840$ F values that are equal to or greater than the observed value of $F = 3.8582$. Thus, if all M arrangements of the $N = 24$ observations listed in Table 9.8 occur with equal chance under the Fisher–Pitman null hypothesis, the exact probability value of $F = 3.8582$ is

$$P(F \ge F_0 | H_0) = \frac{\text{number of } F \text{ values } \ge F_0}{M} = \frac{15{,}840}{279{,}936} = 0.0566 \, ,$$

where F_0 denotes the observed value of test statistic F.

Following Eq. (9.6) on p. 320, the exact expected value of the $M = 279{,}936$ δ test statistic values under the Fisher–Pitman null hypothesis is

$$\mu_\delta = \frac{1}{M} \sum_{i=1}^{M} \delta_i = \frac{4{,}958{,}224{,}209}{279{,}936} = 17{,}711.9921 \, .$$

Following Eq. (9.5) on p. 320, the observed chance-corrected measure of effect size is

$$\Re = 1 - \frac{\delta}{\mu_\delta} = 1 - \frac{17{,}635.1430}{17{,}711.9921} = +0.4339 \times 10^{-2} \, ,$$

indicating approximately chance within-block agreement.

9.6.2 Measures of Effect Size

Given the summary data in Table 9.9, Hays' $\hat{\omega}^2$ measure of effect size is

$$\hat{\omega}^2 = \frac{(g-1)(MS_{Treatments})}{SS_{Total} + MS_{Within\ Blocks}}$$

$$= \frac{(3-1)(639.50 - 178.4048)}{186,448.00 + 236.0417} = 0.4940 \times 10^{-2} \ ,$$

where the mean-square within blocks is

$$MS_{Within\ Blocks} = \frac{SS_{Within\ Blocks}}{n(g-1)} = \frac{3776.6667}{8(3-1)} = 236.0417$$

and the sum-of-squares within blocks is

$$SS_{Within\ Blocks} = SS_{Total} - SS_{Blocks}$$

$$= 186,448.00 - 182,671.3333 = 3776.6667 \ .$$

Pearson's η^2 measure of effect size is

$$\eta^2 = \frac{SS_{Treatments}}{SS_{Total}} = \frac{1279.00}{186,448.00} = 0.6860 \times 10^{-2} \ .$$

Cohen's partial η^2 measure of effect size is

$$\eta^2_{Partial} = \frac{SS_{Treatments}}{SS_{Total} - SS_{Error}} = \frac{1279.00}{186,448.00 - 2497.6667} = 0.6953 \times 10^{-2} \ .$$

And Cohen's f^2 measure of effect size is

$$f^2 = \frac{SS_{Treatments}}{SS_{Total} - SS_{Treatments}} = \frac{1279.00}{186,448.00 - 1279.00} = 0.6813 \times 10^{-2} \ .$$

For comparison, Mielke and Berry's $\Re$ chance-corrected measure of effect size is

$$\Re = 1 - \frac{\delta}{\mu_\delta} = 1 - \frac{17,635.1430}{17,711.9921} = +0.4339 \times 10^{-2} \ .$$

In this case, the five measures of effect size yield about the same magnitude of experimental effect.

9.6.3 An Exact Analysis with $v = 1$

Following Eq. (9.1) on p. 318, for the example data listed in Table 9.8 on p. 333 with $g = 3$ treatments, $b = 8$ blocks, and $N = bg = 24$ observations, the observed value of the permutation test statistic with $v = 1$ is $\delta = 114.0238$. Under the Fisher–Pitman permutation model, the exact probability of an observed δ is the proportion of δ test statistic values computed on all possible, equally-likely arrangements of the $N = 12$ observations listed in Table 9.8 that are equal to or less than the observed value of $\delta = 114.0238$. There are exactly 172,986 δ test statistic values that are equal to or less than the observed value of $\delta = 114.0238$. If all M arrangements of the $N = 24$ observations listed in Table 9.8 occur with equal chance under the Fisher–Pitman null hypothesis, the exact probability value computed on the $M = 279,936$ possible arrangements of the observed data with $b = 8$ blocks preserved for each arrangement is

$$P(\delta \leq \delta_0 | H_0) = \frac{\text{number of } \delta \text{ values } \leq \delta_0}{M} = \frac{163,296}{279,936} = 0.5833 ,$$

where δ_0 denotes the observed value of test statistic δ and M is the number of possible, equally-likely arrangements of the $N = 24$ observations listed in Table 9.8. No comparison is made with Fisher's F-ratio test statistic as F is undefined for ordinary Euclidean scaling.

Following Eq. (9.6) on p. 320, the exact expected value of the $M = 279,936$ δ test statistic values under the Fisher–Pitman null hypothesis is

$$\mu_\delta = \frac{1}{M} \sum_{i=1}^{M} \delta_i = \frac{31,883,815}{279,936} = 113.8968 ,$$

and following Eq. (9.5) on p. 320, the observed chance-corrected measure of effect size is

$$\Re = 1 - \frac{\delta}{\mu_\delta} = 1 - \frac{114.0238}{113.8968} = -0.1114 \times 10^{-2} ,$$

indicating slightly less than chance within-block agreement. No comparisons are made with Hays' $\hat{\omega}^2$, Pearson's η^2, Cohen's partial η^2, or Cohen's f^2 measures of effect size as $\hat{\omega}^2$, η^2, η_{Partial}^2, and f^2 are undefined for ordinary Euclidean scaling.

9.6.4 The Effects of Extreme Values

To illustrate the robustness of ordinary Euclidean scaling with $v = 1$, consider the example data listed in Table 9.8 on p. 333 with changes made to the observations in Block 8. Suppose that an additional 20 points have been added to each of the

Table 9.10 Comparisons of exact permutation probability values with $v = 2$ and $v = 1$ for extreme block values

		Probability	
Change	Block 8	$v = 2$	$v = 1$
+0	375, 350, 382	0.057474	0.583333
+20	395, 370, 402	0.057474	0.583333
+40	415, 390, 422	0.057474	0.583333
+60	435, 410, 442	0.057474	0.583333
+80	455, 430, 462	0.057474	0.583333
+100	475, 450, 482	0.057474	0.583333
+120	495, 470, 502	0.057474	0.583333
+140	515, 490, 522	0.057474	0.583333
+160	535, 510, 542	0.057474	0.583333
+180	555, 530, 562	0.057474	0.583333
+200	575, 550, 582	0.057474	0.583333

$g = 3$ treatment values in Block 8. Block 8 contains the three largest values in each of the $g = 3$ treatments, making it the most extreme of all $b = 8$ blocks. The addition of 20 points increases the three values in Block 8 from $\{375, 350, 382\}$ to $\{395, 370, 402\}$. A reanalysis of the data with the additional 20 points reveals that the probability values for $v = 2$ and $v = 1$ are unaffected by the extra 20 points. In fact, adding an additional 20 points (40 points total) does not alter the probability values. Table 9.10 illustrates the successive addition of 20 points, increasing up to an additional 200 points, demonstrating that the two permutation probability values remain constant. Thus tests under the Fisher–Pitman permutation model with both squared Euclidean scaling with $v = 2$ and ordinary Euclidean scaling with $v = 1$ are shown to be robust to an extreme block of data.

The same pattern holds with Fisher's F-ratio test statistic and asymptotic probability values. Table 9.11 lists the same block data as Table 9.10 with increments of 20 points added to the most extreme block, along with the associated F-ratio test statistic values and asymptotic probability values. The addition of extreme values

Table 9.11 Comparisons of Fisher's F-ratio test statistics and associated asymptotic probability values for extreme block values

Change	Block 8	F-ratio	Probability
+0	375, 350, 382	3.584545	0.055334
+20	395, 370, 402	3.584545	0.055334
+40	415, 390, 422	3.584545	0.055334
+60	435, 410, 442	3.584545	0.055334
+80	455, 430, 462	3.584545	0.055334
+100	475, 450, 482	3.584545	0.055334
+120	495, 470, 502	3.584545	0.055334
+140	515, 490, 522	3.584545	0.055334
+160	535, 510, 542	3.584545	0.055334
+180	555, 530, 562	3.584545	0.055334
+200	575, 550, 582	3.584545	0.055334

Table 9.12 Comparisons of exact permutation probability values with $v = 2$ and $v = 1$ for a single extreme value

Change	Block 8	Probability $v = 2$	Probability $v = 1$
+0	375, 350, 382	0.057474	0.583333
+20	375, 350, 402	0.040431	0.583333
+40	375, 350, 422	0.036912	0.583333
+60	375, 350, 442	0.032968	0.583333
+80	375, 350, 462	0.029635	0.583333
+100	375, 350, 482	0.027449	0.583333
+120	375, 350, 502	0.026299	0.583333
+140	375, 350, 522	0.025524	0.583333
+160	375, 350, 542	0.024945	0.583333
+180	375, 350, 562	0.024291	0.583333
+200	375, 350, 582	0.023823	0.583333

to a block does not change either the value of Fisher's F-ratio test statistic or the asymptotic probability value.

Now consider a different scenario. Suppose that an additional 20 points is added to only one treatment value in Block 8 in Table 9.8 on p. 333. The third value in Block 8 (382) is the largest of the $N = 24$ values. An additional 20 points increases value 382 to 402. In this case, the probability value based on ordinary Euclidean scaling with $v = 1$ is unchanged, remaining at $P = 0.583333$. However, the probability value based on squared Euclidean scaling with $v = 2$ decreases to $P = 0.040431$ from $P = 0.057474$. Table 9.12 illustrates the successive addition of 20 points, increasing up to an additional 200 points, demonstrating that ordinary Euclidean scaling with $v = 1$ under the Fisher–Pitman permutation model is robust to individual extreme values in randomized-blocks designs, while squared Euclidean scaling with $v = 2$ is not robust under the same model. The final probability value based on $v = 2$ of $P = 0.023823$ is less than half of the original probability value of $P = 0.057474$. The difference between the two exact probability values is

$$\Delta_P = 0.057474 - 0.023823 = 0.033651 .$$

For comparison, consider the block data listed in Table 9.13. The data listed in Table 9.13 are the same data listed in Table 9.12, but Table 9.13 also contains the F-ratio test statistic values and associated asymptotic probability values. As is clear from the results given in Table 9.13, Fisher's F-ratio test statistic values are strongly affected by the inclusion of a single extreme value in one block, as are the associated asymptotic probability values. The difference between the two F-ratio test statistics is

$$\Delta_F = 3.584545 - 2.162474 = 1.422071$$

and the difference between the two asymptotic probability values is

$$\Delta_P = 0.151914 - 0.055334 = 0.096580 .$$

Table 9.13 Comparisons of Fisher's F-ratio test statistic values and associated asymptotic probability values for a single extreme value

Change	Block 8	F-ratio	Probability
+0	375, 350, 382	3.584545	0.055334
+20	375, 350, 402	4.126205	0.039017
+40	375, 350, 422	4.097638	0.039726
+60	375, 350, 442	3.793197	0.048265
+80	375, 350, 462	3.434890	0.061132
+100	375, 350, 482	3.109992	0.076284
+120	375, 350, 502	2.838128	0.092321
+140	375, 350, 522	2.615944	0.108329
+160	375, 350, 542	2.434712	0.123762
+180	375, 350, 562	2.285893	0.138331
+200	375, 350, 582	2.162474	0.151914

9.7 Example 4: Exact and Monte Carlo Analyses

For a fourth example of tests for differences, consider the example data given in Table 9.14. It is generally understood that repeated experience with the Graduate Record Examination (GRE) leads to better scores, even without any intervening study. Suppose that eight subjects take the GRE verbal examination on successive Saturday mornings for three weeks. The data with $g = 3$ treatments, $b = 8$ blocks, and $N = 24$ scores are listed in Table 9.14.

Under the Neyman–Pearson population model with treatment means $\bar{x}_{1.} = 552.50$, $\bar{x}_{2.} = 564.3750$, and $\bar{x}_{3.} = 574.3750$, block means $\bar{x}_{.1} = 568.3333$, $\bar{x}_{.2} = 450.00$, $\bar{x}_{.3} = 616.6667$, $\bar{x}_{.4} = 663.3333$, $\bar{x}_{.5} = 436.6667$, $\bar{x}_{.6} = 696.6667$, $\bar{x}_{.7} = 505.00$, and $\bar{x}_{.8} = 573.3333$, grand mean $\bar{x}_{..} = 563.75$, the sum-of-squares total is

$$SS_{\text{Total}} = \sum_{i=1}^{g} \sum_{j=1}^{b} \left(x_{ij} - \bar{x}_{..} \right)^2 = 194{,}512.50 \, ,$$

Table 9.14 Example GRE scores for exact and Monte Carlo analyses with $b = 8$ blocks and $g = 3$ treatments

	Treatment		
Block	1	2	3
1	550	575	580
2	440	440	470
3	610	630	610
4	650	670	670
5	400	460	450
6	700	680	710
7	490	510	515
8	580	550	590

the sum-of-squares treatments is

$$SS_{\text{Treatments}} = b \sum_{i=1}^{g} \left(\bar{x}_{i.} - \bar{x}_{..} \right)^2 = 1918.75 \,,$$

the mean-square treatments is

$$MS_{\text{Treatments}} = \frac{SS_{\text{Treatments}}}{g-1} = \frac{1918.75}{3-1} = 959.3750 \,,$$

the sum-of-squares blocks is

$$SS_{\text{Blocks}} = g \sum_{j=1}^{b} \left(\bar{x}_{.j} - \bar{x}_{..} \right)^2 = 189{,}112.50 \,,$$

the sum-of-squares error is

$$SS_{\text{Error}} = SS_{\text{Total}} - SS_{\text{Blocks}} - SS_{\text{Treatments}}$$

$$= 194{,}512.50 - 189{,}112.50 - 1918.75 = 3481.25 \,,$$

the mean-square error is

$$MS_{\text{Error}} = \frac{SS_{\text{Error}}}{(b-1)(g-1)} = \frac{3481.25}{(8-1)(3-1)} = 248.6607 \,,$$

and the observed value of Fisher's F-ratio test statistic is

$$F = \frac{MS_{\text{Treatments}}}{MS_{\text{Error}}} = \frac{959.3750}{248.6607} = 3.8582 \,.$$

The essential factors, sums of squares (SS), degrees of freedom (df), mean squares (MS), and variance-ratio test statistic (F) are summarized in Table 9.15. Under the Neyman–Pearson null hypothesis, H_0: $\mu_1 = \mu_2 = \cdots = \mu_g$, Fisher's F-ratio test statistic is asymptotically distributed as Snedecor's F with $\nu_1 = g - 1$ and $\nu_2 = (b-1)(g-1)$ degrees of freedom. With $\nu_1 = g - 1 = 3 - 1 = 2$ and $\nu_2 = (b-1)(g-1) = (8-1)(3-1) = 14$ degrees of freedom, the asymptotic probability value of $F = 3.8582$ is $P = 0.0463$, under the assumptions of normality and homogeneity.

Table 9.15 Source table for the GRE data listed in Table 9.13

Factor	SS	df	MS	F
Blocks	189,112.5000			
Treatments	1918.7500	2	959.3750	3.8582
Error	3481.2500	14	248.6607	
Total	194,512.5000			

9.7.1 An Exact Analysis with $v = 2$

For the first analysis of the data in Table 9.14 under the Fisher–Pitman permutation model let $v = 2$, employing squared Euclidean scaling for correspondence with Fisher's F-ratio test statistic. Because there are only

$$M = (g!)^{b-1} = (3!)^{8-1} = 279{,}936$$

possible, equally-likely arrangements in the reference set of all permutations of the $N = 24$ GRE scores listed in Table 9.14, an exact permutation analysis is feasible. Following Eq. (9.1) on p. 318, the observed value of the permutation test statistic is $\delta = 18{,}342.2620$. Based on the expressions given in Eqs. (9.3) and (9.4) on p. 319, the observed values of test statistics F and δ are

$$F = \frac{(b-1)[2SS_{\text{Total}} - g(b-1)\delta]}{g(b-1)\delta - 2SS_{\text{Blocks}}}$$

$$= \frac{(8-1)[2(194{,}512.50) - 3(8-1)(18{,}342.2620)]}{3(8-1)(18{,}342.2620) - 2(189{,}112.50)} = 3.8582$$

and

$$\delta = \frac{2[FSS_{\text{Blocks}} + (b-1)SS_{\text{Total}}]}{g(b-1)(F+b-1)}$$

$$= \frac{2[(3.8582)(189{,}112.50) + (8-1)(194{,}512.50)]}{3(8-1)(3.8582 + 8 - 1)} = 18{,}342.2620 \ .$$

Alternatively, in terms of a randomized-blocks analysis of variance model the observed permutation test statistic is

$$\delta = \frac{2(SS_{\text{Total}} - SS_{\text{Treatments}})}{N - g}$$

$$= \frac{2(194{,}512.50 - 1918.75)}{24 - 3} = 18{,}342.2620 \ .$$

Under the Fisher–Pitman permutation model, the exact probability of an observed δ is the proportion of δ test statistic values computed on all possible, equally-likely arrangements of the $N = 24$ observations listed in Table 9.14 that are equal to or less than the observed value of $\delta = 18{,}342.2620$. There are exactly 12,063 δ test statistic values that are equal to or less than the observed value of $\delta = 18{,}342.2620$. If all M arrangements of the $N = 24$ observations listed in Table 9.14 occur with equal chance under the Fisher–Pitman null hypothesis, the exact probability value of $\delta = 18{,}342.2620$ computed on the $M = 279{,}936$

possible arrangements of the observed data with $b = 8$ blocks preserved for each arrangement is

$$P(\delta \leq \delta_0 | H_0) = \frac{\text{number of } \delta \text{ values } \leq \delta_0}{M} = \frac{12,063}{279,936} = 0.0431,$$

where δ_0 denotes the observed value of test statistic δ and M is the number of possible, equally-likely arrangements of the GRE data listed in Table 9.14.

Alternatively, there are exactly 12,063 F-ratio test statistic values that are equal to or greater than the observed test statistic value of $F = 3.8582$. Thus, if all M arrangements of the $N = 24$ observations listed in Table 9.14 occur with equal chance under the Fisher–Pitman null hypothesis, the exact probability value of $F = 3.8582$ computed on the $M = 279,936$ arrangements of the observed data with $b = 4$ blocks preserved for each arrangement is

$$P(F \geq F_0 | H_0) = \frac{\text{number of } F \text{ values } \geq F_0}{M} = \frac{12,063}{279,936} = 0.0431,$$

where F_0 denotes the observed value of test statistic F.

Following Eq. (9.6) on p. 320, the exact expected value of the $M = 279,936$ δ test statistic values under the Fisher–Pitman null hypothesis is

$$\mu_\delta = \frac{1}{M} \sum_{i=1}^{M} \delta_i = \frac{5,167,818,515}{279,936} = 18,460.7143.$$

Following Eq. (9.5) on p. 320, the observed chance-corrected measure of effect size is

$$\Re = 1 - \frac{\delta}{\mu_\delta} = 1 - \frac{18,342.2620}{18,460.7143} = +0.6416 \times 10^{-2},$$

indicating approximately chance within-block agreement.

9.7.2 Measures of Effect Size

For the GRE data listed in Table 9.14, Hays' $\hat{\omega}^2$ measure of effect size is

$$\hat{\omega}^2 = \frac{(g-1)(MS_{\text{Treatments}})}{SS_{\text{Total}} + MS_{\text{Within Blocks}}}$$

$$= \frac{(3-1)(959.3750 - 248.6607)}{194,512.00 + 337.50} = 0.7295 \times 10^{-2},$$

where the mean-square within blocks is

$$MS_{\text{Within Blocks}} = \frac{SS_{\text{Within Blocks}}}{n(g-1)} = \frac{5400.00}{8(3-1)} = 337.50$$

and the sum-of-squares within blocks is

$$SS_{\text{Within Blocks}} = SS_{\text{Total}} - SS_{\text{Blocks}}$$

$$= 194{,}512.00 - 189{,}112.50 = 5400.00 \ .$$

Pearson's η^2 measure of effect size is

$$\eta^2 = \frac{SS_{\text{Treatments}}}{SS_{\text{Total}}} = \frac{1918.75}{194{,}512.50} = 0.9864 \times 10^{-2} \ ,$$

Cohen's partial η^2 measure of effect size is

$$\eta^2_{\text{Partial}} = \frac{SS_{\text{Treatments}}}{SS_{\text{Total}} - SS_{\text{Error}}} = \frac{1918.75}{194{,}512.00 - 3481.25} = 0.1004 \times 10^{-1} \ ,$$

and Cohen's f^2 measure of effect size is

$$f^2 = \frac{SS_{\text{Treatments}}}{SS_{\text{Total}} - SS_{\text{Treatments}}} = \frac{1918.75}{194{,}512.50 - 1918.75} = 0.9963 \times 10^{-2} \ .$$

For comparison, Mielke and Berry's $\Re$ chance-corrected measure of effect size is

$$\Re = 1 - \frac{\delta}{\mu_\delta} = 1 - \frac{18{,}342.2620}{18{,}460.7143} = +0.6416 \times 10^{-2} \ .$$

Thus, the five measures of effect size yield about the same magnitude of experimental effect for this example analysis.

9.7.3   A Monte Carlo Analysis with $v = 2$

Although there are only $M = 279{,}936$ possible arrangements of the data listed in Table 9.14, making an exact permutation analysis feasible, many computer programs for permutation methods do not provide an option for an exact analysis. Moreover, over-sampling of the M possible arrangements is quite common in the permutation literature because of its efficiency in certain applications; for example, permutation analyses of contingency tables. In this section, over-sampling is demonstrated where $L = 1{,}000{,}000$ random arrangements is greater than the $M = 279{,}936$ possible arrangements.

For the example data listed in Table 9.14 on p. 340 with $v = 2$, the observed value of the permutation test statistic with $v = 2$ is $\delta = 18{,}342.2620$. Under the Fisher–Pitman permutation model, the Monte Carlo probability of an observed δ is the proportion of δ test statistic values computed on the randomly-selected, equally-likely arrangements of the $N = 24$ observations listed in Table 9.14 that are equal to or less than the observed value of $\delta = 18{,}342.2620$. There are exactly 44,421 δ test statistic values that are equal to or less than the observed value of $\delta = 18{,}342.2620$. If all M arrangements of the $N = 24$ observations listed in Table 9.14 occur with equal chance under the Fisher–Pitman null hypothesis, the Monte Carlo probability value computed on a sample of $L = 1{,}000{,}000$ random arrangements of the observed data with $b = 8$ blocks preserved for each arrangement is

$$P(\delta \leq \delta_0 | H_0) = \frac{\text{number of } \delta \text{ values} \leq \delta_0}{L} = \frac{44{,}421}{1{,}000{,}000} = 0.0444,$$

where δ_0 denotes the observed value of test statistic δ and L is the number of randomly-selected, equally-likely arrangements of the GRE data listed in Table 9.14.

Alternatively, there are 44,421 F-ratio test statistic values that are equal to or greater than the observed value of $F = 3.8582$. Thus, if all M arrangements of the $N = 24$ observations listed in Table 9.14 occur with equal chance under the Fisher–Pitman null hypothesis, the Monte Carlo probability value of $F = 3.8582$ is

$$P(F \geq F_0 | H_0) = \frac{\text{number of } F \text{ values} \geq F_0}{L} = \frac{44{,}421}{1{,}000{,}000} = 0.0444,$$

where F_0 denotes the observed value of test statistic F.

The Monte Carlo probability value of $P = 0.0444$ based on $L = 1{,}000{,}000$ randomly-selected arrangements of the observed data compares favorably with the exact probability value of $P = 0.0431$ based on all $M = 279{,}936$ possible arrangements of the observed data.

Following Eq. (9.6) on p. 320, the exact expected value of the $M = 279{,}936$ δ test statistic values under the Fisher–Pitman null hypothesis is

$$\mu_\delta = \frac{1}{M} \sum_{i=1}^{M} \delta_i = \frac{5{,}167{,}818{,}515}{279{,}936} = 18{,}460.7143,$$

and following Eq. (9.5) on p. 320, the observed chance-corrected measure of effect size is

$$\Re = 1 - \frac{\delta}{\mu_\delta} = 1 - \frac{18{,}342.2620}{18{,}460.7143} = +0.6416 \times 10^{-2},$$

indicating approximately chance within-block agreement.

9.7.4   An Exact Analysis with $v = 1$

Consider a second analysis of the example data listed in Table 9.14 on p. 340 under the Fisher–Pitman permutation model with $v = 1$, employing ordinary Euclidean scaling between observations. For the data listed in Table 9.14 with $g = 3$ treatments, $b = 8$ blocks, and $N = bg = (8)(3) = 24$ observations, the observed permutation test statistic with $v = 1$ is $\delta = 116.3095$.

Because there are still only

$$M = (g!)^{b-1} = (3!)^{8-1} = 279{,}936$$

possible, equally-likely arrangements in the reference set of all permutations of the $N = 24$ GRE scores listed in Table 9.14, an exact permutation analysis is feasible.

Under the Fisher–Pitman permutation model, the exact probability of an observed δ is the proportion of δ test statistic values computed on all possible, equally-likely arrangements of the $N = 24$ observations listed in Table 9.14 that are equal to or less than the observed value of $\delta = 116.3095$. There are exactly 186,624 δ test statistic values that are equal to or less than the observed value of $\delta = 116.3095$. If all M arrangements of the $N = 24$ observations listed in Table 9.14 occur with equal chance under the Fisher–Pitman null hypothesis, the exact probability value of $\delta = 116.3095$ computed on the $M = 279{,}936$ possible arrangements of the observed data with $b = 8$ blocks preserved for each arrangement is

$$P(\delta \leq \delta_0 | H_0) = \frac{\text{number of } \delta \text{ values } \leq \delta_0}{M} = \frac{186{,}624}{279{,}936} = 0.6667 \;,$$

where δ_0 denotes the observed value of test statistic δ and M is the number of possible, equally-likely arrangements of the GRE data listed in Table 9.14. No comparison is made with Fisher's F-ratio test statistic as Fisher's F-ratio is undefined for ordinary Euclidean scaling.

Following Eq. (9.6) on p. 320, the exact expected value of the $M = 279{,}936$ δ test statistic values under the Fisher–Pitman null hypothesis is

$$\mu_\delta = \frac{1}{M} \sum_{i=1}^{M} \delta_i = \frac{32{,}514{,}790}{279{,}936} = 116.1508 \;,$$

and following Eq. (9.5) on p. 320, the observed chance-corrected measure of effect size is

$$\Re = 1 - \frac{\delta}{\mu_\delta} = 1 - \frac{116.3095}{116.1508} = -0.1367 \times 10^{-2} \;,$$

indicating slightly less than chance within-block agreement. No comparisons are made with Hays' $\hat{\omega}^2$, Pearson's η^2, Cohen's partial η^2, or Cohen's f^2 measures of effect size as $\hat{\omega}^2$, η^2, η^2_{Partial}, and f^2 are undefined for ordinary Euclidean scaling.

For comparison, a Monte Carlo analysis based on $L = 1,000,000$ randomly-selected arrangements of the observed data listed in Table 9.14 with $v = 1$ yields $\delta = 116.3095$. Under the Fisher–Pitman permutation model, the Monte Carlo probability of an observed δ is the proportion of δ test statistic values computed on the randomly-selected, equally-likely arrangements of the $N = 24$ observations listed in Table 9.14 that are equal to or less than the observed value of $\delta = 116.3095$. There are exactly 666,384 δ test statistic values that are equal to or less than the observed value of $\delta = 116.3095$. If all M arrangements of the $N = 24$ observations listed in Table 9.14 occur with equal chance under the Fisher–Pitman null hypothesis, the Monte Carlo probability value of $\delta = 116.3095$ computed on a sample of $L = 1,000,000$ randomly-selected arrangements of the observed data with $b = 8$ blocks preserved for each arrangement is

$$P(\delta \leq \delta_0 | H_0) = \frac{\text{number of } \delta \text{ values} \leq \delta_0}{L} = \frac{666,384}{1,000,000} = 0.6664 \, ,$$

where δ_0 denotes the observed value of test statistic δ and L is the number of randomly-selected, equally-likely arrangements of the GRE data listed in Table 9.14.

It is perhaps interesting that, for the example data listed in Table 9.14, the asymptotic probability value of $F = 3.8582$ with $v_1 = 2$ and $v_2 = 14$ degrees of freedom is $P = 0.0463$, the exact permutation probability value of $\delta = 18,342.2620$ with $v = 2$ is $P = 0.0431$, the Monte Carlo probability value of $\delta = 18,342.2620$ based on $L = 1,000,000$ random arrangements of the observed data is $P = 0.0444$, but the exact permutation probability value of $\delta = 116.3095$ with $v = 1$ is $P = 0.6667$. Thus the difference in exact probability values between analyses based on $v = 1$ and $v = 2$ is

$$\Delta_P = 0.6667 - 0.0431 = 0.6236 \, ,$$

which is a considerable discrepancy.

To be sure, the set of example data listed in Table 9.14 is rather innocuous—nothing unusual or extreme immediately presents itself. However, two values are somewhat extreme and it is extreme values that usually account for large differences in probability values based on squared Euclidean scaling with $v = 2$ and ordinary Euclidean scaling with $v = 1$. The two somewhat extreme values are $x_{6,1} = 700$ in Treatment 1 and $x_{6,3} = 710$ in Treatment 3. The value of 700 is 147.50 points above the average of Treatment 1 ($\bar{x}_{1.} = 552.50$) and 1.42 standard deviations above the average value in Treatment 1. The value of 710 is 135.6250 points above the average of Treatment 3 ($\bar{x}_{3.} = 574.3750$) and 1.48 standard deviations above the average value in Treatment 3.

The effects of these two values can be revealed by reducing the two values and re-analyzing the revised data. Consider reducing value $x_{6,1} = 700$ to $x_{6,1} = 600$, which with a standard score of $+0.46$ is closer to the mean of $\bar{x}_{.1} = 552.50$, and also reducing value $x_{6,3} = 710$ to $x_{6,3} = 600$, which with a standard score of $+0.28$ is closer to the mean of $\bar{x}_{.3} = 574.3750$. The result is to bring the probability values closer together, with an exact probability value based on squared Euclidean scaling with $v = 2$ of $P = 0.0799$, an exact probability value based on ordinary Euclidean scaling with $v = 1$ of $P = 0.2716$, and a difference between the two exact probability values of

$$\Delta_P = 0.2716 - 0.0799 = 0.1917$$

instead of a difference of

$$\Delta_P = 0.6667 - 0.0431 = 0.6236 .$$

The effects of the two extreme values can further be revealed by eliminating the two values. When the two values are eliminated—set equal to zero—and re-analyzed, the exact probability value based on squared Euclidean scaling with $v = 2$ is $P = 0.2651$ and the exact probability value based on ordinary Euclidean scaling with $v = 1$ is $P = 0.3914$ with a difference between the two exact probability values of only

$$\Delta_P = 0.3914 - 0.2651 = 0.1263 .$$

Table 9.16 lists the raw GRE scores from Table 9.14 on p. 340 along with associated standard scores, given in parentheses. To emphasize that the standard scores $+1.48$ and $+1.42$ are extreme relative to other scores listed in Table 9.16, a listing of the 13 positive standard scores in order is

Standard score: $+ 1.48, +1.42, +1.27, +1.27, +1.04, +0.94,$

$+ 0.72, +0.55, +0.39, +0.27, +0.17, +0.16, +0.12 .$

Table 9.16 Example data from Table 9.14 with raw GRE scores and associated standard scores (in parentheses)

Block	Treatment		
	1	2	3
1	550 (-0.02)	575 ($+0.12$)	580 ($+0.06$)
2	440 (-1.09)	440 (-1.36)	470 (-1.14)
3	610 ($+0.55$)	630 ($+0.72$)	610 ($+0.39$)
4	650 ($+0.94$)	670 ($+1.16$)	670 ($+1.04$)
5	400 (-1.47)	460 (-1.14)	450 (-1.36)
6	700 ($+1.42$)	680 ($+1.27$)	710 ($+1.48$)
7	490 (-0.60)	510 (-0.52)	515 (-0.65)
8	580 ($+0.27$)	550 (-0.16)	590 ($+0.17$)

9.8 Example 5: Rank-Score Permutation Analyses

It is often necessary to analyze rank-score data when the required parametric assumptions of randomized-blocks designs cannot be met. However, with permutation methods it is never necessary to convert raw-score data to ranks [2]. The conventional approach to multi-sample rank-score data is Friedman's two-way analysis of variance for ranks [3].

9.8.1 The Friedman Analysis of Variance for Ranks

Let b denote the number of blocks and g denote the number of objects to be ranked. Then Friedman's test statistic is given by

$$\chi_r^2 = \frac{12}{bg(g+1)} \sum_{i=1}^{g} R_i^2 - 3b(g+1) \, ,$$

where R_i for $i = 1, \ldots, g$ is the sum of the rank scores for the ith object and there are no tied rank scores. A number of statistics are either identical, related, or equivalent to Friedman's χ_r^2 test statistic. Among these are Kendall and Babington Smith's coefficient of concordance, the average value of all pairwise Spearman's rank-order correlation coefficients, and the Wallis rank-order correlation ratio.

To illustrate Friedman's analysis of variance for ranks, consider the rank scores listed in Table 9.17; that is, rank scores r_{ij} for $i = 1, \ldots, g$ and $j = 1, \ldots, b$. For the rank-score data listed in Table 9.17, the sum of the squared rank scores is

$$\sum_{i=1}^{g} R_i^2 = 4^2 + 14^2 + 15^2 + 13^2 + 11^2 + 6^2 = 763 \, ,$$

Table 9.17 Example data for the Friedman analysis of variance for ranks with $b = 3$ blocks and $g = 6$ objects

Object	Block 1	2	3	R
1	1	1	2	4
2	6	5	3	14
3	3	6	6	15
4	4	4	5	13
5	5	2	4	11
6	2	3	1	6
Sum				63

and the observed value of Friedman's test statistic is

$$\chi_r^2 = \frac{12}{bg(g+1)} \sum_{i=1}^{g} R_i^2 - 3b(g+1)$$

$$= \frac{12}{(3)(6)(6+1)} \, 763 - (3)(3)(6+1) = 9.6667 \, .$$

Friedman's χ_r^2 test statistic is asymptotically distributed as Pearson's chi-squared under the Neyman–Pearson null hypothesis with $g - 1$ degrees of freedom. Under the Neyman–Pearson null hypothesis, the observed value of $\chi_r^2 = 9.6667$ with $g - 1 = 6 - 1 = 5$ degrees of freedom yields an asymptotic probability value of $P = 0.0853$.

9.8.2 An Exact Analysis with $v = 2$

For the first analysis of the rank-score data listed in Table 9.17 under the Fisher–Pitman permutation model let $v = 2$, employing squared Euclidean scaling between the pairs of rank scores for correspondence with Friedman's χ_r^2 test statistic, and let

$$x_{ij}' = (x_{1ij}, x_{2ij}, x_{3ij}, \ldots, x_{rij})$$

denote a transposed vector of r measurements associated with the ith treatment and jth block. Then the permutation test statistic is given by

$$\delta = \left[g \binom{b}{2} \right]^{-1} \sum_{i=1}^{g} \sum_{j=1}^{b-1} \sum_{k=j+1}^{b} \Delta(x_{ij}, x_{ik}) \, , \qquad (9.14)$$

where $\Delta(x, y)$ is a symmetric distance-function value of two points $x' = (x_1, x_2, \ldots, x_r)$ and $y' = (y_1, y_2, \ldots, y_r)$ in an r-dimensional Euclidean space. In the context of a randomized-block design,

$$\Delta(x, y) = \sum_{i=1}^{r} |x_i - y_i|^v \, ,$$

where $v > 0$.

For the rank-score data listed in Table 9.17 there are only

$$M = (g!)^{b-1} = (6!)^{3-1} = 518{,}400$$

possible, equally-likely arrangements in the reference set of all permutations of the rank-score data listed in Table 9.17, making an exact permutation analysis feasible. For the rank scores listed in Table 9.17 let $v = 2$, employing squared Euclidean scaling between the pairs of rank scores for correspondence with Friedman's χ_r^2 test statistic, the observed value of the permutation test statistic with $v = 2$ is $\delta = 3.1111$.

Under the Fisher–Pitman permutation model, the exact probability of an observed δ is the proportion of δ test statistic values computed on all possible, equally-likely arrangements of the $N = 18$ rank scores listed in Table 9.17 that are equal to or less than the observed value of $\delta = 3.1111$. There are exactly 29,047 δ test statistic values that are equal to or less than $\delta = 3.1111$. If all M arrangements of the $N = 18$ rank scores listed in Table 9.17 occur with equal chance under the Fisher–Pitman null hypothesis, the exact probability of $\delta = 3.1111$ computed on the $M = 518,400$ possible arrangements of the observed rank scores with $b = 3$ blocks preserved for each arrangement is

$$P(\delta \le \delta_0|H_0) = \frac{\text{number of } \delta \text{ values} \le \delta_0}{M} = \frac{29,047}{518,400} = 0.0560 ,$$

where δ_0 denotes the observed value of test statistic δ and M is the number of possible, equally-likely arrangements of the $N = 18$ rank scores listed in Table 9.17. The functional relationships between test statistics χ_r^2 and δ with $v = 2$ are given by

$$\chi_r^2 = \frac{b(g^2 - 1) - 6(b - 1)\delta}{g + 1} \tag{9.15}$$

and

$$\delta = \frac{b(g^2 - 1) - (g + 1)\chi_r^2}{6(b - 1)} . \tag{9.16}$$

Following Eq. (9.15) for the $N = 18$ rank scores listed in Table 9.17, the observed value of test statistic χ_r^2 with respect to the observed value of test statistic δ is

$$\chi_r^2 = \frac{3(6^2 - 1) - 6(3 - 1)(3.1111)}{6 + 1} = 9.6667$$

and following Eq. (9.16), the observed value of test statistic δ with respect to the observed value of test statistic χ_r^2 is

$$\delta = \frac{3(6^2 - 1) - (6 + 1)(9.6667)}{6(3 - 1)} = 3.1111 .$$

Following Eq. (9.6) on p. 320, the exact expected value of the $M = 518,400 \, \delta$ test statistic values under the Fisher–Pitman null hypothesis is

$$\mu_\delta = \frac{1}{M} \sum_{i=1}^{M} \delta_i = \frac{3,024,000}{518,400} = 5.8333 \; .$$

Alternatively, in terms of a randomized-blocks analysis of variance model the exact expected value of test statistic δ is

$$\mu_\delta = \frac{2SS_{\text{Total}}}{N} = \frac{2(52.50)}{18} = 5.8333 \; ,$$

where

$$SS_{\text{Total}} = \sum_{i=1}^{g} \sum_{j=1}^{b} r_{ij}^2 - \left(\sum_{i=1}^{g} \sum_{j=1}^{b} r_{ij} \right)^2 \Big/ bg$$

$$= 273 - (63)^2/(3)(6) = 52.50 \; .$$

Following Eq. (9.5) on p. 320, the observed chance-corrected measure of effect size is

$$\Re = 1 - \frac{\delta}{\mu_\delta} = 1 - \frac{3.1111}{5.8333} = +0.4667 \; ,$$

indicating approximately 47% within-block agreement above what is expected by chance. No comparisons are made with Hays' $\hat{\omega}^2$, Pearson's η^2, Cohen's partial η^2, or Cohen's f^2 measures of effect size as $\hat{\omega}^2$, η^2, η_{Partial}^2, and f^2 are undefined for rank-score data.

9.8.3   An Exact Analysis with $v = 1$

For a second analysis of the rank-score data listed in Table 9.17 under the Fisher–Pitman permutation model let $v = 1$, employing ordinary Euclidean scaling between the rank scores. For the rank scores listed in Table 9.17 there are still only

$$M = (g!)^{b-1} = (6!)^{3-1} = 518,400$$

possible, equally-likely arrangements in the reference set of all permutations of the rank-score data listed in Table 9.17, making an exact permutation analysis feasible. For the $N = 18$ rank scores listed in Table 9.17 the observed value of the permutation test statistic with $v = 1$ is $\delta = 1.4444$.

Under the Fisher–Pitman permutation model, the exact probability of an observed δ is the proportion of δ test statistic values computed on all possible, equally-likely arrangements of the $N = 18$ rank scores listed in Table 9.17 that are equal to or less than the observed value of $\delta = 1.4444$. There are exactly 55,528 δ test statistic values that are equal to or greater than $\delta = 1.4444$. If all M arrangements of the $N = 18$ rank scores listed in Table 9.17 occur with equal chance under the Fisher–Pitman null hypothesis, the exact probability of $\delta = 1.4444$ computed on the $M = 518{,}400$ possible arrangements of the observed rank scores with $b = 3$ blocks preserved for each arrangement is

$$P(\delta \le \delta_0 | H_0) = \frac{\text{number of } \delta \text{ values} \le \delta_0}{M} = \frac{55{,}528}{518{,}400} = 0.1071 \,,$$

where δ_0 denotes the observed value of test statistic δ and M is the number of possible, equally-likely arrangements of the $N = 18$ rank scores listed in Table 9.17. No comparison is made with Friedman's χ_r^2 analysis of variance for ranks as χ_r^2 is undefined for ordinary Euclidean scaling.

Following Eq. (9.6) on p. 320, the exact expected value of the $M = 518{,}400$ δ test statistic values under the Fisher–Pitman null hypothesis is

$$\mu_\delta = \frac{1}{M} \sum_{i=1}^{M} \delta_i = \frac{1{,}008{,}000}{518{,}400} = 1.9444$$

and following Eq. (9.5) on p. 320, the observed chance-corrected measure of effect size is

$$\Re = 1 - \frac{\delta}{\mu_\delta} = 1 - \frac{1.4444}{1.9444} = +0.2571 \,,$$

indicating approximately 26% within-block agreement above what is expected by chance. No comparisons are made with Hays' $\hat{\omega}^2$, Pearson's η^2, Cohen's partial η^2, or Cohen's f^2 measures of effect size as $\hat{\omega}^2$, η^2, η_{Partial}^2, and f^2 are undefined for rank-score data.

9.9 Example 6: Multivariate Permutation Analyses

It is oftentimes necessary to test for differences among $g \ge 3$ treatment groups where $r \ge 2$ measurements scores have been obtained from each of $b \ge 2$ blocks. To illustrate the analysis of randomized blocks with multivariate measurements, consider the data listed in Table 9.18 wherein each of two observers is asked to estimate distance and elevation in meters of 12 distant objects.

Table 9.18 Example data
with $g = 12$ objects, $b = 2$
blocks, and $r = 2$
measurements

Object	Observer A		Observer B	
	Distance	Elevation	Distance	Elevation
1	120	10	125	10
2	80	15	85	20
3	100	5	95	10
4	150	20	140	15
5	75	10	60	5
6	50	5	60	10
7	50	20	50	25
8	20	20	25	15
9	90	15	90	15
10	95	25	90	20
11	100	25	90	20
12	70	5	70	5

9.9.1 A Monte Carlo Analysis with $v = 2$

For the example data listed in Table 9.18 with $g = 12$ treatments (objects), $b = 2$
blocks (observers), $r = 2$ measurements, and $N = bg = (2)(12) = 24$ multivariate
observations, the observed value of the permutation test statistic with $v = 2$ is
$\delta = 72.9167$. There are

$$M = (g!)^{b-1} = (12!)^{2-1} = 479{,}001{,}600$$

possible, equally-likely arrangements in the reference set of all permutations of the
multivariate data listed in Table 9.18, making an exact permutation analysis impractical and a Monte Carlo analysis advisable. Under the Fisher–Pitman permutation
model, the Monte Carlo probability value of an observed δ is the proportion of δ test
statistic values computed on the randomly-selected, equally-likely arrangements of
the $N = 24$ multivariate observations listed in Table 9.18 that are equal to or less
than the observed value of $\delta = 72.9167$.

For the example data listed in Table 9.18 and $L = 1{,}000{,}000$ random
arrangements of the observed data, there are exactly four δ test statistic values that
are equal to or less than the observed value of $\delta = 72.9167$. If all M arrangements
of the $N = 24$ observations listed in Table 9.18 occur with equal chance under the
Fisher–Pitman null hypothesis, the Monte Carlo probability value of $\delta = 72.9167$
computed on $L = 1{,}000{,}000$ random arrangements of the observed data with $b = 2$
blocks preserved for each arrangement is

$$P(\delta \leq \delta_0 | H_0) = \frac{\text{number of } \delta \text{ values} \leq \delta_0}{L} = \frac{4}{1{,}000{,}000} = 0.4000 \times 10^{-5} \, ,$$

where δ_o denotes the observed value of test statistic δ and L is the number of randomly-selected, equally-likely arrangements of the distance-elevation data listed in Table 9.18.

When the probability value is very small, as it is in this case, Monte Carlo permutation methods are not very precise with only $L = 1,000,000$ random arrangements of the observed data. A reanalysis of the multivariate data listed in Table 9.18 with $L = 100,000,000$ random arrangements yields a probability value of

$$P(\delta \leq \delta_o | H_0) = \frac{\text{number of } \delta \text{ values } \leq \delta_o}{L} = \frac{5}{100,000,000} = 0.5000 \times 10^{-7} .$$

Following Eq. (9.6) on p. 320, the exact expected value of test statistic δ under the Fisher–Pitman null hypothesis is

$$\mu_\delta = \frac{1}{M} \sum_{i=1}^{M} \delta_i = \frac{1,001,246,506,445}{479,001,600} = 2090.2780$$

and following Eq. (9.5) on p. 320, the observed chance-corrected measure of effect size is

$$\Re = 1 - \frac{\delta}{\mu_\delta} = 1 - \frac{72.9167}{2,090.2780} = +0.9651 ,$$

indicating approximately 97% within-block agreement above what is expected by chance. No comparisons are made with Hays' $\hat{\omega}^2$, Pearson's η^2, Cohen's partial η^2, or Cohen's f^2 measures of effect size as $\hat{\omega}^2$, η^2, η^2_{Partial}, and f^2 are undefined for multivariate data.

9.9.2 An Exact Analysis with $v = 2$

Although an exact permutation analysis with $M = 479,001,600$ possible arrangements of the observed data is not practical for the example data listed in Table 9.18, it is not impossible. For an exact permutation analysis with $v = 2$, the observed value of δ is $\delta = 72.9167$. There are exactly 20 δ test statistic values that are equal to or less than the observed value of $\delta = 72.9167$. If all M arrangements of the observed data occur with equal chance under the Fisher–Pitman null hypothesis, the exact probability value computed on the $M = 479,001,600$ possible arrangements of the observed data with $b = 2$ blocks preserved for each arrangement is

$$P(\delta \leq \delta_o | H_0) = \frac{\text{number of } \delta \text{ values } \leq \delta_o}{M} = \frac{20}{479,001,600} = 0.4175 \times 10^{-7} ,$$

where δ_o denotes the observed value of test statistic δ and M is the number of possible, equally-likely arrangements of the distance-elevation data listed in Table 9.18.

Following Eq. (9.6) on p. 320, the exact expected value of test statistic δ under the Fisher–Pitman null hypothesis is

$$\mu_\delta = \frac{1}{M} \sum_{i=1}^{M} \delta_i = \frac{0.1001 \times 10^{13}}{479{,}001{,}600} = 2090.2780$$

and following Eq. (9.5) on p. 320 the observed chance-corrected measure of effect size is

$$\Re = 1 - \frac{\delta}{\mu_\delta} = 1 - \frac{72.9167}{2090.2780} = +0.9651 \, ,$$

indicating approximately 97% within-block agreement above what is expected by chance. No comparisons are made with Hays' $\hat{\omega}^2$, Pearson's η^2, Cohen's partial η^2, or Cohen's f^2 measures of effect size as $\hat{\omega}^2$, η^2, η^2_{Partial}, and f^2 are undefined for multivariate data.

9.9.3 A Monte Carlo Analysis with $v = 1$

For the data listed in Table 9.18 with $v = 1$, the observed value of δ is $\delta = 7.1305$. Since there are still

$$M = (g!)^{b-1} = (12!)^{2-1} = 479{,}001{,}600$$

possible, equally-likely arrangements in the reference set of all permutations of the multivariate data listed in Table 9.18, a Monte Carlo analysis is preferred. Under the Fisher–Pitman permutation model, the Monte Carlo probability value of an observed δ is the proportion of δ test statistic values computed on the randomly-selected, equally-likely arrangements of the $N = 24$ multivariate observations listed in Table 9.18 that are equal to or less than the observed value of $\delta = 7.1305$. For the data listed in Table 9.18 and $L = 1{,}000{,}000$ random arrangements of the data, there are exactly three δ test statistic values that are equal to or less than the observed value of $\delta = 7.1305$. If all M arrangements of the $N = 24$ multivariate observations listed in Table 9.18 occur with equal chance under the Fisher–Pitman null hypothesis, the Monte Carlo probability value of $\delta = 7.1305$ is

$$P(\delta \le \delta_o | H_0) = \frac{\text{number of } \delta \text{ values} \le \delta_o}{L} = \frac{3}{1{,}000{,}000} = 0.3000 \times 10^{-5} \, ,$$

where δ_0 denotes the observed value of test statistic δ and L is the number of randomly-selected, equally-likely arrangements of the distance-elevation data listed in Table 9.18.

Following Eq. (9.6) on p. 320, the exact expected value of test statistic δ under the Fisher–Pitman null hypothesis is

$$\mu_\delta = \frac{1}{M} \sum_{i=1}^{M} \delta_i = \frac{17{,}916{,}053{,}734}{479{,}001{,}600} = 37.4029$$

and following Eq. (9.5) on p. 320, the observed chance-corrected measure of effect size is

$$\Re = 1 - \frac{\delta}{\mu_\delta} = 1 - \frac{7.1305}{37.4029} = +0.8094 \,,$$

indicating approximately 81% within-block agreement above that is expected by chance. No comparisons are made with Hays' $\hat{\omega}^2$, Pearson's η^2, Cohen's partial η^2, or Cohen's f^2 measures of effect size as $\hat{\omega}^2$, η^2, η^2_{Partial}, and f^2 are undefined for multivariate data.

9.9.4 An Exact Analysis with $v = 1$

For an exact permutation analysis with $v = 1$, the observed value of δ is $\delta = 7.1305$. There are exactly four δ test statistic values that are equal to or less than the observed value of $\delta = 7.1305$. If all M arrangements of the $N = 24$ multivariate observations listed in Table 9.18 occur with equal chance under the Fisher–Pitman null hypothesis, the exact probability value of δ computed on the $M = 479{,}001{,}600$ possible arrangements of the observed data with $b = 2$ blocks reserved for each arrangement is

$$P(\delta \le \delta_0 | H_0) = \frac{\text{number of } \delta \text{ values } \le \delta_0}{M}$$

$$= \frac{4}{479{,}001{,}600} = 0.8351 \times 10^{-8} \,,$$

where δ_0 denotes the observed value of test statistic δ and M is the number of possible, equally-likely arrangements of the distance-elevation data listed in Table 9.18.

Following Eq. (9.6) on p. 320, the exact expected value of test statistic δ under the Fisher–Pitman null hypothesis is

$$\mu_\delta = \frac{1}{M} \sum_{i=1}^{M} \delta_i = \frac{17{,}916{,}053{,}734}{479{,}001{,}600} = 37.4029$$

and following Eq. (9.5) on p. 320 the observed chance-corrected measure of effect size is

$$\Re = 1 - \frac{\delta}{\mu_\delta} = 1 - \frac{7.1305}{37.4029} = +0.8094 \,,$$

indicating approximately 81% within-block agreement above what is expected by chance. No comparisons are made with Hays' $\hat{\omega}^2$, Pearson's η^2, Cohen's partial η^2, or Cohen's f^2 measures of effect size as $\hat{\omega}^2$, η^2, η^2_{Partial}, and f^2 are undefined for multivariate data.

9.10 Summary

This chapter examined statistical methods for multiple dependent samples where the null hypothesis under the Neyman–Pearson population model posits no experimental differences among the $g \geq 3$ populations that the g random samples are presumed to represent. Under the Neyman–Pearson population model of statistical inference the conventional randomized-blocks analysis of variance and four measures of effect size were described and illustrated: Fisher's F test statistic, and Hays' $\hat{\omega}^2$, Pearson's η^2, Cohen's η^2_{Partial}, and Cohen's f^2 measures of effect size, respectively.

Under the Fisher–Pitman permutation model of statistical inference, test statistic δ and associated measure of effect size $\Re$ were described and illustrated for randomized-blocks designs. For tests of $g \geq 3$ dependent samples, test statistic δ was demonstrated to be applicable to both ordinary Euclidean scaling functions with $v = 1$ and squared Euclidean scaling functions with $v = 2$. Effect size measure, $\Re$, was shown to be applicable to either $v = 1$ or $v = 2$ without modification with a chance-corrected interpretation.

Six examples illustrated permutation-based test statistics δ and $\Re$ for randomized-blocks designs. In the first example, a small sample of $N = 8$ observations in $g = 2$ treatment groups and $b = 4$ blocks was utilized to describe and illustrate the calculation of test statistics δ and $\Re$ for randomized-blocks designs. The second example with $N = 24$ observations in $g = 4$ treatment groups and $b = 6$ blocks demonstrated the chance-corrected measure of effect size, $\Re$, for randomized-blocks designs and compared $\Re$ to the four conventional measures of effect size for $g \geq 3$ dependent samples: Hays' $\hat{\omega}^2$, Pearson's η^2, Cohen's partial η^2, and Cohen's f^2. The third example with $N = 24$ observations in $g = 3$ treatment groups and $b = 8$ blocks illustrated the effects of extreme values on analyses based on $v = 1$ for ordinary Euclidean scaling and $v = 2$ for squared Euclidean scaling. The fourth example with $N = 24$ observations in $g = 3$ treatment groups and $b = 8$ blocks compared exact and Monte Carlo permutation statistical methods for randomized-blocks designs, illustrating the accuracy and efficiency of Monte Carlo analyses. The fifth example with $N = 18$ observations in $g = 6$ treatment groups and $b = 3$ blocks illustrated an application of permutation statistical methods to univariate rank-score data, comparing a permutation analysis of rank-score data with Friedman's g-sample analysis of variance for ranks. In the sixth example, both test statistic δ and effect-size measure $\Re$ were extended to multivariate data with $N = 48$ observations in $g = 12$ treatment groups, $b = 2$ blocks, and $r = 2$ measurements.

Chapter 10 continues the presentation of permutation statistical methods, examining permutation alternatives to simple linear correlation and regression. Research designs that utilize correlation and regression have a long history, are taught in every introductory class, and are among the most popular tests in the contemporary research literature.

References

1. Carroll, A.E.: A measured look at a study that alarmed some drinkers. N.Y. Times **167**, A12 (2018)
2. Feinstein, A.R.: Clinical biostatistics XXIII: the role of randomization in sampling, testing, allocation, and credulous idolatry (Part 2). Clin. Pharmacol. Ther. **14**, 898–915 (1973)
3. Friedman, M.: The use of ranks to avoid the assumption of normality implicit in the analysis of variance. J. Am. Stat. Assoc. **32**, 675–701 (1937)
4. Hotelling, H., Pabst, M.R.: Rank correlation and tests of significance involving no assumption of normality. Ann. Math. Stat. **7**, 29–43 (1936)
5. Kennedy, J.J.: The eta coefficient in complex ANOVA designs. Educ. Psych. Meas. **30**, 885–889 (1970)
6. Levine, T.R., Hullett, C.R.: Eta squared, partial eta squared, and misreporting of effect size in communication research. Hum. Commun. Res. **28**, 612–625 (2002)
7. Mielke, P.W., Berry, K.J.: Permutation Methods: A Distance Function Approach, 2nd edn. Springer, New York (2007)
8. Pedhazur, E.J.: Multiple Regression in Behavioral Research: Explanation and Prediction, 3rd edn. Harcourt, Fort Worth (1997)
9. Richardson, J.T.E.: Eta squared and partial eta squared as measures of effect size in educational research. Educ. Res. Rev. **6**, 135–147 (2011)
10. Sechrest, L., Yeaton, W.H.: Magnitude of experimental effects in social science research. Eval. Rev. **6**, 579–600 (1982)
11. Wood, A.M., Kaptage, S., Butterworth, A.S., Willeit, P., Warnakula, S., Bolton, T., et al.: Risk thresholds for alcohol consumption: combined analysis of individual-participant data for 599 912 current drinkers in 83 prospective studies. Lancet **391**, 1513–1523 (2018)

Chapter 10
Correlation and Regression

Abstract This chapter introduces permutation methods for measures of correlation and regression, the best-known of which is Pearson's product-moment correlation coefficient. Included in this chapter are six example analyses illustrating computation of exact permutation probability values for correlation and regression, calculation of measures of effect size for measures of correlation and regression, the effects of extreme values on conventional (ordinary least squares) and permutation (least absolute deviation) correlation and regression, exact and Monte Carlo permutation procedures for measures of correlation and regression, application of permutation methods to correlation and regression with rank-score data, and analysis of multiple correlation and regression. Included in this chapter are permutation versions of ordinary least squares correlation and regression, least absolute deviation correlation and regression, Spearman's rank-order correlation coefficient, Kendall's rank-order correlation coefficient, Spearman's footrule measure of correlation, and a permutation-based alternative for the conventional measures of effect size for correlation and regression: Pearson's r^2.

This chapter presents exact and Monte Carlo permutation statistical methods for measures of linear correlation and regression. Also presented in this chapter is a permutation-based measure of effect size for a variety of measures of linear correlation and regression. Simple linear correlation coefficients between two variables constitute the foundation for a large family of advanced analytic techniques and are taught in every introductory course.

In this chapter, permutation statistical methods for measures of linear correlation and regression are illustrated with six example analyses. The first example utilizes a small set of observations to illustrate the computation of exact permutation methods for measures of linear correlation, wherein the permutation test statistic, δ, is developed and compared with Pearson's conventional product-moment correlation coefficient. The second example develops a permutation-based measure of effect size as a chance-corrected alternative to Pearson's squared product-moment correlation coefficient. The third example compares permutation statistical methods

© Springer Nature Switzerland AG 2019

K. J. Berry et al., *A Primer of Permutation Statistical Methods*,
https://doi.org/10.1007/978-3-030-20933-9_10

based on ordinary and squared Euclidean scaling functions, with an emphasis on the analysis of data sets containing extreme values. Ordinary least squares (OLS) regression, based on squared Euclidean scaling, and least absolute deviation (LAD) regression, based on ordinary Euclidean scaling, are compared and contrasted. The fourth example utilizes a larger data set for providing comparisons of exact permutation methods and Monte Carlo permutation methods, demonstrating the efficiency of Monte Carlo statistical methods for correlation analyses. The fifth example illustrates the application of permutation statistical methods to univariate rank-score data, comparing permutation statistical methods with Spearman's rank-order correlation coefficient, Kendall's rank-order correlation coefficient, and Spearman's footrule measure of rank-order correlation. The sixth example illustrates the application of permutation statistical methods to multivariate correlation and regression. Both OLS and LAD multivariate linear regression are described and compared for multivariate observations.

10.1   Introduction

The most popular measure of linear correlation between two interval-level variables, say, x and y, is Pearson's r_{xy} product-moment correlation coefficient wherein the Neyman–Pearson null hypothesis (H_0) posits a value for a population parameter, such as a population correlation coefficient; that is, H_0: $\rho_{xy} = \theta$, where θ is a specified value between -1 and $+1$. For example, the null hypothesis might stipulate that the correlation in the population from which a bivariate sample has been drawn is H_0: $\rho_{xy} = 0$. In this chapter the null hypothesis, H_0: $\rho_{xy} = 0$, is used exclusively for two reasons. First, most introductory courses in statistical methods restrict their discussions to H_0: $\rho_{xy} = 0$. Null hypotheses such as H_0: $\rho_{xy} \neq 0$ are usually treated in more advanced courses. Second, Fisher's normalizing transformation for r_{xy} when $\rho_{xy} \neq 0$ has been found to be unsatisfactory unless either the population correlation coefficient $\rho_{xy} = 0$ or the population is known to be bivariate normal [4].

The problem is easy to illustrate. Consider a population in which the product-moment correlation is equal to zero; that is, $\rho_{xy} = 0$, such as depicted in Fig. 10.1. Random sampling from a population in which $\rho_{xy} = 0$ produces a symmetric, discrete sampling distribution of r_{xy} values that can be approximated by Student's t distribution with $N - 2$ degrees of freedom, such as depicted in Fig. 10.2.

Now consider a population in which the product-moment correlation is not equal to zero; that is, $\rho_{xy} = +0.60$, such as depicted in Fig. 10.3. Random sampling from a population in which $\rho_{xy} = +0.60$ produces an negatively-skewed, discrete sampling distribution of r_{xy} values that cannot be approximated by Student's t distribution with $N - 2$ degrees of freedom, such as depicted in Fig. 10.4.

Fig. 10.1 Simulated
scatterplot of a population
with $\rho_{xy} = 0.00$

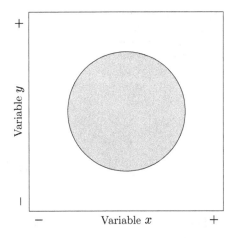

Fig. 10.2 Simulated discrete
permutation distribution of
r_{xy} from a population with
$\rho_{xy} = +0.00$

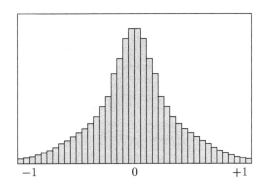

Fig. 10.3 Simulated
scatterplot of a population
with $\rho_{xy} = +0.60$

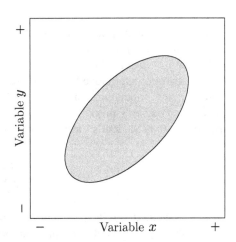

Fig. 10.4 Simulated discrete permutation distribution of r_{xy} from a population with $\rho_{xy} = +0.60$

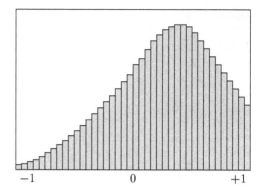

For simple linear correlation with two interval-level variables and N paired observations, Pearson's product-moment correlation coefficient is given by

$$
r_{xy} = \frac{\displaystyle\sum_{i=1}^{N}(x_i - \bar{x})(y_i - \bar{y})}{\sqrt{\left[\displaystyle\sum_{i=1}^{N}(x_i - \bar{x})^2\right]\left[\displaystyle\sum_{i=1}^{N}(y_i - \bar{y})^2\right]}} ,
$$

where $\bar{x}$ and $\bar{y}$ denote the arithmetic means of variables x and y given by

$$
\bar{x} = \frac{1}{N}\sum_{i=1}^{N}x_i \quad \text{and} \quad \bar{y} = \frac{1}{N}\sum_{i=1}^{N}y_i ,
$$

respectively, x_i and y_i denote the ith observed sample values for $i = 1, \ldots, N$, and N is the number of bivariate observations.

Under the Neyman–Pearson population model the null hypothesis is H_0: $\rho_{xy} = \theta$ and the two-tail alternative hypothesis is H_1: $\rho_{xy} \neq \theta$, where θ is a hypothesized value for the population correlation coefficient. The conventional test of significance for Pearson's product-moment correlation coefficient with null hypothesis, H_0: $\rho_{xy} = 0$, is Student's t test statistic given by

$$
t = r_{xy}\sqrt{\frac{N-2}{1-r_{xy}^2}} ,
$$

which is assumed to follow Student's t distribution with $N - 2$ degrees of freedom, under the assumptions of normality and homogeneity. The permissible probability of a type I error is denoted by α and if the observed value of t is more extreme than the critical values of $\pm t$ that define α, the null hypothesis is rejected with a probability of type I error equal to or less than α. The test of significance does not determine whether or not the null hypothesis is true, but only provides the probability that, if the null hypothesis is true, the sample has been drawn from a population with the value specified under the null hypothesis.

The assumptions underlying Pearson's product-moment correlation coefficient are (1) the observations are independent, (2) the data are a random sample from a well-defined population with $\rho_{xy} = 0$, (3) the relationship between the predictor variable and the criterion variable is linear, (4) homogeneity of variance, and (5) the target variables x and y are distributed bivariate normal in the population.

10.1.1 A Permutation Approach

Consider a simple linear correlation analysis between two variables under the Fisher–Pitman permutation model of statistical inference. As discussed in previous chapters, the permutation model differs from the Neyman–Pearson population model in several ways. Under the Fisher–Pitman permutation model there is no null hypothesis specifying a population parameter. Instead, the Fisher–Pitman null hypothesis simply states that all possible arrangements of the observed data occur with equal chance [5]. Also, there is no alternative hypothesis under the permutation model and no specified α level. Moreover, there is no requirement of random sampling, no degrees of freedom, and no assumption of normality or homogeneity. Finally, the Fisher–Pitman permutation statistical model provides exact probability values.

A permutation alternative to a conventional correlation analysis for two variables is easily defined. Let x_i and y_i denote the paired sample values for $i = 1, \ldots, N$. The permutation test statistic is given by

$$\delta = S_x^2 + S_y^2 - 2|r_{xy}|S_x S_y + (\bar{x} - \bar{y})^2 ,$$

where the sample means for variables x and y are given by

$$\bar{x} = \frac{1}{N} \sum_{i=1}^{N} x_i \quad \text{and} \quad \bar{y} = \frac{1}{N} \sum_{i=1}^{N} y_i ,$$

respectively, and the sample variances for variables x and y are given by

$$S_x^2 = \frac{1}{N} \sum_{i=1}^{N} (x_i - \bar{x})^2 \quad \text{and} \quad S_y^2 = \frac{1}{N} \sum_{i=1}^{N} (y_i - \bar{y})^2 ,$$

respectively.[1]

---

[1] Note that whereas a permutation approach eschews estimated population parameters and degrees of freedom, the summations are divided by N, not $N - 1$. Thus S_x^2 and S_y^2 denote the sample variances, not the estimated population variances.

Under the Fisher–Pitman null hypothesis, the exact probability value of an observed δ is the proportion of δ test statistic values calculated on all possible arrangements of the observed data that are equal to or less than the observed value of δ; that is,

$$P(\delta \leq \delta_0 | H_0) = \frac{\text{number of } \delta \text{ values } \leq \delta_0}{M},$$

where δ_0 denotes the observed value of test statistic δ and M is the number of possible, equally-likely arrangements in the reference set of all permutations of the observed data.

10.2   Example 1: The Relationship Between r_{xy} and δ

An example will serve to illustrate the relationships between test statistics r_{xy} and δ for a simple correlation analysis. Consider the small set of data listed in Table 10.1 with $N = 4$ bivariate observations. For the example bivariate observations listed in Table 10.1, the sample means for variables x and y are

$$\bar{x} = \frac{1}{N} \sum_{i=1}^{N} x_i = \frac{24 + 31 + 55 + 43}{4} = 38.25$$

and

$$\bar{y} = \frac{1}{N} \sum_{i=1}^{N} y_i = \frac{20 + 36 + 49 + 35}{4} = 35.00 ,$$

respectively, the sample product-moment correlation coefficient is

$$r_{xy} = \frac{\sum_{i=1}^{N} (x_i - \bar{x})(y_i - \bar{y})}{\sqrt{\left[\sum_{i=1}^{N} (x_i - \bar{x})^2 \right] \left[\sum_{i=1}^{N} (y_i - \bar{y})^2 \right]}}$$

$$= \frac{+441.00}{\sqrt{(558.75)(422.00)}} = +0.9082 ,$$

Table 10.1 Example correlation data on $N = 4$ bivariate observations

Object	Variable	
	x	y
1	24	20
2	31	36
3	55	49
4	43	35

and Student's t test statistic is

$$t = r_{xy}\sqrt{\frac{N-2}{1-r_{xy}^2}} = +0.9082\sqrt{\frac{4-2}{1-(+0.9082)^2}} = +3.0684 \ .$$

Under the Neyman–Pearson null hypothesis, H_0: $\rho_{xy} = 0$, test statistic t is asymptotically distributed as Student's t with $N - 2$ degrees of freedom. With $N - 2 = 4 - 2 = 2$ degrees of freedom, the asymptotic two-tail probability value of $t = +3.0684$ is $P = 0.0918$, under the assumptions of linearity, normality, and homogeneity.

10.2.1 An Exact Permutation Analysis

Now consider the bivariate data listed in Table 10.1 under the Fisher–Pitman permutation model. For the example bivariate data listed in Table 10.1, the sample means are $\bar{x} = 38.25$ and $\bar{y} = 35.00$, the sample variances are $S_x^2 = 139.6875$ and $S_y^2 = 105.50$, the sample standard deviations are $S_x = 11.8189$ and $S_y = 10.2713$, the sample product-moment correlation coefficient is $r_{xy} = +0.9082$, and the observed permutation test statistic is

$$\delta = S_x^2 + S_y^2 - 2|r_{xy}|S_x S_y + (\bar{x} - \bar{y})^2 = 139.6875 + 105.50$$

$$- 2(0.9082)(11.8189)(10.2713) + (38.25 - 35.00)^2 = 35.25 \ . \qquad (10.1)$$

Note that in Eq. (10.1), S_x, S_x^2, S_y, S_y^2, $\bar{x}$, $\bar{y}$, and the constant 2 are all invariant under permutation, leaving only $|r_{xy}|$ to be calculated for each arrangement of the observed data.

An exact permutation analysis requires exhaustive shuffles of either the $N = 4$ x values or the $N = 4$ y values while holding the other set of values constant. For the example data listed in Table 10.1 there are only

$$M = N! = 4! = 24$$

possible, equally-likely arrangements in the reference set of all permutations of the bivariate data listed in Table 10.1, making an exact permutation analysis feasible. Under the Fisher–Pitman permutation model, the exact probability of an observed δ is the proportion of δ test statistic values computed on all possible, equally-likely arrangements of the $N = 4$ bivariate observations listed in Table 10.1 that are equal to or less than the observed value of $\delta = 35.25$. Table 10.2 lists the $M = 24$ arrangements of the example data listed in Table 10.1 with the x values shuffled and the associated values for r_{xy} and δ, ordered by the $|r_{xy}|$ values from largest ($|r_1| = 0.9432$) to smallest ($|r_{24}| = 0.1524$) and by the δ values from smallest

Table 10.2 All $M = 24$ possible, equally-likely arrangements of the bivariate data listed in Table 10.1

Arrangement	Variable x	Variable y	$|r_{xy}|$	δ
1*	55, 31, 24, 43	20, 36, 49, 35	0.9432	26.75
2*	24, 43, 55, 31	20, 36, 49, 35	0.9329	29.25
3*	55, 43, 24, 31	20, 36, 49, 35	0.9185	32.75
4*	24, 31, 55, 43	20, 36, 49, 35	0.9082	35.25
5	55, 24, 31, 43	20, 36, 49, 35	0.7558	72.25
6	31, 43, 55, 24	20, 36, 49, 35	0.7167	81.75
7	55, 43, 31, 24	20, 36, 49, 35	0.7167	81.75
8	31, 24, 55, 43	20, 36, 49, 35	0.6775	91.25
9	24, 55, 43, 31	20, 36, 49, 35	0.6116	107.25
10	43, 31, 24, 55	20, 36, 49, 35	0.5725	116.75
11	24, 31, 43, 55	20, 36, 49, 35	0.5622	119.25
12	43, 55, 24, 31	20, 36, 49, 35	0.5231	128.75
13	55, 24, 43, 31	20, 36, 49, 35	0.4098	156.25
14	31, 55, 43, 24	20, 36, 49, 35	0.3954	159.75
15	55, 31, 43, 24	20, 36, 49, 35	0.3954	159.75
16	43, 24, 31, 55	20, 36, 49, 35	0.3851	162.25
17	31, 24, 43, 55	20, 36, 49, 35	0.3316	175.25
18	43, 31, 55, 24	20, 36, 49, 35	0.3213	177.75
19	43, 55, 31, 24	20, 36, 49, 35	0.3213	177.75
20	43, 24, 55, 31	20, 36, 49, 35	0.3068	181.25
21	24, 55, 31, 43	20, 36, 49, 35	0.2657	191.25
22	24, 43, 31, 55	20, 36, 49, 35	0.2409	197.25
23	31, 43, 24, 55	20, 36, 49, 35	0.1771	212.75
24	31, 55, 24, 43	20, 36, 49, 35	0.1524	218.75

($\delta_1 = 29.25$) to largest ($\delta_{24} = 218.75$). For test statistic δ there are four δ test statistic values that are equal to or less than the observed value of $\delta = 35.25$ ($\delta_1 = 26.75$, $\delta_2 = 29.25$, $\delta_3 = 32.75$, and $\delta_4 = 35.25$). The arrangements yielding the four smallest δ values are indicated with asterisks in Table 10.2. If all M arrangements of the $N = 4$ bivariate observations listed in Table 10.1 occur with equal chance under the Fisher–Pitman null hypothesis, the exact probability value of $\delta = 35.25$ computed on the $M = 24$ possible arrangements of the observed data with $N = 4$ bivariate observations preserved for each arrangement is

$$P(\delta \leq \delta_o) = \frac{\text{number of } \delta \text{ values} \leq \delta_o}{M} = \frac{4}{24} = 0.1667 \,,$$

where δ_o denotes the observed value of δ and M is the number of possible, equally-likely arrangements of the $N = 4$ bivariate observations listed in Table 10.1.

Alternatively, since test statistics δ and r_{xy} are equivalent under the Fisher–Pitman null hypothesis, there are four $|r_{xy}|$ values that are equal to or greater than the observed value of $|r_{xy}| = 0.9082$ ($|r_1| = 0.9432$, $|r_2| = 0.9329$, $|r_3| = 0.9185$, and $|r_4| = 0.9082$) yielding an exact probability value for $|r_{xy}| = 0.9082$ of

$$P(|r_{xy}| \geq |r_0|) = \frac{\text{number of } |r_{xy}| \text{ values } \geq |r_0|}{M} = \frac{4}{24} = 0.1667 \,,$$

where $|r_0|$ denotes the observed value of $|r_{xy}|$. There is a considerable difference between the asymptotic probability value for r_{xy} based on Student's t distribution ($P = 0.0918$) and the exact permutation probability value for δ ($P = 0.1667$). The actual difference between the two probability values is

$$\Delta_P = 0.1667 - 0.0918 = 0.0749 \,.$$

The difference is most probably due to the very small number of arrangements of the observed data. A continuous mathematical function such as Student's t cannot be expected to provide a precise fit to only 24 data points of which only 21 are different.

10.3 Example 2: Measures of Effect Size

Measures of effect size express the practical or clinical significance of a sample correlation coefficient, as contrasted with the statistical significance of the correlation coefficient. For an illustration of the measurement of effect size, consider the example data listed in Table 10.3 with $N = 11$ bivariate observations. The standard measure of effect size is simply the squared Pearson product-moment correlation between variables x and y. For the example bivariate data listed in Table 10.3, the

Table 10.3 Example correlation data on $N = 11$ bivariate observations

Object	Variable	
	x	y
1	11	4
2	18	11
3	12	1
4	27	16
5	15	5
6	21	9
7	25	10
8	15	2
9	18	8
10	23	7
11	12	3

sample means for variables x and y are

$$\bar{x} = \frac{1}{N} \sum_{i=1}^{N} x_i = \frac{11 + 18 + \cdots + 12}{11} = 17.9091$$

and

$$\bar{y} = \frac{1}{N} \sum_{i=1}^{N} y_i = \frac{4 + 11 + \cdots + 3}{11} = 6.9091 \,,$$

respectively, the sample product-moment correlation coefficient is

$$r_{xy} = \frac{\displaystyle\sum_{i=1}^{N} \left(x_i - \bar{x}\right)\left(y_i - \bar{y}\right)}{\sqrt{\left[\displaystyle\sum_{i=1}^{N} \left(x_i - \bar{x}\right)^2\right]\left[\displaystyle\sum_{i=1}^{N} \left(y_i - \bar{y}\right)^2\right]}}$$

$$= \frac{+209.9091}{\sqrt{(302.9091)(200.9091)}} = +0.8509 \,,$$

the squared product-moment measure of effect size is

$$r_{xy}^2 = (+0.8509)^2 = 0.7240 \,,$$

and Student's t test statistic is

$$t = r_{xy}\sqrt{\frac{N-2}{1-r_{xy}^2}} = +0.8509\sqrt{\frac{11-2}{1-(+0.8509)^2}} = +4.8592 \,.$$

Under the Neyman–Pearson null hypothesis, H_0: $\rho_{xy} = 0$, test statistic t is asymptotically distributed as Student's t with $N - 2$ degrees of freedom. With $N - 2 = 11 - 2 = 9$ degrees of freedom, the asymptotic two-tail probability value of $t = +4.8592$ is $P = 0.8969 \times 10^{-3}$, under the assumptions of linearity, normality, and homogeneity.

10.3.1   An Exact Permutation Analysis

Now consider the example data listed in Table 10.3 under the Fisher–Pitman permutation model. For the example data listed in Table 10.3, the sample means are $\bar{x} = 17.9091$ and $\bar{y} = 6.9091$, the sample variances are $S_x^2 = 27.5372$ and $S_y^2 = 18.2645$, the sample standard deviations are $S_x = 5.2476$ and $S_y = 4.2737$, the sample product-moment correlation coefficient is $r_{xy} = +0.8509$, and the observed permutation test statistic is

$$\delta = S_x^2 + S_y^2 - 2|r_{xy}|S_x S_y + (\bar{x} - \bar{y})^2 = 27.5372 + 18.2645$$

$$- 2(0.8509)(5.2476)(4.2737) + (17.9091 - 6.9091)^2 = 128.6364 .$$

An exact permutation analysis requires shuffling of either the $N = 11$ x values or the $N = 11$ y values while holding the other set of values constant. For the example data listed in Table 10.3 there are

$$M = N! = 11! = 39{,}916{,}800$$

possible, equally-likely arrangements in the reference set of all permutations of the observed bivariate data, making an exact permutation analysis feasible.

The exact expected value of the $M = 39{,}916{,}800$ δ test statistic values under the Fisher–Pitman null hypothesis is

$$\mu_\delta = \frac{1}{M} \sum_{i=1}^{M} \delta_i = \frac{6{,}658{,}188{,}218}{39{,}916{,}800} = 166.8017 .$$

Alternatively, the exact expected value of test statistic δ is

$$\mu_\delta = S_x^2 + S_y^2 + (\bar{x} - \bar{y})^2$$

$$= 27.5372 + 18.2645 + (17.9091 - 6.9091)^2 = 166.8017 .$$

The observed chance-corrected measure of effect size is

$$\Re = 1 - \frac{\delta}{\mu_\delta} = 1 - \frac{128.6364}{166.8017} = +0.2288 ,$$

indicating approximately 23% agreement between the x and y values above what is expected by chance.

Under the Fisher–Pitman permutation model, the exact probability of an observed δ is the proportion of δ test statistic values computed on all possible, equally-likely arrangements of the $N = 11$ bivariate observations that are equal to or less than the observed value of $\delta = 128.6364$. There are exactly 35,216 δ test statistic values that are equal to or less than the observed value of $\delta = 128.6364$. If all M arrangements of the $N = 11$ bivariate observations listed in Table 10.3 occur with equal chance under the Fisher–Pitman null hypothesis, the exact probability value of $\delta = 128.6364$ computed on the $M = 39{,}916{,}800$ possible arrangements of the observed data with $N = 11$ bivariate observations preserved for each arrangement is

$$P(\delta \le \delta_0 | H_0) = \frac{\text{number of } \delta \text{ values } \le \delta_0}{M} = \frac{35{,}216}{39{,}916{,}800} = 0.8822 \times 10^{-3} \; ,$$

where δ_0 denotes the observed value of test statistic δ and M is the number of possible, equally-likely arrangements of the $N = 11$ bivariate observations listed in Table 10.3. In this example there are 39,916,800 data points to be fit by Student's t distribution and there are no extreme values. Thus the asymptotic probability value ($P = 0.8969 \times 10^{-3}$) and the exact permutation probability value ($P = 0.8822 \times 10^{-3}$) are similar, with a difference between the probability values of only

$$\Delta_P = 0.8969 \times 10^{-3} - 0.8822 \times 10^{-3} = 0.1459 \times 10^{-4} \; .$$

10.4   Example 3: Analyses with $v = 2$ and $v = 1$

Ordinary least squares (OLS) linear regression and correlation have long been recognized as useful tools in many areas of research. The optimal properties of OLS linear regression and correlation are well known when the errors are normally distributed. However, in practice the assumption of normality is rarely justified. Least absolute deviation (LAD) regression and correlation are often superior to OLS linear regression and correlation when the errors are not normally distributed. Estimators of OLS regression parameters can be severely affected by unusual values in the criterion variable, in one or more of the predictor variables, or both. In contrast, LAD regression is less sensitive to the effects of unusual variables because the errors are not squared [3]. The effect of extreme values on OLS and LAD regression and correlation is analogous to the effect of extreme values on the mean and median as measures of location.

Consider N paired x_i and y_i observed values for $i = 1, \ldots, N$. For the OLS regression equation given by

$$\hat{y}_i = \hat{\alpha}_{yx} + \hat{\beta}_{yx} x_i \; ,$$

where $\hat{y}_i$ is the ith of N predicted criterion values and x_i is the ith of N predictor values, $\hat{\alpha}_{yx}$ and $\hat{\beta}_{ys}$ are the OLS parameter estimators of the population intercept (α_{yx}) and population slope (β_{yx}), respectively, and are given by

$$\hat{\beta}_{yx} = \frac{\sum\limits_{i=1}^{N} (x_i - \bar{x})(y_i - \bar{y})}{\sum\limits_{i=1}^{N} (x_i - \bar{x})^2}$$

and

$$\hat{\alpha}_{yx} = \bar{y} - \hat{\beta}_{yx}\bar{x} \ ,$$

where $\bar{x}$ and $\bar{y}$ are the sample means of variables x and y, respectively. Estimators of OLS regression parameters minimize the sum of the squared differences between the observed (y_i) and predicted ($\hat{y}_i$) criterion values for $i = 1, \ldots, N$; that is,

$$\sum_{i=1}^{N} |y_i - \hat{y}_i|^v \ ,$$

where for OLS regression based on a squared Euclidean scaling function, $v = 2$.

For the LAD regression equation given by

$$\tilde{y}_i = \tilde{\alpha}_{yx} + \tilde{\beta}_{yx}x_i \ ,$$

where $\tilde{y}_i$ is the ith of N predicted criterion values and x_i is the ith of N predictor values, $\tilde{\alpha}_{yx}$ and $\tilde{\beta}_{yx}$ are the LAD parameter estimators of the population intercept (α_{yx}) and population slope (β_{yx}), respectively.[2]

Unlike OLS regression, no simple expressions can be given for LAD regression estimators $\tilde{\alpha}_{yx}$ and $\tilde{\beta}_{yx}$. However, values for $\tilde{\alpha}_{yx}$ and $\tilde{\beta}_{yx}$ may be found through an efficient linear programming algorithm, such as provided by Barrodale and Roberts [1, 2]. In contrast to estimators of OLS regression parameters, estimators of LAD regression parameters minimize the sum of the absolute differences between the observed (y_i) and predicted ($\tilde{y}_i$) criterion values for $i = 1, \ldots, N$; that is,

$$\sum_{i=1}^{N} |y_i - \tilde{y}_i|^v \ ,$$

where for LAD regression based on ordinary Euclidean scaling, $v = 1$.

For LAD regression it is convenient to have a measure of agreement, not product-moment correlation, between the observed and predicted y values. Let the permutation test statistic be given by

$$\delta = \frac{1}{N} \sum_{i=1}^{N} |y_i - \tilde{y}_i|^v$$

---

[2]In this section, a caret($\wedge$) over a symbol such as $\hat{\alpha}$ or $\hat{\beta}$ indicates an OLS regression model predicted value of a corresponding population parameter, while a tilde ($\sim$) over a symbol such as $\tilde{\alpha}$ or $\tilde{\beta}$ indicates a LAD regression model predicted value of a corresponding population parameter.

Table 10.4 Example
bivariate correlation data on
$N = 10$ subjects

Subject	x	y
1	14	25
2	8	23
3	5	21
4	2	10
5	1	12
6	3	11
7	9	19
8	2	13
9	3	13
10	9	16

and let $v = 1$ for correspondence with LAD regression. Then the exact expected
value of test statistic δ under the Fisher–Pitman null hypothesis is given by

$$\mu_\delta = \frac{1}{N^2} \sum_{i=1}^{N} \sum_{j=1}^{N} |y_i - \tilde{y}_j|^v,$$

and a chance-corrected measure of agreement between the observed y_i values and
the LAD predicted $\tilde{y}_i$ values for $i = 1, \ldots, N$ is given by

$$\Re = 1 - \frac{\delta}{\mu_\delta}.$$

10.4.1   An Example OLS Regression Analysis

To illustrate the relative differences between OLS and LAD regression, consider
the small example set of bivariate values listed in Table 10.4 for $N = 10$
subjects. For the bivariate data listed in Table 10.4 the OLS estimate of the
population slope is $\hat{\beta}_{yx} = +1.0673$, the OLS estimate of the population intercept is
$\hat{\alpha}_{yx} = +10.3229$, and the Pearson product-moment correlation coefficient is $r_{xy} =$
$+0.8414$. Table 10.5 lists the $N = 10$ observed values for variables x and y, the
OLS predicted y values ($\hat{y}$), the residual errors ($\hat{e}$), and the squared residual errors
($\hat{e}^2$). Under the Neyman–Pearson population model Pearson's product-moment
correlation coefficient is asymptotically distributed as Student's t under the null
hypothesis, H_0: $\rho_{xy} = 0$, with $N - 2$ degrees of freedom.[3] For the $N = 10$ bivariate

---

[3]One degree of freedom is lost due to the sample estimate ($\hat{\alpha}_{yx}$) of the population intercept and
one degree of freedom is lost due to the sample estimate ($\hat{\beta}_{yx}$) of the population slope.

Table 10.5 Observed x and y values with associated predicted values ($\hat{y}$), residual errors ($\hat{e}$), and squared residual errors ($\hat{e}^2$) from the bivariate correlation data listed in Table 10.4

Subject	x	y	$\hat{y}$	$\hat{e}$	$\hat{e}^2$
1	14	25	25.2656	−0.2656	0.0705
2	8	23	18.8616	+4.1384	17.1264
3	5	21	15.6596	+5.3404	28.5199
4	2	10	12.4576	−2.4576	6.0398
5	1	12	11.3903	+0.6097	0.3718
6	3	11	13.5249	−2.5249	6.3753
7	9	19	19.9289	−0.9289	0.8629
8	2	13	12.4576	+0.5424	0.2942
9	3	13	13.5249	−0.5249	0.2756
10	9	16	19.9289	−3.9289	15.4365
Sum	56	163	163.0000	0.0000	75.3728

observations listed in Table 10.4 with $N - 2 = 10 - 2 = 8$ degrees of freedom Student's test statistic,

$$t = r_{xy}\sqrt{\frac{N-2}{1-r_{xy}^2}} = +0.8414\sqrt{\frac{10-2}{1-(+0.8414)^2}} = +4.4039 \, ,$$

yields an asymptotic two-tail probability value of $P = 0.2275 \times 10^{-2}$, under the assumptions of linearity, normality, and homogeneity.

10.4.2 An Example LAD Regression Analysis

For the bivariate data listed in Table 10.4, the LAD estimate of the population intercept is $\tilde{\alpha}_{yx} = +9.7273$, the LAD estimate of the population slope is $\tilde{\beta}_{yx} = +1.0909$, the observed permutation test statistic is

$$\delta = \frac{1}{N}\sum_{i=1}^{N}|y_i - \tilde{y}_i| = \frac{20.6364}{10} = 2.0636 \, ,$$

the exact expected value of test statistic δ under the Fisher–Pitman null hypothesis is

$$\mu_\delta = \frac{1}{N^2}\sum_{i=1}^{N}\sum_{j=1}^{N}|y_i - \tilde{y}_j| = \frac{533.8182}{10^2} = 5.3382 \, ,$$

Table 10.6 Observed x and y values with associated predicted values ($\tilde{y}$), residual errors ($\tilde{e}$), and absolute residual errors ($|\tilde{e}|$) from the bivariate correlation data listed in Table 10.4

Subject	x	y	$\tilde{y}$	$\tilde{e}$	$|\tilde{e}|$
1	14	25	25.0000	0.0000	0.0000
2	8	23	18.4545	+4.5455	4.5455
3	5	21	15.1818	+5.8182	5.8182
4	2	10	11.9090	−1.9091	1.9091
5	1	12	10.8182	+1.1818	1.1818
6	3	11	13.0000	−2.0000	2.0000
7	9	19	19.5455	−0.5455	0.5455
8	2	13	11.9090	+1.0909	1.0909
9	3	13	13.0000	0.0000	0.0000
10	9	16	19.5455	−3.5455	3.5455
Sum	56	163	158.3636	+4.6364	20.6364

and the chance-corrected measure of agreement between the observed y values and the LAD predicted $\tilde{y}$ values is

$$\Re = 1 - \frac{\delta}{\mu_\delta} = 1 - \frac{2.0636}{5.3382} = +0.6134 \,,$$

indicating approximately 61% agreement between the observed and predicted values of variable y.

Table 10.6 lists the $N = 10$ observed values of variables x and y, the predicted y values ($\tilde{y}$), the residual errors ($\tilde{e}$), and the absolute residual errors ($|\tilde{e}|$).

Since there are only

$$M = N! = 10! = 3{,}628{,}800$$

possible, equally-likely arrangements in the reference set of all permutations of the bivariate data listed in Table 10.4, an exact permutation analysis is possible. Under the Fisher–Pitman permutation model, the exact probability of an observed δ is the proportion of δ test statistic values computed on all possible, equally-likely arrangements of the $N = 10$ bivariate observations listed in Table 10.4 that are equal to or less than the observed value of $\delta = 2.0636$. Alternatively, the exact probability value of an observed $\Re$ agreement coefficient is the proportion of $\Re$ values computed on all possible, equally-likely arrangements of the $N = 10$ bivariate observations listed in Table 10.4 that are equal to or greater than the observed value of $\Re = +0.6134$. There are exactly 15,533 $\Re$ test statistic values that are equal to or greater than the observed value of $\Re = +0.6134$.

If all M arrangements of the $N = 10$ bivariate observations listed in Table 10.4 occur with equal chance under the Fisher–Pitman null hypothesis, the exact probability value of $\Re = +0.6134$ computed on the $M = 3{,}628{,}800$ possible arrangements of the observed data with $N = 10$ bivariate observations preserved for each arrangement is

$$P(\Re \geq \Re_0 | H_0) = \frac{\text{number of } \Re \text{ values } \geq \Re_0}{M} = \frac{15{,}533}{3{,}628{,}800} = 0.4280 \times 10^{-2},$$

where $\Re_0$ denotes the observed value of test statistic $\Re$.

Alternatively, since $\mu_\delta = 5.3382$ is a constant,

$$P(\delta \leq \delta_0 | H_0) = \frac{\text{number of } \delta \text{ values } \leq \delta_0}{M} = \frac{15{,}533}{3{,}628{,}800} = 0.4280 \times 10^{-2},$$

where δ_0 denotes the observed value of test statistic δ and M is the number of possible, equally-likely arrangements of the $N = 10$ bivariate observations listed in Table 10.4.

10.4.3   The Effects of Extreme Values

For the example bivariate data listed in Table 10.4 on p. 374, the exact probability value based on LAD regression and ordinary Euclidean scaling with $v = 1$ is $P = 0.4280 \times 10^{-2}$ and the asymptotic probability value based on OLS regression and squared Euclidean scaling with $v = 2$ is $P = 0.2275 \times 10^{-2}$. In this case the difference between the asymptotic and exact probability values is only

$$\Delta_P = 0.4280 \times 10^{-2} - 0.2275 \times 10^{-2} = 0.2006 \times 10^{-2}.$$

The small difference in probability values is due to the fact that there are no extreme values in the data listed in Table 10.4 on p. 374. OLS analyses based on squared Euclidean scaling with $v = 2$ are mean-based and LAD analyses based on ordinary Euclidean scaling with $v = 1$ are median-based. Consequently, LAD regression analyses are highly resistant to extreme values.

Extreme values are common in applied research. To demonstrate the difference between OLS analyses based on squared Euclidean scaling with $v = 2$ and LAD analyses based on ordinary Euclidean scaling with $v = 1$ when the data contain an extreme value, consider the bivariate data listed in Table 10.7. The data listed in Table 10.7 are the same data listed in Table 10.4 on p. 374 with one alteration: the value of $y_2 = 23$ has been increased to $y_2 = 90$, thereby providing an extreme value.

For the bivariate data listed in Table 10.4 on p. 374 without an extreme value ($y_2 = 23$), the OLS sample correlation coefficient is $r_{xy} = +0.8414$, Student's t test statistic is $t = +4.4039$, and the asymptotic probability value to six decimal places is $P = 0.002275$. For the bivariate data listed in Table 10.7 with an extreme value ($y_2 = 90$), the OLS sample correlation coefficient is $r_{xy} = +0.3636$, Student's t test statistic is $t = +1.1042$, and the asymptotic probability value is $P = 0.301606$.

Table 10.7 Example
bivariate LAD correlation
data on $N = 10$ subjects with
an extreme value included

Subject	x	y
1	14	25
2	8	90
3	5	21
4	2	10
5	1	12
6	3	11
7	9	19
8	2	13
9	3	13
10	9	16

The difference between the two OLS correlation coefficients is

$$\Delta_{r_{xy}} = 0.8414 - 0.3636 = 0.4778$$

and the difference between the two OLS probability values is

$$\Delta_P = 0.301606 - 0.002275 = 0.299331 .$$

For the bivariate data listed in Table 10.4 on p. 374 without an extreme value
($y_2 = 23$), the LAD agreement measure is $\Re = +0.6134$ and the exact probability
value to six decimal places is $P = 0.004280$. For the bivariate data listed in
Table 10.7 with an extreme value ($y_2 = 90$), the LAD agreement measure is
$\Re = +0.2696$ and the exact probability value is $P = 0.006317$. The difference
between the two LAD agreement measures is

$$\Delta_\Re = 0.6134 - 0.2696 = 0.3438$$

and the difference between the two LAD probability values is

$$\Delta_P = 0.006317 - 0.004280 = 0.002037 .$$

The difference between the two LAD agreement measures ($\Delta_\Re = 0.3438$)
is considerably smaller than the difference between the two OLS correlation
coefficients ($\Delta_{r_{xy}} = 0.4778$) and the difference between the two LAD probability
values ($\Delta_P = 0.002037$) is almost two orders of magnitude smaller than the
difference between the two OLS probability values ($\Delta_P = 0.299331$). While the
LAD regression analysis of the data listed in Table 10.7 is clearly affected by the
presence of an extreme value, LAD regression based on ordinary Euclidean scaling
with $v = 1$ is a robust procedure relative to OLS regression based on squared
Euclidean scaling with $v = 2$ when extreme values are present.

10.5 Example 4: Exact and Monte Carlo Analyses

As sample sizes become large, the number of possible arrangements of the observed data makes exact permutation methods impractical. For example, for a sample size of $N = 20$ there are

$$M = N! = 20! = 2{,}432{,}902{,}008{,}176{,}640{,}000$$

possible, equally-likely arrangements in the reference set of all permutations of the observed data to be analyzed. Far too many arrangements to be practical. Monte Carlo permutation methods examine a random sample of all M possible arrangements of the observed data, providing efficient and accurate results. Provided that the probability value is not too small, $L = 1{,}000{,}000$ random arrangements are usually sufficient to ensure three decimal places of accuracy [6].

For a fourth, larger example of bivariate correlation, consider the data on $N = 12$ objects listed in Table 10.8 under the Neyman–Pearson population model. For the example data listed in Table 10.8 with $N = 12$ bivariate observations, the means of variables x and y are

$$\bar{x} = \frac{1}{N} \sum_{i=1}^{N} x_i = \frac{9 + 10 + \cdots + 8}{12} = 17.3333$$

and

$$\bar{y} = \frac{1}{N} \sum_{i=1}^{N} y_i = \frac{21 + 25 + \cdots + 18}{12} = 6.9167 \,,$$

Table 10.8 Example correlation data on $N = 12$ bivariate observations

	Variable	
Object	x	y
1	9	21
2	10	25
3	2	15
4	4	11
5	5	15
6	16	27
7	1	12
8	11	18
9	7	11
10	3	12
11	7	23
12	8	18

respectively, and Pearson's product-moment correlation coefficient between variables x and y is

$$
r_{xy} = \frac{\sum_{i=1}^{N}(x_i - \bar{x})(y_i - \bar{y})}{\sqrt{\left[\sum_{i=1}^{N}(x_i - \bar{x})^2\right]\left[\sum_{i=1}^{N}(y_i - \bar{y})^2\right]}}
$$

$$
= \frac{+209.3333}{\sqrt{[(346.6667)(200.9167)]}} = +0.7932 .
$$

The conventional test of significance for Pearson's product-moment correlation coefficient is given by

$$
t = r_{xy}\sqrt{\frac{N-2}{1-r_{xy}^2}} .
$$

Under the Neyman–Pearson null hypothesis, H_0: $\rho_{xy} = 0$, test statistic t is asymptotically distributed as Student's t with $N - 2$ degrees of freedom.

For the example data listed in Table 10.8,

$$
t = r_{xy}\sqrt{\frac{N-2}{1-r_{xy}^2}} = +0.7932\sqrt{\frac{12-2}{1-(+0.7932)^2}} = +4.1188
$$

and with $N - 2 = 12 - 2 = 10$ degrees of freedom the asymptotic two-tail probability value is $P = 0.2081\times10^{-2}$, under the assumptions of linearity, normality, and homogeneity.

10.5.1   A Monte Carlo Permutation Analysis

Now consider the data listed in Table 10.8 under the Fisher–Pitman permutation model. For the example data listed in Table 10.8 with $N = 12$ bivariate observations, the sample means are $\bar{x} = 6.9167$ and $\bar{y} = 17.3333$, the sample variances are $S_x^2 = 16.7431$ and $S_y^2 = 28.8889$, the sample standard deviations are $S_x = 4.0918$ and $S_y = 5.3748$, the sample product-moment correlation coefficient is $r_{xy} = +0.7932$, and the observed permutation test statistic is

$$
\delta = S_x^2 + S_y^2 - 2|r_{xy}|S_x S_y + (\bar{x} - \bar{y})^2 = 16.7431 + 28.8889
$$

$$
- 2(0.7932)(4.0918)(5.3748) + (6.9167 - 17.3333)^2 = 119.25 .
$$

A permutation analysis of correlation requires shuffling either the $N = 12$ x values or the $N = 12$ y values, while holding the other variable constant. Even with the small sample of $N = 12$ bivariate observations, there are

$$M = N! = 12! = 479{,}001{,}600$$

possible, equally-likely arrangements in the reference set of all permutations of the example data listed in Table 10.8, making an exact permutation analysis impractical. Under the Fisher–Pitman permutation model, the Monte Carlo probability of an observed δ is the proportion of δ test statistic values computed on the randomly-selected, equally-likely arrangements of the $N = 12$ bivariate observations listed in Table 10.8 that are equal to or less than the observed value of $\delta = 119.25$. Based on $L = 1{,}000{,}000$ random arrangements of the $N = 12$ bivariate observations listed in Table 10.8, there are exactly 1868 δ test statistic values that are equal to or less than the observed value of $\delta = 119.25$.

If all M arrangements of the $N = 12$ bivariate observations listed in Table 10.8 occur with equal chance under the Fisher–Pitman null hypothesis, the Monte Carlo probability value of $\delta = 119.25$ computed on $L = 1{,}000{,}000$ random arrangements of the observed data with $N = 12$ bivariate observations preserved for each arrangement is

$$P(\delta \leq \delta_0 | H_0) = \frac{\text{number of } \delta \text{ values } \leq \delta_0}{L} = \frac{1868}{1{,}000{,}000} = 0.1868 \times 10^{-2} \,,$$

where δ_0 denotes the observed value of test statistic δ and L is the number of randomly-selected, equally-likely arrangements of the $N = 12$ bivariate observations listed in Table 10.8.

10.5.2   An Exact Permutation Analysis

While $M = 479{,}001{,}600$ possible arrangements may make an exact permutation analysis impractical, it is not impossible. There are exactly 896,384 δ test statistic values that are equal to or less than the observed value of $\delta = 119.25$. If all M arrangements of the $N = 12$ bivariate observations listed in Table 10.8 occur with equal chance under the Fisher–Pitman null hypothesis, the exact probability value of $\delta = 119.25$ computed on the $M = 479{,}001{,}600$ possible arrangements of the observed data with $N = 12$ bivariate observations preserved for each arrangement is

$$P(\delta \leq \delta_0) = \frac{\text{number of } \delta \text{ values } \leq \delta_0}{M} = \frac{896{,}384}{479{,}001{,}600} = 0.1871 \times 10^{-2} \,,$$

where δ_0 denotes the observed value of test statistic δ and M is the number of possible, equally-likely arrangements of the $N = 12$ bivariate observations listed in Table 10.8. Alternatively,

$$P(|r_{xy}| \geq |r_o|) = \frac{\text{number of } |r_{xy}| \text{ values } \geq |r_o|}{M}$$

$$= \frac{896,384}{479,001,600} = 0.1871 \times 10^{-2} ,$$

where $|r_o|$ denotes the observed value of $|r_{xy}|$.

The difference between the exact probability value based on all $M = 479,001,600$ possible arrangements of the example data listed in Table 10.8 and the Monte Carlo probability value based on $L = 1,000,000$ random arrangements of the example data is only

$$\Delta_P = 0.001871 - 0.001868 = 0.000003 .$$

To illustrate the accuracy of Monte Carlo permutation methods, Table 10.9 lists 10 independent Monte Carlo analyses of the bivariate data listed in Table 10.8 each initialized with a different seed and each analysis based on $L = 1,000,000$ random arrangements of the observed data, comparing the Monte Carlo probability values with the exact probability value based on all $M = 479,001,600$ possible arrangements of the observed data. The exact probability value is $P = 0.001871$, the average of the 10 Monte Carlo probability values listed in Table 10.9 is $P = 0.001868$, and the difference between the average of the 10 Monte Carlo probability values and the exact probability value is

$$\Delta_P = 0.001868 - 0.001871 = 0.000003 ,$$

Table 10.9 Ten independent Monte Carlo runs on the data listed in Table 10.8 based on $L = 1,000,000$ random arrangements for each run

Run	Seed	Monte Carlo probability	Exact probability	Difference
1	11	0.001912	0.001871	+0.000041
2	13	0.001809	0.001871	−0.000062
3	17	0.001900	0.001871	+0.000029
4	19	0.001896	0.001871	+0.000025
5	23	0.001916	0.001871	+0.000045
6	29	0.001861	0.001871	−0.000010
7	31	0.001809	0.001871	−0.000062
8	37	0.001847	0.001871	−0.000024
9	41	0.001851	0.001871	−0.000020
10	43	0.001883	0.001871	+0.000012

demonstrating the accuracy and efficiency of Monte Carlo permutation statistical methods. Finally, it should be noted that not only are all the differences listed in Table 10.9 very small, but half of the differences are positive and half are negative.

10.6   Example 5: Rank-Score Permutation Analyses

It is not uncommon for researchers to analyze data consisting of rank scores. The correlation coefficients for untied rank-score data most often found in the literature are Spearman's rank-order correlation coefficient given by

$$r_s = 1 - \frac{6 \sum\limits_{i=1}^{N} d_i^2}{N(N^2 - 1)} , \tag{10.2}$$

where for variables x and y, $d_i = x_i - y_i$ for $i = 1, \ldots, N$ bivariate observations, and Kendall's rank-order correlation coefficient given by

$$\tau = \frac{2S}{N(N - 1)} ,$$

where S denotes the number of concordant pairs of rank scores (C) minus the number of discordant pairs (D).[4]

10.6.1   Spearman's Rank-Order Correlation Coefficient

Consider Spearman's rank-order correlation coefficient for N bivariate rank scores under the Neyman–Pearson population model. An example set of data is given in Table 10.10 with $N = 11$ bivariate rank scores.

Following Eq. (10.2) for the data listed in Table 10.10, Spearman's rank-order correlation coefficient is

$$r_s = 1 - \frac{6 \sum\limits_{i=1}^{N} d_i^2}{N(N^2 - 1)} = 1 - \frac{6(138)}{11(11^2 - 1)} = +0.3727 .$$

Under the Neyman–Pearson null hypothesis, H_0: $\rho_{xy} = 0$, Spearman's r_s test statistic is asymptotically distributed as Student's t with $N - 2$ degrees of freedom.

---

[4]For simplification and clarity the formulæ and examples are limited to untied rank-score data.

Table 10.10 Average weekly spending in dollars on alcohol (x) and tobacco (y) in $N = 11$ Confederate states in 1863

State	Alcohol (x)	Tobacco (y)	Rank x	Rank y	d	d^2
Florida	6.57	2.73	1	11	−10	100
Georgia	6.20	4.48	2	2	0	0
Alabama	6.15	4.51	3	1	+2	4
Mississippi	6.08	3.87	4	4	0	0
Louisiana	5.91	3.54	5	6	−1	1
Arkansas	5.61	3.72	6	5	+1	1
Missouri	5.34	4.21	7	3	+4	16
South Carolina	5.11	2.88	8	10	−2	4
North Carolina	4.87	3.41	9	7	+2	4
Texas	4.49	3.29	10	8	+2	4
Virginia	4.41	3.11	11	9	+2	4
Sum					0	138

For the $N = 11$ bivariate rank scores listed in Table 10.10 with $N - 2 = 11 - 2 = 9$ degrees of freedom,

$$t = r_s \sqrt{\frac{N-2}{1-r_s^2}} = +0.3727 \sqrt{\frac{11-2}{1-(+0.3727)^2}} = +1.2050$$

yielding an asymptotic two-tail probability value of $P = 0.2589$, under the assumption of normality.

10.6.2   An Exact Permutation Analysis

For an analysis of the bivariate correlation data listed in Table 10.10 under the Fisher–Pitman permutation model let the differences between the rank scores be squared for correspondence with Spearman's rank-order correlation coefficient. Let $d_i = x_i - y_i$ for $i = 1, \ldots, N$, then the permutation test statistic is given by

$$\delta = \frac{1}{N} \sum_{i=1}^{N} d_i^2 . \tag{10.3}$$

Following Eq. (10.3), for the rank-score data listed in Table 10.10 with $N = 11$ bivariate observations the observed value of the permutation test statistic is

$$\delta = \frac{1}{N} \sum_{i=1}^{N} d_i^2 = \frac{138}{11} = 12.5455 .$$

Because there are only

$$M = N! = 11! = 39{,}916{,}800$$

possible, equally-likely arrangements in the reference set of all permutations of the alcohol and tobacco data listed in Table 10.10, an exact permutation analysis is feasible. Under the Fisher–Pitman permutation model, the exact probability of an observed δ is the proportion of δ test statistic values computed on all possible, equally-likely arrangements of the $N = 11$ rank scores listed in Table 10.10 that are equal to or less than the observed value of $\delta = 12.5455$.[5] There are exactly 10,400,726 δ test statistic values that are equal to less than the observed value of $\delta = 12.5455$. If all M arrangements of the $N = 11$ bivariate rank scores listed in Table 10.10 occur with equal chance under the Fisher–Pitman null hypothesis, the exact probability value of $\delta = 12.5455$ computed on the $M = 39{,}916{,}800$ possible arrangements of the observed data with $N = 11$ bivariate observations preserved for each arrangement is

$$P(\delta \leq \delta_0 | H_0) = \frac{\text{number of } \delta \text{ values} \leq \delta_0}{M} = \frac{10{,}400{,}726}{39{,}916{,}800} = 0.2606 \,,$$

where δ_0 denotes the observed value of test statistic δ and M is the number of possible, equally-likely arrangements of the $N = 11$ bivariate rank scores listed in Table 10.10.

10.6.3   The Relationship Between r_s and δ

The functional relationships between test statistics δ and r_s are given by

$$\delta = \frac{(N^2 - 1)(1 - r_s)}{6} \quad \text{and} \quad r_s = 1 - \frac{6\delta}{N^2 - 1} \,. \tag{10.4}$$

Following the first expression given in Eq. (10.4), the observed value of test statistic δ with respect to the observed value of Spearman's r_s is

$$\delta = \frac{(N^2 - 1)(1 - r_s)}{6} = \frac{(11^2 - 1)(1 - 0.3727)}{6} = 12.5455$$

---

[5]Note that in Eq. (10.3) N is a constant, so only the sum-of-squared differences need be calculated for each arrangement of the observed data.

and, following the second expression in Eq. (10.4), the observed value of Spearman's r_s with respect to the observed value of test statistic δ is

$$r_s = 1 - \frac{6\delta}{N^2 - 1} = 1 - \frac{6(12.5455)}{11^2 - 1} = +0.3727 .$$

Because test statistics δ and r_s are equivalent under the Fisher–Pitman null hypothesis, the exact probability value of Spearman's $r_s = +0.3727$ is identical to the exact probability value of $\delta = 12.5455$; that is,

$$P(\delta \leq \delta_o) = \frac{\text{number of } \delta \text{ values } \leq \delta_o}{M} = \frac{10,400,726}{39,916,800} = 0.2606$$

and

$$P(|r_s| \geq |r_o|) = \frac{\text{number of } |r_s| \text{ values } \geq |r_o|}{M} = \frac{10,400,726}{39,916,800} = 0.2606 ,$$

where δ_o and r_o denote the observed values of δ and r_s, respectively, and M is the number of possible, equally-likely arrangements of the $N = 11$ bivariate rank scores listed in Table 10.10.

The exact expected value of the $M = 39,916,800$ δ test statistic values under the Fisher–Pitman null hypothesis is

$$\mu_\delta = \frac{1}{M} \sum_{i=1}^{M} \delta_i = \frac{798,336,000}{39,916,800} = 20.00 .$$

Alternatively, the exact expected value of test statistic δ is

$$\mu_\delta = \frac{N^2 - 1}{6} = \frac{11^2 - 1}{6} = 20.00 .$$

Then the observed chance-corrected measure of effect size is

$$\Re = 1 - \frac{\delta}{\mu_\delta} = 1 - \frac{12.5455}{20.00} = +0.3727 ,$$

indicating approximately 37% agreement between the x and y rank-score values above what is expected by chance.

When the N rank-score values in variable y are a simple permutation of the rank-score values in variable x it can easily be shown that Mielke and Berry's $\Re$ measure of effect size and Spearman's r_s rank-order correlation coefficient are equivalent under the Neyman–Pearson population model with squared Euclidean scaling; that is, $\Re = +0.3727$ and $r_s = +0.3727$. Specifically, given

$$\delta = \frac{(N^2 - 1)(1 - r_s)}{6} \quad \text{and} \quad \mu_\delta = \frac{N^2 - 1}{6} \ ,$$

then

$$\Re = 1 - \frac{\delta}{\mu_\delta} = 1 - \frac{(N^2 - 1)(1 - r_s)}{6} \times \frac{6}{N^2 - 1} = 1 - (1 - r_s) = r_s \ .$$

10.6.4 Kendall's Rank-Order Correlation Coefficient

A popular alternative to Spearman's r_s rank-order correlation coefficient is Kendall's τ rank-order correlation coefficient given by

$$\tau = \frac{S}{\binom{N}{2}} = \frac{2S}{N(N - 1)} \ ,$$

where $S = C - D$, C denotes the number of concordant pairs of the observed data, and D denotes the number of discordant pairs of the observed data. To illustrate the difference between concordant and discordant pairs, consider the example data with $N = 4$ bivariate rank scores listed in Table 10.11. There are

$$M = \binom{N}{2} = \binom{4}{2} = \frac{4(4 - 1)}{2} = 6$$

possible, equally-likely arrangements in the reference set of all permutations of the example data listed in Table 10.11 to be considered. The first (x, y) pair is $x_1 = 1$ and $x_2 = 2$, and $y_1 = 2$ and $y_2 = 3$. Since $x_1 = 1$ is less than $x_2 = 2$ and $y_1 = 2$ is less than $y_2 = 3$, the first (x, y) pair is considered to be *concordant* as the values of variables x and y are in the same order for the pair.

The next (x, y) pair is $x_1 = 1$ and $x_3 = 3$, and $y_1 = 2$ and $y_3 = 1$. Since $x_1 = 1$ is less than $x_3 = 3$ but $y_1 = 2$ is greater than $y_3 = 1$, the second (x, y)

Table 10.11 Example rank-score data on $N = 4$ bivariate observations

Object	Variable	
	x	y
1	1	2
2	2	3
3	3	1
4	4	4

Table 10.12 Calculation of concordant (C) and discordant (D) pairs for the example rank-score data listed in Table 10.11

Pair	Variable x	y	C	D
1	1 < 2	2 < 3	1	
2	1 < 3	2 > 1		1
3	1 < 4	2 < 4	1	
4	2 < 3	3 > 1		1
5	2 < 4	3 < 4	1	
6	3 < 4	1 < 4	1	
Sum			4	2

pair is considered to be *discordant* as the values of variables x and y are not in the same order for the pair. Table 10.12 illustrates the calculation of the six concordant (C) and discordant (D) pairs for the rank-score data listed in Table 10.11. For the six (x, y) pairs listed in Table 10.12, the number of concordant pairs is $C = 4$, the number of discordant pairs is $D = 2$, and Kendall's $S = C - D = 4 - 2 = +2$. When M becomes large the calculations can become cumbersome. Table 10.13 illustrates the calculation of Kendall's S for the rank-score data listed in Table 10.12 on p. 388 with $N = 11$ bivariate pairs.

The process illustrated in Table 10.13 is straightforward. Determine the value for Kendall's S by arranging the values of variable x in their natural order and arranging the values of variable y corresponding to the values of variable x, as in Table 10.13. Starting with the first value of variable y on the left (11), count the number of rank scores to the right of 11 that are smaller than 11 and score each as (-1); these (-1) values represent the disagreements in order. For the calculations listed in Table 10.13 there are 10 values that are smaller than 11. Next count the number of rank scores to the right of 11 that are larger than 11 and score each as $(+1)$; these $(+1)$ values

Table 10.13 Example calculations for determining the value of Kendall's S test statistic

x	1	2	3	4	5	6	7	8	9	10	11	
y	11	2	1	4	6	5	3	10	7	8	9	Sum
		−1	−1	−1	−1	−1	−1	−1	−1	−1	−1	−10
			−1	+1	+1	+1	+1	+1	+1	+1	+1	+7
				+1	+1	+1	+1	+1	+1	+1	+1	+8
					+1	+1	−1	+1	+1	+1	+1	+5
						−1	−1	+1	+1	+1	+1	+2
							−1	+1	+1	+1	+1	+3
								+1	+1	+1	+1	+4
									−1	−1	−1	−3
										+1	+1	+2
											+1	+1
												0
Sum												+19

represent the agreements in order. In this case there are no values larger than 11. Sum the 10 (-1) and zero $(+1)$ values and place the sum at the end of the first row.

The next y value is 2. Count the number of rank scores to the right of 2 that are smaller than 2 and score each as (-1); there is only one value (1) that is smaller than 2. Next count the number of rank scores to the right of 2 that are larger than 2 and score each as $(+1)$; there are eight values that are larger than 2. Sum the one (-1) and eight $(+1)$ values and place the sum at the end of the second row. Continue the procedure for all ranks in variable y, summing the results. The final sum is the value for Kendall's S. Alternatively, there are 37 $(+1)$ values in Table 10.13; these are the concordant pairs (C). There are 18 (-1) values in Table 10.13; these are the discordant pairs (D). Then, $S = C - D = 37 - 18 = +19$.

For the rank-score data listed in Table 10.10 on p. 384 with $N = 11$ untied rank scores, Kendall's rank-order correlation coefficient is

$$\tau = \frac{2S}{N(N-1)} = \frac{2(+19)}{11(11-1)} = +0.3455 \ .$$

In testing the significance of the association between paired ranks it is more convenient to apply a test directly to S rather than τ as the number of pairs, $N(N-1)/2$, is a constant. Kendall's S is asymptotically distributed $N(0, 1)$ with mean of zero and variance given by

$$\sigma_S^2 = \frac{N(N-1)(2N+5)}{18}$$

as $N \to \infty$. Since the normal distribution is an approximation to the discrete sampling distribution of S, a correction for continuity should be applied. For the rank-score data listed in Table 10.10 on p. 384, the normal deviate with continuity correction applied is

$$z = \frac{|S| - 1}{\left[N(N-1)(2N+5)/18\right]^{1/2}}$$

$$= \frac{19 - 1}{\left\{11(11-1)[(2)(11)+5]/18\right\}^{1/2}} = +1.4013 \ ,$$

yielding an asymptotic two-tail probability value of $P = 0.1611$, under the assumption of normality.

10.6.5 An Exact Permutation Analysis

Consider an analysis of the correlation data listed in Table 10.10 on p. 384 with $N = 11$ bivariate observations under the Fisher–Pitman permutation model. There are

$$M = N! = 11! = 39{,}916{,}800$$

possible, equally-likely arrangements in the reference set of all permutations of the example data listed in Table 10.10, making an exact permutation analysis feasible. Under the Fisher–Pitman permutation model, the exact probability of an observed value of Kendall's S is the proportion of S test statistic values computed on all possible, equally-likely arrangements of the $N = 11$ bivariate rank scores listed in Table 10.10 that are equal to or greater than the observed value of $S = +19$. There are exactly 6,436,200 S test statistic values that are equal to or greater than the observed value of $S = +19$. If all M arrangements of the $N = 11$ bivariate rank scores listed in Table 10.10 occur with equal chance under the Fisher–Pitman null hypothesis, the exact probability value of $S = 19$ computed on the $M = 39{,}916{,}800$ possible arrangements of the observed data with $N = 11$ bivariate observations preserved for each arrangement is

$$P(|S| \geq |S_o|) = \frac{\text{number of } |S| \text{ values } \geq |S_o|}{M} = \frac{6{,}436{,}200}{39{,}916{,}800} = 0.1612 \, ,$$

where S_o denotes the observed value of Kendall's S and M is the number of possible, equally-likely arrangements of the $N = 11$ bivariate observations listed in Table 10.10.

10.6.6 Spearman's Footrule Correlation Coefficient

While Charles Spearman is most often remembered for his contributions to factor analysis and his development of the rank-order correlation coefficient given by

$$r_s = 1 - \frac{6 \sum_{i=1}^{2} d_i^2}{N(N^2 - 1)} \, ,$$

which was discussed in Sect. 10.6.1, Spearman also developed a lesser-known correlation coefficient that he called the "footrule" given by

$$\mathcal{R} = 1 - \frac{3 \sum_{i=1}^{N} |x_i - y_i|}{N^2 - 1} \, ,$$

where x_i and y_i denote the ith observed rank-score values for $i = 1, \ldots, N$ and N is the number of bivariate rank scores.

Table 10.14 Example
bivariate rank-score
correlation data with $N = 8$
pairs of data

Pair	x	y	$x - y$	$|x - y|$
1	8	7	+1	1
2	6	6	0	0
3	2	4	-2	2
4	4	2	+2	2
5	7	8	-1	1
6	5	5	0	0
7	1	3	-2	2
8	3	1	+2	2
Sum				10

To illustrate Spearman's footrule measure of correlation, consider the example
data listed in Table 10.14 with $N = 8$ bivariate untied rank-score observations.
For the $N = 8$ bivariate rank-score observations listed in Table 10.14, Spearman's
footrule is

$$\mathcal{R} = 1 - \frac{3 \sum_{i=1}^{N} |x_i - y_i|}{N^2 - 1} = 1 - \frac{3(10)}{8^2 - 1} = +0.5238 \ .$$

For comparison, Spearman's rank-order correlation coefficient calculated on the
rank-score data listed in Table 10.14 is $r_s = +0.7857$ and Kendall's rank-order
correlation coefficient is $\tau = +0.6429$.
   Since there are only

$$M = N! = 8! = 40{,}320$$

possible, equally-likely arrangements in the reference set of all permutations of the
observed x and y rank scores listed in Table 10.14, an exact permutation analysis
is feasible. Under the Fisher–Pitman permutation model, the exact probability of an
observed $\mathcal{R}$ is the proportion of $\mathcal{R}$ test statistic values computed on all possible,
equally-likely arrangements of the $N = 8$ bivariate rank scores listed in Table 10.14
that are equal to or greater than the observed value of $\mathcal{R} = +0.5238$. There are
exactly 1248 $\mathcal{R}$ test statistic values that are equal to or greater than the observed
value of $\mathcal{R} = +0.5238$. If all M arrangements of the $N = 8$ rank scores listed in
Table 10.14 occur with equal chance under the Fisher–Pitman null hypothesis, the
exact probability value of $\mathcal{R} = +0.5238$ computed on the $M = 40{,}320$ possible
arrangements of the observed data with $N = 8$ bivariate rank scores preserved for
each arrangement is

$$P(\mathcal{R} \geq \mathcal{R}_o | H_0) = \frac{\text{number of } \mathcal{R} \text{ values} \geq \mathcal{R}_o}{M} = \frac{1248}{40{,}320} = 0.0310 \ ,$$

where $\mathcal{R}_o$ denotes the observed value of Spearman's $\mathcal{R}$ and M is the number of possible, equally-likely arrangements of the $N = 8$ bivariate rank scores listed in Table 10.14.

10.6.7 The Relationship Between Statistics $\mathcal{R}$ and $\mathfrak{R}$

It can easily be demonstrated that Spearman's $\mathcal{R}$ footrule measure and Mielke and Berry's $\mathfrak{R}$ measure of effect size are equivalent measures under the Fisher–Pitman permutation model with ordinary Euclidean scaling. Let

$$\delta = \frac{1}{N} \sum_{i=1}^{N} |x_i - y_i| \tag{10.5}$$

denote an average distance function based on all possible paired absolute differences among values of the two rankings and let

$$\mu_\delta = \frac{1}{N^2} \sum_{i=1}^{N} \sum_{j=1}^{N} |x_i - y_j| \tag{10.6}$$

denote the expected value of test statistic δ. Then Spearman's footrule measure is given by

$$\mathcal{R} = 1 - \frac{\delta}{\mu_\delta}, \tag{10.7}$$

which is also the equation for Mielke and Berry's $\mathfrak{R}$ measure of effect size.

The calculation of test statistics δ, μ_δ, and $\mathfrak{R}$ can be illustrated and compared with Spearman's $\mathcal{R}$ footrule measure using an example set of data. Consider the small set of rank-score data listed in Table 10.15 with $N = 5$ bivariate observations. Table 10.16 illustrates the calculation of Spearman's footrule measure for the rank-score data listed in Table 10.15. Given the calculations listed in Table 10.16, the

Table 10.15 Bivariate rank scores assigned to $N = 5$ objects

Object	x	y
1	5	4
2	2	1
3	1	2
4	3	3
5	4	5

Table 10.16 Detailed calculations for Spearman's footrule measure with $N = 5$ bivariate observations

Pair	i	x_i	y_i	$x_i - y_i$	$|x_i - y_i|$
1	1	5	4	-1	1
2	2	2	1	$+1$	1
3	3	1	2	-1	1
4	4	3	3	0	0
5	5	4	5	-1	1

Table 10.17 Calculation of $|x_i - y_i|$ for $i = 1, \ldots, N$ for δ

Pair	i	x_i	y_i	$|x_i - y_i|$
1	1	5	4	$|5 - 4| = 1$
2	2	2	1	$|2 - 1| = 1$
3	3	1	2	$|1 - 2| = 1$
4	4	3	3	$|3 - 3| = 0$
5	5	4	5	$|4 - 5| = 1$

observed value of Spearman's footrule measure is

$$
\mathcal{R} = \frac{3 \sum\limits_{i=1}^{N} |x_i - y_i|}{N^2 - 1} = \frac{3(1 + 1 + 1 + 0 + 1)}{5^2 - 1} = +0.50 \;.
$$

Table 10.17 illustrates the calculation of δ for the rank-score data listed in Table 10.15. Given the calculations listed in Table 10.17, the observed value of test statistic δ is

$$
\delta = \frac{1}{N} \sum\limits_{i=1}^{N} |x_i - y_i| = \frac{1 + 1 + 1 + 0 + 1}{5} = 0.80 \;.
$$

Table 10.18 illustrates the calculation of μ_δ for the rank-score data listed in Table 10.15. Given the calculations listed in Table 10.18, the exact expected value of the $N^2 \, \delta$ test statistic values under the Fisher–Pitman null hypothesis is

$$
\mu_\delta = \frac{1}{N^2} \sum\limits_{i=1}^{N} \sum\limits_{j=1}^{N} |x_i - y_j| = \frac{1 + 0 + 2 + \cdots + 2 + 0 + 1}{5^2} = 1.60 \;.
$$

Then the chance-corrected measure of agreement is

$$
\mathfrak{R} = 1 - \frac{\delta}{\mu_\delta} = 1 - \frac{0.80}{1.60} = +0.50 \;,
$$

Table 10.18 Calculation of $|x_i - y_j|$ for $i, j = 1, \ldots, N$ for μ_δ

Pair	i	j	$|x_i - y_j|$	Pair	i	j	$|x_i - y_j|$
1	1	2	$|1-2|=1$	14	3	5	$|3-5|=2$
2	1	1	$|1-1|=0$	15	3	4	$|3-4|=1$
3	1	3	$|1-3|=2$	16	4	2	$|4-2|=2$
4	1	5	$|1-5|=4$	17	4	1	$|4-1|=3$
5	1	4	$|1-4|=3$	18	4	3	$|4-3|=1$
6	2	2	$|2-2|=0$	19	4	5	$|4-5|=1$
7	2	1	$|2-1|=1$	20	4	4	$|4-4|=0$
8	2	3	$|2-3|=1$	21	5	2	$|5-2|=3$
9	2	5	$|2-5|=3$	22	5	1	$|5-1|=4$
10	2	4	$|2-4|=2$	23	5	3	$|5-3|=2$
11	3	2	$|3-2|=1$	24	5	5	$|5-5|=0$
12	3	1	$|3-1|=2$	25	5	4	$|5-4|=1$
13	3	3	$|2-5|=0$				

indicating 50% agreement above that expected by chance. Thus, the equivalence between

$$R = 1 - \frac{3\sum_{i=1}^{N}|x_i - y_i|}{N^2 - 1} \quad \text{and} \quad \Re = 1 - \frac{\delta}{\mu_\delta}$$

is demonstrated.

10.6.8 A More Rigorous Proof

In this section a proof is offered that mathematically establishes the equivalence of Spearman's footrule measure and Mielke and Berry's chance-corrected measure of effect size. Consider the expected value of test statistic δ as defined in Eq. (10.6) and given by

$$\mu_\delta = \frac{1}{N^2} \sum_{i=1}^{N} \sum_{j=1}^{N} |x_i - y_j|.$$

Then,

$$\mu_\delta = \frac{2}{N^2} \sum_{i=1}^{N-1} \sum_{j=i+1}^{N} (j - i)$$

$$= \frac{1}{N^2} \sum_{i=1}^{N-1} \left[N(N+1) + i^2 - i(2N+1) \right]$$

$$= \frac{N(N-1)}{6N^2}\left[6(N+1)+(2N-1)-3(2N+1)\right]$$

$$= \frac{N-1}{6N}\left[2(N+1)\right]$$

$$= \frac{N^2-1}{3N}$$

The chance-corrected measure of effect size defined in Eq. (10.7) on p. 392 is

$$\Re = 1 - \frac{\delta}{\mu_\delta} \ .$$

Therefore,

$$\delta = \mu_\delta(1 - \Re) \ .$$

Given the permutation test statistic defined in Eq. (10.5) on p. 392; that is,

$$\delta = \frac{1}{N} \sum_{i=1}^{N} |x_i - y_i| \ ,$$

and substituting δ into Spearman's footrule measure

$$R = 1 - \frac{3\sum_{i=1}^{N} |x_i - y_i|}{N^2 - 1}$$

yields

$$R = 1 - \frac{3N\delta}{N^2 - 1}$$

and substituting $\mu_\delta(1 - \Re)$ for δ yields

$$R = 1 - \frac{3N\mu_\delta(1 - \Re)}{N^2 - 1} \ .$$

Finally, substituting $(N^2 - 1)/3N$ for μ_δ yields

$$R = 1 - \frac{3N\left(\dfrac{N^2 - 1}{3N}\right)(1 - \Re)}{N^2 - 1} = 1 - (1 - \Re) = \Re \ .$$

10.7   Example 6: Multivariate Permutation Analyses

Many introductory textbooks in statistics include a brief introduction to multiple correlation, usually limiting the discussion to two predictors for simplicity. The OLS multiple regression equation is given by

$$\hat{y} = \hat{\beta}_0 + \hat{\beta}_1 x_1 + \hat{\beta}_2 x_2 + \cdots + \hat{\beta}_p x_p \, ,$$

where $\hat{y}$ denotes the predicted value of the criterion variable, $x_1, \, x_2, \, \ldots, \, x_p$ denote p predictor variables, $\hat{\beta}_1, \, \hat{\beta}_2, \, \ldots, \, \hat{\beta}_p$ denote the OLS regression weights for each of the p predictor variables, and $\hat{\beta}_0$ is the estimate of the population intercept. The assumptions underlying OLS multiple regression are (1) the observations are independent, (2) a linear relationship exists between the criterion variable and the predictor variables, (3) multivariate normality, (4) no multicollinearity among the variables, and (5) the variances of the error terms are similar across the values of the p predictor variables; that is, homogeneity.

10.7.1   A Conventional OLS Multivariate Analysis

To illustrate multiple correlation analyses with OLS and LAD regression, consider the example data listed in Table 10.19 with $p = 2$ predictors where variable y is Hours of Housework done by husbands per week, variable x_1 is Number of Children in the family, and variable x_2 is husband's Years of Education for $N = 12$ families. For the multivariate data listed in Table 10.19, the unstandardized OLS regression coefficients are

$$\hat{\beta}_0 = +2.5260 \, , \quad \hat{\beta}_1 = +0.6356 \, , \quad \text{and} \quad \hat{\beta}_2 = -0.0649 \, ,$$

Table 10.19 Example multivariate correlation data on $N = 12$ families with $p = 2$ predictors

Family	x_1	x_2	y
A	1	12	1
B	1	14	2
C	1	16	3
D	1	16	5
E	2	18	3
F	2	16	1
G	3	12	5
H	3	12	0
I	4	10	6
J	4	12	3
K	5	10	7
L	5	16	4

Table 10.20 Observed x and y values with associated predicted values ($\hat{y}$), residual errors ($\hat{e}$), and squared residual errors ($\hat{e}^2$) for the multivariate correlation data listed in Table 10.19

Family	x_1	x_2	y	$\hat{y}$	$\hat{e}$	$\hat{e}^2$
A	1	12	1	2.3823	−1.3823	1.9108
B	1	14	2	2.2525	−0.2525	0.0638
C	1	16	3	2.1226	+0.8774	0.7698
D	1	16	5	2.1226	+2.8774	8.2795
E	2	18	3	2.6283	+0.3717	0.1382
F	2	16	1	2.7581	−1.7582	3.0911
G	3	12	5	3.6534	+1.3466	1.8132
H	3	12	0	3.6534	−3.6534	13.3477
I	4	10	6	4.4189	+1.5811	2.5000
J	4	12	3	4.2889	−1.2890	1.6615
K	5	10	7	5.0544	+1.9456	3.7853
L	6	16	4	4.6648	−0.6648	0.4420
Sum	32	164	40	40.0000	0.0000	37.8028

and the observed squared OLS multiple correlation coefficient is $R^2 = 0.2539$. Table 10.20 lists the $N = 12$ observed values for variables x and y, the predicted y values ($\hat{y}$), the residual errors ($\hat{e}$), and the squared residual errors ($\hat{e}^2$).

The summary statistics given in Table 10.20 suggest an alternative method to determine the value of the multiple correlation coefficient. Define

$$R^2 = r_{y\hat{y}}^2 = \frac{\left[N \sum_{i=1}^{N} y\hat{y} - \left(\sum_{i=1}^{N} y_i \right) \left(\sum_{i=1}^{N} \hat{y} \right) \right]^2}{\left[N \sum_{i=1}^{N} y_i^2 - \left(\sum_{i=1}^{N} y_i \right)^2 \right] \left[N \sum_{i=1}^{N} \hat{y}_i^2 - \left(\sum_{i=1}^{N} \hat{y}_i \right)^2 \right]}. \qquad (10.8)$$

For the multivariate data listed in Table 10.19, $N = 12$,

$$\sum_{i=1}^{N} y_i = 40.00, \quad \sum_{i=1}^{N} y_i^2 = 184.00 \quad \sum_{i=1}^{N} \hat{y}_i = 40.00, \quad \sum_{i=1}^{N} \hat{y}_i^2 = 146.1984,$$

and

$$\sum_{i=1}^{N} y\hat{y} = 146.1984.$$

Then following Eq. (10.8),

$$R^2 = r_{y\hat{y}}^2 = \frac{[12(146.1984) - (40)(40)]^2}{[12(184.00) - (40)^2][12(146.1984) - (40)^2]]} = 0.2539.$$

If, under the Neyman–Pearson population model the null hypothesis posits the population correlation is zero; that is, H_0: $R_{y \cdot x_1, x_2} = 0$, the conventional OLS test of significance is given by

$$F = \frac{R^2(N - p - 1)}{p(1 - R^2)} \ ,$$

which is asymptotically distributed as Snedecor's F with $v_1 = p$ and $v_2 = N - p - 1$ degrees of freedom. For the multivariate data listed in Table 10.19,

$$F = \frac{R^2(N - p - 1)}{p(1 - R^2)} = \frac{0.2539(12 - 2 - 1)}{2(1 - 0.2539)} = 1.5313$$

and with $v_1 = p = 2$ and $v_2 = N - p - 1 = 12 - 2 - 1 = 9$ degrees of freedom, the asymptotic probability value of $F = 1.5313$ is $P = 0.2677$, under the assumptions of linearity, normality, and homogeneity.

10.7.2 A Monte Carlo Permutation Analysis

Because there are

$$M = N! = 12! = 479{,}001{,}600$$

possible, equally-likely arrangements in the reference set of all permutations of the family data listed in Table 10.19, a Monte Carlo permutation analysis is most appropriate. Under the Fisher–Pitman permutation model, the Monte Carlo probability of an observed R^2 is the proportion of R^2 test statistic values computed on the randomly-selected, equally-likely arrangements of the $N = 12$ multivariate observations listed in Table 10.19 that are equal to or greater than the observed value of $R^2 = 0.2539$. Based on $L = 1{,}000{,}000$ randomly-selected arrangements of the $N = 12$ multivariate observations listed in Table 10.19, there are exactly 268,026 R^2 test statistic values that are equal to greater than the observed value of $R^2 = 0.2539$.

If all M arrangements of the $N = 12$ multivariate observations listed in Table 10.19 occur with equal chance under the Fisher–Pitman null hypothesis, the Monte Carlo probability value of $R^2 = 0.2539$ computed on $L = 1{,}000{,}000$ randomly-selected arrangements of the observed data with $N = 12$ multivariate observations preserved for each arrangement is

$$P(R^2 \geq R_0^2 | H_0) = \frac{\text{number of } R^2 \text{ values} \geq R_0^2}{L} = \frac{268{,}026}{1{,}000{,}000} = 0.2680 \ ,$$

where R_o^2 denotes the observed value of R^2 and L is the number of randomly-selected, equally-likely arrangements of the multivariate observations listed in Table 10.19.

10.7.3   An Exact Permutation Analysis

While $M = 479{,}001{,}600$ possible arrangements may make an exact permutation analysis impractical, it is not impossible. There are exactly $128{,}420{,}329$ R^2 test statistic values that are equal to or greater than the observed value of $R^2 = 0.2539$. If all M arrangements of the $N = 12$ multivariate observations listed in Table 10.19 occur with equal chance under the Fisher–Pitman null hypothesis, the exact probability value of $R^2 = 0.2539$ computed on the $M = 479{,}001{,}600$ possible arrangements of the observed data with $N = 12$ multivariate observations preserved for each arrangement is

$$P\left(R^2 \geq R_o^2 | H_0\right) = \frac{\text{number of } R^2 \text{ values} \geq R_o^2}{M} = \frac{128{,}420{,}329}{479{,}001{,}600} = 0.2681 \, ,$$

where R_o^2 denotes the observed value of R^2 and M is the number of possible, equally-likely arrangements of the multivariate observations listed in Table 10.19.

10.7.4   A LAD Multivariate Regression Analysis

Now consider a LAD regression analysis of the multivariate data listed in Table 10.19 on p. 396. Table 10.21 lists the $N = 12$ observed values for variables x_1, x_2, and y, the predicted y values ($\tilde{y}$), the residual errors ($\tilde{e}$), and the absolute residual errors ($|\tilde{e}|$).

For the family data listed in Table 10.19, the LAD regression coefficients are

$$\tilde{\beta}_0 = +4.7500 \, , \quad \tilde{\beta}_1 = +0.2500 \, , \quad \text{and} \quad \tilde{\beta}_2 = -0.1250 \, ,$$

the observed permutation test statistic is

$$\delta = \frac{1}{N} \sum_{i=1}^{N} \left| y_i - \tilde{y}_i \right| = \frac{1}{N} \sum_{i=1}^{N} |\tilde{e}| = \frac{18}{12} = 1.50 \, ,$$

Table 10.21 Observed x and
y values with associated
predicted values ($\tilde{y}$), residual
errors ($\tilde{e}$), and absolute errors
($|\tilde{e}|$) for the multivariate
correlation data listed in
Table 10.19

Family	x_1	x_2	y	$\tilde{y}$	$\tilde{e}$	$|\tilde{e}|$
A	1	12	1	3.5000	−2.5000	2.5000
B	1	14	2	3.2500	−1.2500	1.2500
C	1	16	3	3.0000	0.0000	0.0000
D	1	16	5	3.0000	+2.0000	2.0000
E	2	18	3	3.0000	0.0000	0.0000
F	2	16	1	3.2500	−2.2500	2.2500
G	3	12	5	4.0000	+1.0000	1.0000
H	3	12	0	4.0000	−4.0000	4.0000
I	4	10	6	4.5000	+1.5000	1.5000
J	4	12	3	4.2500	−1.2500	1.2500
K	5	10	7	4.7500	+2.2500	2.2500
L	6	16	4	4.0000	0.0000	0.0000
Sum	32	164	40	44.5000	−4.5000	18.0000

the exact expected value of test statistic δ under the Fisher–Pitman null hypothesis is

$$
\mu_\delta = \frac{1}{N^2} \sum_{i=1}^{N} \sum_{j=1}^{N} |y_i - \tilde{y}_j|
$$

$$
= \frac{|1 - 3.50| + |1 - 3.25| + |1 - 3.00| + \cdots + |4 - 4.75| + |4 - 4.00|}{12^2}
$$

$$
= \frac{260}{144} = 1.8056 \, ,
$$

and the observed LAD measure of agreement between the y and $\tilde{y}$ values is

$$
\Re = 1 - \frac{\delta}{\mu_\delta} = 1 - \frac{1.5000}{1.8056} = +0.1692 \, ,
$$

indicating approximately 17% agreement between the observed and predicted y
values.

There are

$$
M = N! = 12! = 479{,}001{,}600
$$

possible, equally-likely arrangements in the reference set of all permutations of the
family data listed in Table 10.19, making an exact permutation analysis impractical.
Under the Fisher–Pitman permutation model, the Monte Carlo probability of an
observed $\Re$ is the proportion of $\Re$ test statistic values computed on the randomly-
selected, equally-likely arrangements of the $N = 12$ multivariate observations

listed in Table 10.19 that are equal to or greater than the observed value of $\mathfrak{R} = +0.1692$. Based on $L = 1{,}000{,}000$ randomly-selected arrangements of the $N = 12$ multivariate observations listed in Table 10.19, there are exactly 37,824 $\mathfrak{R}$ test statistic values that are equal to greater than the observed value of $\mathfrak{R} = +0.1692$.

If all M arrangements of the $N = 12$ multivariate observations listed in Table 10.19 occur with equal chance under the Fisher–Pitman null hypothesis, the Monte Carlo probability value of $\mathfrak{R} = +0.1692$ computed on $L = 1{,}000{,}000$ randomly-selected arrangements of the observed data with $N = 12$ multivariate observations preserved for each arrangement is

$$P\left(\mathfrak{R} \geq \mathfrak{R}_0 | H_0\right) = \frac{\text{number of } \mathfrak{R} \text{ values } \geq \mathfrak{R}_0}{L} = \frac{37{,}824}{1{,}000{,}000} = 0.0378 \,,$$

where $\mathfrak{R}_0$ denotes the observed value of $\mathfrak{R}$ and L is the number of randomly-selected, equally-likely arrangements of the $N = 12$ multivariate observations listed in Table 10.19.

10.7.5 An Exact Permutation Analysis

Now consider an exact permutation analysis of the $M = 479{,}001{,}600$ arrangements of the family data listed in Table 10.19. If all M arrangements of the $N = 12$ multivariate observations listed in Table 10.19 occur with equal chance under the Fisher–Pitman null hypothesis, the exact probability value of $\mathfrak{R} = +0.1692$ computed on the $M = 479{,}001{,}600$ possible arrangements of the observed data with $N = 12$ multivariate observations preserved for each arrangement is

$$P\left(\mathfrak{R} \geq \mathfrak{R}_0 | H_0\right) = \frac{\text{number of } \mathfrak{R} \text{ values } \geq \mathfrak{R}_0}{M} = \frac{18{,}117{,}645}{479{,}001{,}600} = 0.0378 \,,$$

where $\mathfrak{R}_0$ denotes the observed value of $\mathfrak{R}$ and M is the number of possible, equally-likely arrangements of the $N = 12$ multivariate observations listed in Table 10.19.

10.7.6 Analyses with an Extreme Value

Suppose that the husband in Family "L" in Table 10.19 on p. 396 was a stay-at-home house-husband and instead of contributing just 4 h of housework per week, he actually contributed 40 h, as in Table 10.22.

Table 10.22 Example
multivariate correlation data
on $N = 12$ families with
$p = 2$ predictors, where the
husband in family L
contributed 40 h of
housework per week

Family	x_1	x_2	y
A	1	12	1
B	1	14	2
C	1	16	3
D	1	16	5
E	2	18	3
F	2	16	1
G	3	12	5
H	3	12	0
I	4	10	6
J	4	12	3
K	5	10	7
L	5	16	40

10.7.7   An Ordinary Least Squares (OLS) Analysis

For the multivariate data listed in Table 10.22, the unstandardized OLS regression
coefficients are

$$\hat{\beta}_0 = -41.6558 , \quad \hat{\beta}_1 = +5.7492 , \quad \text{and} \quad \hat{\beta}_2 = +2.3896 ,$$

and the observed squared OLS multiple correlation coefficient is $R^2 = 0.5786$.
    There are

$$M = N! = 12! = 479{,}001{,}600$$

possible, equally-likely arrangements in the reference set of all permutations of the
family data listed in Table 10.22, making an exact permutation analysis impractical.
Under the Fisher–Pitman permutation model, the Monte Carlo probability of an
observed R^2 is the proportion of R^2 test statistic values computed on the randomly-
selected, equally-likely arrangements of the observed data that are equal to or greater
than the observed value of $R^2 = 0.5786$. Based on $L = 1{,}000{,}000$ randomly-
selected arrangements of the $N = 12$ multivariate observations listed in Table 10.22,
there are exactly 15,215 R^2 test statistic values that are equal to greater than the
observed value of $R^2 = 0.5786$.
    If all M arrangements of the $N = 12$ multivariate observations listed in
Table 10.22 occur with equal chance under the Fisher–Pitman null hypothesis, the
Monte Carlo probability value of $R^2 = 0.5786$ computed on $L = 1{,}000{,}000$
random arrangements of the observed data with $N = 12$ multivariate observations
preserved for each arrangement is

$$P\left(R^2 \geq R_0^2 | H_0\right) = \frac{\text{number of } R^2 \text{ values} \geq R_0^2}{L} = \frac{15{,}215}{1{,}000{,}000} = 0.0152 ,$$

where R_o^2 denotes the observed value of R^2 and L is the number of randomly-selected, equally-likely arrangements of the $N = 12$ multivariate observations listed in Table 10.22.

Although an exact permutation analysis of $M = 479{,}001{,}600$ arrangements of the family data listed in Table 10.22 may be impractical, it is not impossible. If all M arrangements of the $N = 12$ multivariate observations listed in Table 10.22 occur with equal chance under the Fisher–Pitman null hypothesis, the exact probability value of $R^2 = 0.5786$ computed on the $M = 479{,}001{,}600$ possible arrangements of the observed data with $N = 12$ multivariate observations preserved for each arrangement is

$$P\left(R^2 \geq R_o^2 | H_0\right) = \frac{\text{number of } R^2 \text{ values} \geq R_o^2}{M} = \frac{7{,}328{,}725}{479{,}001{,}600} = 0.0153 \, ,$$

where R_o^2 denotes the observed value of R^2 and M is the number of possible, equally-likely arrangements of the $N = 12$ multivariate observations listed in Table 10.22.

For comparison,

$$F = \frac{R^2(N - p - 1)}{p(1 - R^2)} = \frac{0.5786(12 - 2 - 1)}{2(1 - 0.5786)} = 6.1785 \, ,$$

where F is asymptotically distributed as Snedecor's F with $v_1 = p$ and $v_2 = N - p - 1$ degrees of freedom. With $v_1 = p = 2$ and $v_2 = N - p - 1 = 12 - 2 - 1 = 9$ degrees of freedom, the asymptotic probability value of $F = 6.1785$ is $P = 0.0205$, under the assumptions of linearity, normality, and homogeneity.

10.7.8 A Least Absolute Deviation (LAD) Analysis

For the multivariate family data listed in Table 10.22 on p. 402, the LAD regression coefficients are

$$\tilde{\beta}_0 = -6.75 \, , \quad \tilde{\beta}_1 = +1.75 \, , \quad \tilde{\beta}_2 = +0.50 \, ,$$

the observed permutation test statistic is $\delta = 3.9583$, the exact expected value of δ under the Fisher–Pitman null hypothesis is $\mu_\delta = 5.4687$, and the LAD chance-corrected measure of agreement between the observed y values and the predicted $\tilde{y}$ values is

$$\mathfrak{R} = 1 - \frac{\delta}{\mu_\delta} = 1 - \frac{3.9583}{5.4687} = +0.2762 \, ,$$

indicating approximately 28% agreement between the observed and predicted y values.

There are

$$M = N! = 12! = 479{,}001{,}600$$

possible, equally-likely arrangements in the reference set of all permutations of the family data listed in Table 10.22, making an exact permutation analysis impractical. Under the Fisher–Pitman permutation model, the Monte Carlo probability of an observed $\Re$ is the proportion of $\Re$ test statistic values computed on the randomly-selected, equally-likely arrangements of the observed data that are equal to or greater than the observed value of $\Re = +0.2762$. Based on $L = 1{,}000{,}000$ randomly-selected arrangements of the $N = 12$ multivariate observations listed in Table 10.22, there are exactly 3409 $\Re$ test statistic values that are equal to greater than the observed value of $\Re = +0.2762$.

If all M arrangements of the $N = 12$ multivariate observations listed in Table 10.22 occur with equal chance under the Fisher–Pitman null hypothesis, the Monte Carlo probability value of $\Re = +0.2762$ computed on $L = 1{,}000{,}000$ randomly-selected arrangements of the observed data with $N = 12$ multivariate observations preserved for each arrangement is

$$P\left(\Re \geq \Re_0 | H_0\right) = \frac{\text{number of } \Re \text{ values } \geq \Re_0}{L}$$

$$= \frac{3409}{1{,}000{,}000} = 0.3409 \times 10^{-2},$$

where $\Re_0$ denotes the observed value of $\Re$ and L is the number of randomly-selected, equally-likely arrangements of the $N = 12$ multivariate observations listed in Table 10.22.

For comparison, consider an exact permutation analysis of the $M = 479{,}001{,}600$ arrangements of the observed data. If all M arrangements of the $N = 12$ multivariate observations listed in Table 10.22 occur with equal chance under the Fisher–Pitman null hypothesis, the exact probability value of $\Re = +0.2762$ computed on the $M = 479{,}001{,}600$ possible arrangements of the observed data with $N = 12$ multivariate observations preserved for each arrangement is

$$P\left(\Re \geq \Re_0 | H_0\right) = \frac{\text{number of } \Re \text{ values } \geq \Re_0}{M}$$

$$= \frac{163{,}234{,}242}{479{,}001{,}600} = 0.3408 \times 10^{-2},$$

where $\Re_0$ denotes the observed value of $\Re$ and M is the number of possible, equally-likely arrangements of the $N = 12$ multivariate observations listed in Table 10.22.

The results of the comparison of the OLS and LAD regression analyses with $y_{12} = 4$ and $y_{12} = 40$ h of housework by the husband in family "L" are summarized

Table 10.23 Comparison of OLS and LAD analyses for the data given in Table 10.19 with 4 h of housework for the husband in family L and the data given in Table 10.22 with 40 h of housework for the husband in family L

| Hours | OLS analysis | | LAD analysis | |
	R^2	Probability	$\Re$	Probability
4	0.2539	0.2681	0.1692	0.0378
40	0.5786	0.0153	0.2762	0.0034
$|\Delta|$	0.3247	0.2528	0.1070	0.0344

in Table 10.23. The value of 40 h of housework by the husband in family "L" is, by any definition, an extreme value. It is readily apparent that the extreme value of 40 h had a profound impact on the results of the OLS analysis. The OLS multiple correlation coefficient more than doubled from $R^2 = 0.2539$ to $R^2 = 0.5786$, yielding a difference between the two OLS multiple correlation coefficients of

$$\Delta_{R^2} = 0.5786 - 0.2539 = 0.3247 \,,$$

and the corresponding exact probability value decreased from $P = 0.2681$ to $P = 0.0153$, yielding a difference between the two OLS probability values of

$$\Delta_P = 0.2681 - 0.0153 = 0.2528 \,.$$

The impact of 40 h of housework on the LAD analysis is more modest with the LAD chance-corrected measure of agreement increasing only slightly from $\Re = 0.1692$ to $\Re = 0.2762$, yielding a difference between the two LAD multiple correlation coefficients of

$$\Delta_{\Re} = 0.2762 - 0.1692 = 0.1070 \,,$$

and the exact probability value decreasing from $P = 0.0378$ to $P = 0.0034$, yielding a difference between the two LAD probability values of only

$$\Delta_P = 0.0378 - 0.0034 = 0.0344 \,.$$

10.8 Summary

Under the Neyman–Pearson population model of statistical inference, this chapter examined product-moment linear correlation and regression, including both simple and multiple linear correlation and regression. The conventional measure of effect size for simple OLS correlation and regression is Pearson's r_{xy}^2. Under the Fisher–Pitman permutation model of statistical inference, test statistics δ and associated measure of effect size $\Re$ were developed and illustrated for simple correlation and regression.

As in previous chapters, six examples illustrated statistics δ and $\Re$ for measures of linear correlation and regression. In the first example, a small sample of $N = 4$ bivariate observations was utilized to describe and simplify the calculation of statistics δ and $\Re$ for linear correlation and regression. The second example developed the permutation-based, chance-corrected measure of effect size, $\Re$, and related the permutation measure to Pearson's r_{xy}^2 measure of effect size. The third example with $N = 10$ bivariate observations illustrated the effects of extreme values on both ordinary least squares (OLS) regression based on squared Euclidean scaling with $v = 2$ and least absolute deviation (LAD) regression based on ordinary Euclidean scaling with $v = 1$. The fourth example with $N = 12$ bivariate observations compared exact and Monte Carlo probability procedures. A Monte Carlo permutation procedure was shown to be an accurate and efficient alternative to the calculation of an exact probability value, provided the probability value is not too small. The fifth example with $N = 11$ bivariate rank scores applied permutation statistical methods to rank-score correlation data, comparing permutation statistical methods to Spearman's rank-order correlation coefficient, Kendall's rank-order correlation coefficient, and Spearman's footrule correlation coefficient. The sixth example extended statistics δ and $\Re$ to multivariate correlation data. An example with $N = 12$ multivariate observations was analyzed with both OLS and LAD regression. A final example containing an extreme value provided a comparison of the two regression models when extreme values occur.

Chapter 11 concludes the presentation of permutation statistical methods with analyses of contingency tables. Six examples illustrate various permutation procedures applied to the analysis of contingency tables. The first example is devoted to goodness-of-fit tests. The second example considers contingency tables in which two nominal-level (categorical) variables have been cross-classified. The third example considers contingency tables in which two ordinal-level (ranked) variables have been cross-classified. The fourth example considers contingency tables in which one nominal-level variable and one ordinal-level variable have been cross-classified. The fifth example considers contingency tables in which one nominal-level variable and one interval-level variable have been cross-classified. The sixth example considers contingency tables in which one ordinal-level variable and one interval-level variable have been cross-classified.

References

1. Barrodale, I., Roberts, F.D.K.: A improved algorithm for discrete ℓ_1 linear approximation. J. Numer. Anal. **10**, 839–848 (1973)
2. Barrodale, I., Roberts, F.D.K.: Solution of an overdetermined system of equations in the ℓ_1 norm. Commun. ACM **17**, 319–320 (1974)

3. Berry, K.J., Mielke, P.W.: Least sum of absolute deviations regression: distance, leverage, and influence. Percept. Motor Skill. **86**, 1063–1070 (1998)
4. Berry, K.J., Mielke, P.W.: A Monte Carlo investigation of the Fisher Z transformation for normal and nonnormal distributions. Psychol. Rep. **87**, 1101–1114 (2000)
5. Hotelling, H., Pabst, M.R.: Rank correlation and tests of significance involving no assumption of normality. Ann. Math. Stat. **7**, 29–43 (1936)
6. Johnston, J.E., Berry, K.J., Mielke, P.W.: Permutation tests: precision in estimating probability values. Percept. Motor Skill. **105**, 915–920 (2007)

Chapter 11
Contingency Tables

Abstract This chapter introduces permutation methods for the analysis of contingency tables. Included in this chapter are six example analyses illustrating computation of permutation methods for goodness-of-fit tests, analysis of contingency tables composed of two nominal-level (categorical) variables, analysis of contingency tables composed of two ordinal-level (ranked) variables, analysis of contingency tables composed of one nominal-level variable and one ordinal-level variable, analysis of contingency tables composed of one nominal-level variable and one interval-level variable, and analysis of contingency tables composed of one ordinal-level variable and one interval-level variable. Included in this chapter are permutation versions of Pearson chi-squared goodness-of-fit test, Pearson's chi-squared test of independence, Cramér's symmetrical measure of nominal association, Goodman and Kruskal's τ_a and τ_b asymmetric measures of association for two categorical variables, Goodman and Kruskal's G measure of association for two ranked variables, Somers' d_{yx} and d_{xy} asymmetric measures of association for two ranked variables, Freeman's θ measure of association for a categorical independent variable and a ranked dependent variable, Pearson's point-biserial correlation coefficient for one dichotomous variable and one interval-level variable, and Jaspen's correlation coefficient for one ranked variable and one interval-level variable.

This chapter introduces exact and Monte Carlo permutation statistical methods for selected measures of relationship among nominal-, ordinal-, and interval-level variables, commonly called contingency table analysis. The analysis of contingency tables with their associated measures of effect size and tests of significance constitutes a substantial portion of nonparametric statistical methods.

In this last chapter, exact and Monte Carlo permutation statistical methods for the analysis of contingency tables are illustrated with six types of analyses. The first section of the chapter considers permutation statistical methods applied to conventional goodness-of-fit tests; for example, Pearson's chi-squared goodness-of-fit test. The second section is devoted to permutation statistical methods for analyzing contingency tables composed of two cross-classified nominal-level (categorical)

© Springer Nature Switzerland AG 2019

K. J. Berry et al., *A Primer of Permutation Statistical Methods*,
https://doi.org/10.1007/978-3-030-20933-9_11

variables; for example, Pearson's symmetric chi-squared test of independence for two categorical variables and Goodman and Kruskal's t_a and t_b asymmetric measures of association for two categorical variables. The third section utilizes permutation statistical methods for analyzing contingency tables composed of two cross-classified ordinal-level (ranked) variables; for example, Goodman and Kruskal's symmetric G measure of association for two ranked variables and Somers' d_{yx} and d_{xy} asymmetric measures of association for two ranked variables. The fourth section is the first of three sections utilizing permutation statistical methods for analyzing contingency tables composed of two cross-classified mixed-level variables. In this fourth section permutation statistical methods are utilized for analyzing contingency tables composed of one nominal-level (categorical) variable cross-classified with one ordinal-level (ranked) variable; for example, Freeman's θ measure for one categorical independent variable and one ranked dependent variable. The fifth section utilizes permutation statistical methods for analyzing contingency tables composed of one nominal-level variable cross-classified with one interval-level variable; for example, Pearson's point-biserial correlation coefficient for one dichotomous variable and one interval-level variable. The sixth section utilizes permutation statistical methods for analyzing contingency tables composed of one ordinal-level variable cross-classified with one interval-level variable; for example, Jaspen's correlation coefficient for one ranked variable and one interval-level variable.[1]

There exist a vast array of measures of association and correlation. The few measures described here illustrate the application of permutation statistical methods to the analysis of two-way contingency tables at various levels of measurement and were selected for their popularity in the research literature and inclusion in various introductory textbooks. For a more comprehensive treatment of permutation statistical methods applied to measures of association and correlation see a 2018 book on *The Measurement of Association* by the authors [2].

11.1 Goodness-of-Fit Tests

Goodness-of-fit tests are essential for determining how well observed data conform to hypothetical models. When at all reasonable, exact goodness-of-fit tests are preferred over asymptotic tests. More specifically, goodness-of-fit tests are designed to compare the observed values in k discrete, unordered categories with values that are expected to occur under chance conditions. For example, for a fair coin the expectation for 100 independent trials is 50 heads and 50 tails over many, many trials of 100 tosses. The observed values, say 60 heads and 40 tails, are then compared with expected values under the null hypothesis, H_0: $p(H) = p(T) = 0.50$.

---

[1]There is never any reason to relate a higher-level independent variable with a lower-level dependent variable due to the loss of information from the independent variable.

The most popular goodness-of-fit test for k discrete, unordered categories is Pearson's chi-squared test, although Wald's likelihood-ratio test is occasionally encountered in the contemporary literature. Utilizing the conventional notation presented in many introductory textbooks, Pearson's chi-squared goodness-of-fit test for k discrete, unordered categories is given by

$$\chi^2 = \sum_{i=1}^{k} \frac{O_i^2}{E_i} - N \,,$$

where O_i and E_i denote the observed and expected frequency values, respectively, for $i = 1, \ldots, k$. Under the Neyman–Pearson null hypothesis, H_0: $O_i = E_i$ for $i = 1, \ldots, k$, χ^2 is asymptotically distributed as Pearson's χ^2 with $k - 1$ degrees of freedom, under the assumption of normality.[2]

Consider the random assignment of N objects to k discrete, unordered categories where the probability that any one of the N objects occurs in the ith category is $p_i > 0$ for $i = 1, \ldots, k$. Then the probability that O_i objects occur in the ith category for $i = 1, \ldots, k$ is the multinomial probability given by

$$P(O_1, O_2, \ldots, O_k | p_1, p_2, \ldots, p_k, N) = \frac{N!}{\displaystyle\prod_{i=1}^{k} O_i!} \prod_{i=1}^{k} p_i^{O_i} \,,$$

where

$$\sum_{i=1}^{k} O_i = N \quad \text{and} \quad \sum_{i=1}^{k} p_i = 1 \,.$$

11.1.1 Example 1

Two example analyses will serve to illustrate the permutation approach to goodness-of-fit-tests. For the first analysis under the Neyman–Pearson population model of statistical inference, consider a small example set of data with $k = 3$ unordered categories, $N = 6$ total objects, $O_1 = 5$ objects in the first category, $O_2 = 1$ object in the second category, and $O_3 = 0$ objects in the third category. The observed and expected frequencies along with the associated theoretical proportions are listed in Table 11.1. For the example data listed in Table 11.1 with $N = 6$ observations,

---

[2]Pearson's χ^2 test statistic is one of several test statistics that utilizes a lower-case Greek letter for both the sample test statistic and the population parameter.

Category number	Observed frequency	Expected frequency	Theoretical proportion
1	5	2	0.3333
2	1	2	0.3333
3	0	2	0.3333
Sum	6	6	1.0000

Table 11.1 Example data for Pearson's chi-squared goodness-of-fit test statistic with $k = 3$ discrete, unordered categories and $N = 6$ observations

Pearson's chi-squared goodness-of-fit test statistic is

$$\chi^2 = \sum_{i=1}^{k} \frac{O_i^2}{E_i} - N = \frac{5^2}{2} + \frac{1^2}{2} + \frac{0^2}{2} - 6 = 7.00 \ .$$

Under the Neyman–Pearson null hypothesis, H_0: $O_i = E_i$ for $i = 1, \ldots, k$, χ^2 is asymptotically distributed as Pearson's χ^2 with $k - 1$ degrees of freedom. With $k - 1 = 3 - 1 = 2$ degrees of freedom, the asymptotic probability value of $\chi^2 = 7.00$ is $P = 0.0302$, under the assumption of normality.

11.1.2 An Exact Permutation Analysis

For the example data listed in Table 11.1 under the Fisher–Pitman permutation model of statistical inference there are exactly

$$M = \binom{N + k - 1}{k - 1} = \binom{6 + 3 - 1}{3 - 1} = \binom{8}{2} = 28$$

possible, equally-likely arrangements in the reference set of all permutations of the example data listed in Table 11.1. Table 11.2 lists the $M = 28$ arrangements of the observed data, the associated χ^2 values, and the multinomial point probability values to six decimal places, ordered by the χ^2 values from lowest ($\chi_1^2 = 0.00$) to highest ($\chi_{28}^2 = 12.00$). The exact probability value of $\chi^2 = 7.00$ is the sum of the multinomial point probability values associated with values of χ^2 that are equal to or greater than the observed χ^2 value. There are only nine arrangements of the observed data with χ^2 test statistic values that are equal to or greater than the observed value of $\chi^2 = 7.00$: six values of $\chi^2 = 7.00$ and three values of $\chi^2 = 12.00$, all in rows indicated with asterisks in Table 11.2. Thus if all M arrangements of the $N = 6$ observations listed in Table 11.1 occur with equal chance under the Fisher–Pitman null hypothesis, the exact probability value of $\chi^2 = 7.00$ computed on the $M = 28$ possible arrangements of the observed data with $k = 4$ categories preserved for each arrangement is

$$P = 6(0.008230) + 3(0.001372) = 0.053496 \ .$$

Table 11.2 Example discrete probability distribution for the data given in Table 11.1 with χ^2 test statistic values and associated multinomial probability values

Order	Frequencies	χ^2 value	Probability
1	2 2 2	0.00	0.123457
2	3 2 1	1.00	0.082305
3	3 1 2	1.00	0.082305
4	2 3 1	1.00	0.082305
5	2 1 3	1.00	0.082305
6	1 3 2	1.00	0.082305
7	1 2 3	3.00	0.082305
8	3 3 0	3.00	0.027435
9	3 0 3	3.00	0.027435
10	0 3 3	3.00	0.027435
11	4 1 1	3.00	0.041152
12	1 4 1	3.00	0.041152
13	1 1 4	3.00	0.041152
14	4 2 0	4.00	0.020576
15	4 0 2	4.00	0.020576
16	2 4 0	4.00	0.020576
17	2 0 4	4.00	0.020576
18	0 4 2	4.00	0.020576
19	0 2 4	4.00	0.020576
20*	5 1 0	7.00	0.008230
21*	5 0 1	7.00	0.008230
22*	1 5 0	7.00	0.008230
23*	1 0 5	7.00	0.008230
24*	0 5 1	7.00	0.008230
25*	0 1 5	7.00	0.008230
26*	6 0 0	12.00	0.001372
27*	0 6 0	12.00	0.001372
28*	0 0 6	12.00	0.001372
Sum			1.000000

There is a substantial difference between the exact probability value of $P = 0.0535$ and the asymptotic probability value of $P = 0.0302$; that is,

$$\Delta_P = 0.0535 - 0.0302 = 0.0233 \ .$$

With the sparse data given in Table 11.1 there are only $M = 28$ possible arrangements of cell frequencies given the marginal frequency totals and it would be unreasonable to expect a continuous mathematical function such as Pearson's χ^2 to fit such a small discrete distribution consisting of only six different values with any precision.

Fig. 11.1 Punnett square depicting RYRY, RYRy, RYrY, RYry, RyRY, RyrY, rYRY, rYRy, and ryRY hybrids with nine black circles, RyRy, Ryry, and ryRy hybrids with three dark gray circles, rYrY, rYry, and ryrY hybrids with three light gray circles, and the sole ryry hybrid with a single white circle

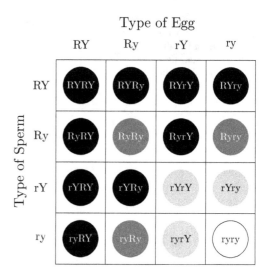

11.1.3   Example 2

Gregor Mendel (1822–1884) is notable for his studies of hybridization utilizing the common garden pea while he resided in the Augustinian monastery of St. Thomas at Brünn in Austrian Silesia.[3,4] In one of his many studies of garden peas, Mendel crossed hybrid plants producing round yellow peas with hybrid plants producing wrinkled green peas. To produce his hybrids, Mendel carefully brushed the pollen of one pea plant onto the pistils of another plant. The first generation, as expected, produced all round yellow peas—both dominant characteristics. However, the second generation yielded four varieties of peas: round yellow, wrinkled yellow, round green, and wrinkled green.[5]

Figure 11.1 displays the different varieties of peas in a Punnett square where RY denotes round yellow peas, Ry denotes round green peas, rY denotes wrinkled yellow peas, and ry denotes wrinkled green peas.[6] In the Punnett diagram in Fig. 11.1, the round-yellow hybrids, RYRY, RYRy, RYrY, RYry, RyRY, RyrY, rYRY, rYRy, and ryRY, are indicated by nine black circles (●), the round-green hybrids, RyRy, Ryry, and ryRy, are indicated by three dark gray circles (●), the wrinkled-

---

[3]Presently the region of Silesia is located largely in Poland with smaller parts in the Czech Republic and in Germany.

[4]Mendel's birth name was Johann, but he adopted the name Gregor when he entered the monastery in 1843 at the age of 21.

[5]Mendel was elected abbot of the monastery in 1868 at the age of 46, the administrative duties of which precluded any further research. Mendel passed away in 1884 at the age of 62.

[6]More technically, RY denotes round and yellow, Ry denotes round and not yellow, rY denotes not-round and yellow, and ry denotes not-round and not-yellow.

Table 11.3 Mendel's second-generation hybridization frequency data for $N = 556$ common garden peas

Category	Ratio	Frequency Observed	Expected
RY	9	315	312.75
Ry	3	101	104.25
rY	3	108	104.25
ry	1	32	34.75
Sum		556	556.00

yellow hybrids, rYrY, rYry, and ryrY, are indicated by three light gray circles (◉), and the single wrinkled-green ryry hybrid is indicated by a white circle (○).

Mendel's 15 double-hybrid plants produced a sample of $N = 556$ peas. Mendel's data for the $N = 556$ second-generation hybrids are listed in Table 11.3, along with the expected values which approximate the ratios 9:3:3:1.

For Mendel's hybridization data listed in Table 11.3, Pearson's chi-squared goodness-of-fit test statistic is

$$\chi^2 = \sum_{i=1}^{k} \frac{O_i^2}{E_i} - N = \frac{315^2}{312.75} + \frac{101^2}{104.25} + \frac{108^2}{104.25} + \frac{32^2}{34.75} - 556 = 0.4700 \,.$$

Under the Neyman–Pearson null hypothesis, H_0: $O_i = E_i$ for $i = 1, \ldots, k$, χ^2 is asymptotically distributed as Pearson's χ^2 with $k - 1$ degrees of freedom. With $k - 1 = 4 - 1 = 3$ degrees of freedom, the asymptotic probability value of $\chi^2 = 0.4700$ is $P = 0.9254$, under the assumption of normality.

In a 1936 paper published in *Annals of Science*, R.A. Fisher, Galton Professor of Eugenics at University College, London, re-examined Mendel's hybridization data, questioned Mendel's recording of his observations, and concluded that the very close agreement between Mendel's observed and expected series was unlikely to have arisen by chance [4]. Fisher submitted his paper at Christmas time in 1936 to *Annals of Science* with a comment to the editor, Dr. Douglas McKie:

> I had not expected to find the strong evidence which has appeared that the data had been cooked. This makes my paper far more sensational than ever I had intended... (quoted in Box [3, p. 297]).

11.1.4 An Exact Permutation Analysis

Under the Fisher–Pitman permutation model, the exact probability value of an observed chi-squared value of $\chi^2 = 7.00$ is given by the sum of the multinomial point probability values associated with the values of χ^2 that are equal to or greater than the observed χ^2 value. For the Mendel hybridization data listed in Table 11.3

under the permutation model there are

$$M = \binom{N+k-1}{k-1} = \binom{556+4-1}{4-1} = \binom{559}{3} = 28{,}956{,}759$$

possible, equally-likely arrangements in the reference set of all permutations of Mendel's hybridization data listed in Table 11.3, making an exact permutation analysis feasible. If all M arrangements of the $N = 556$ observations listed in Table 11.3 occur with equal chance under the Fisher–Pitman null hypothesis, the exact probability value of the observed chi-squared value of $\chi^2 = 0.4700$ computed on the $M = 28{,}956{,}759$ possible arrangements of the observed data with $k = 4$ categories preserved for each arrangement is $P = 0.9381$; that is, the sum of the multinomial probability values associated with values of $\chi^2 = 0.4700$ or greater.

11.1.5 A Measure of Effect Size

A chi-squared test of goodness-of-fit and its associated probability value provide no information as to the closeness of the fit between the observed and theoretical values, only whether they are statistically significant under the Neyman–Pearson population-model null hypothesis. Measures of effect size are essential in such cases as they index the magnitude of the fit between the observed and expected frequencies and indicate the practical significance of the research. A maximum-corrected measure of effect size is easily specified for a chi-squared goodness-of-fit test [1].

Define

$$q = \min(E_1, E_2, \ldots, E_k)$$

for k disjoint, unordered categories. Then with q determined, the maximum value of χ^2 is given by

$$\chi^2_{\max} = \frac{N(N-q)}{q} \tag{11.1}$$

and a maximum-corrected measure of effect size for Pearson's chi-squared goodness-of-fit test is given by

$$ES(\chi^2) = \frac{\chi^2_0}{\chi^2_{\max}} ,$$

where χ^2_0 denotes the observed value of χ^2 [8].

Table 11.4 Maximum arrangement of cell frequencies for Mendel's second-generation hybridization frequency data with $N = 556$ observations

Category	Ratio	Frequency	
		Observed	Expected
RY	9	0	312.75
Ry	3	0	104.25
rY	3	0	104.25
ry	1	556	34.75
Sum		556	556.00

For Mendel's hybridization data listed in Table 11.3, the minimum expected frequency value is

$$q = \min(E_1, E_2, E_3, E_4) = \min(312.75, 104.25, 104.25, 34.75) = 34.75 ,$$

and the maximum possible Pearson's χ^2 test statistic value given $k = 4$, $q = 34.75$, and $N = 556$ is

$$\chi^2_{\max} = \frac{N(N - q)}{q} = \frac{556(566 - 34.75)}{34.75} = 8340 .$$

To illustrate the function of Eq. (11.1) imagine that all $N = 556$ observations are concentrated in the one category with the smallest expected value and the remaining $k - 1$ categories contain zero observations. In this case all $N = 556$ observations are concentrated in the last category with the minimum expected value of $E_4 = 34.75$, such as depicted in Table 11.4. Then the maximum value of Pearson's chi-squared goodness-of-fit test statistic is

$$\chi^2_{\max} = \sum_{i=1}^{k} \frac{O_i^2}{E_i} - N$$

$$= \frac{0^2}{312.75} + \frac{0^2}{104.25} + \frac{0^2}{104.25} + \frac{556^2}{34.75} - 556 = 8340 ,$$

and the maximum-corrected measure of effect size is

$$ES(\chi^2) = \frac{\chi^2}{\chi^2_{\max}} = \frac{0.4700}{8340} = 0.5636 \times 10^{-4} ,$$

indicating that the observed value of $\chi^2 = 0.4700$ is an insignificantly small proportion of the maximum possible χ^2 value, given the expected values $E_1 = 312.75$, $E_2 = 104.25$, $E_3 = 104.25$, and $E_4 = 34.75$.

11.2   Contingency Measures: Nominal by Nominal

The most popular test for the cross-classification of two nominal-level (categorical) variables is Pearson's chi-squared test of independence, which is presented in every introductory textbook. Utilizing the conventional notation presented in many introductory textbooks for a contingency table with r rows and c columns, Pearson's chi-squared test statistic is given by

$$\chi^2 = N \left(\sum_{i=1}^{r} \sum_{j=1}^{c} \frac{O_{ij}^2}{R_i C_j} - 1 \right) , \tag{11.2}$$

where O_{ij} denotes the observed frequency in the ith row and jth column for $i = 1, \ldots, r$ and $j = 1, \ldots, c$, R_i denotes a row marginal frequency total for $i = 1, \ldots, r$, C_j denotes a column marginal frequency total for $j = 1, \ldots, c$, and N denotes the total number of values in the observed contingency table.

11.2.1   Example 1

Two examples will serve to illustrate Pearson's chi-squared test of independence for an $r \times c$ contingency table. For an analysis under the Neyman–Pearson population model, consider the sparse example data given in Table 11.5 with $r = 3$ rows, $c = 3$ columns, and $N = 9$ observations. Under the Neyman–Pearson population model, the chi-squared test statistic value for the example data given in Table 11.5 is

$$\chi^2 = N \left(\sum_{i=1}^{r} \sum_{j=1}^{c} \frac{O_{ij}^2}{R_i C_j} - 1 \right)$$

$$= 9 \left[\frac{0^2}{(2)(2)} + \frac{0^2}{(2)(3)} + \frac{2^2}{(2)(4)} + \frac{0^2}{(3)(2)} + \frac{3^2}{(3)(3)} + \frac{0^2}{(3)(4)} \right.$$

$$\left. + \frac{2^2}{(4)(2)} + \frac{0^2}{(4)(3)} + \frac{2^2}{(4)(4)} - 1 \right] = 11.2500 .$$

Table 11.5 Example data for Pearson's chi-squared test of independence with $r = 3$ rows, $c = 3$ columns, and $N = 9$ cross-classified observations

	Column			
Row	1	2	3	Total
1	0	0	2	2
2	0	3	0	3
3	2	0	2	4
Total	2	3	4	9

Under the Neyman–Pearson null hypothesis, H_0: $O_{ij} = E_{ij}$ for $i = 1, \ldots, r$ and $j = 1, \ldots, c$, where the expected cell values are given by

$$E_{ij} = \frac{O_{ij}}{R_i C_j}$$

for $i = 1, \ldots, r$ and $j = 1, \ldots, c$, χ^2 is asymptotically distributed as Pearson's χ^2 with $(r-1)(c-1)$ degrees of freedom. With $(r-1)(c-1) = (3-1)(3-1) = 4$ degrees of freedom, the asymptotic probability value of $\chi^2 = 11.2500$ is $P = 0.0239$, under the assumption of normality.

11.2.2 A Measure of Effect Size

The fact that a chi-squared statistical test produces a low probability value indicates only that there are differences among the response measurement scores between the two variables that (possibly) cannot be attributed to error. The obtained probability value does not indicate whether these differences are of any practical value. Measures of effect size express the practical or clinical significance of an obtained chi-squared value, as contrasted with the statistical significance of a chi-squared value. The most popular measure of effect size for Pearson's chi-squared test of independence is Cramér's V given by

$$V = \sqrt{\frac{\chi^2}{N\left[\min(r-1, c-1)\right]}} \ .$$

For the example data given in Table 11.6 with $\chi^2 = 11.2500$, Cramér's measure of effect size is

$$V = \sqrt{\frac{11.2500}{9\left[\min(3-1, 3-1)\right]}} = \sqrt{\frac{11.2500}{18.00}} = 0.7906 \ .$$

For a critical evaluation of Cramér's V measure of effect size, see a discussion in *The Measurement of Association* by the authors [2, pp. 80–82].

Occasionally in the contemporary literature, Cohen's measure of effect size for a chi-squared test of independence is encountered. Cohen's measure is given by

$$w = \sqrt{\frac{\chi^2}{N}} \ .$$

Table 11.6 All $M = 39$ arrangements of the frequency data given in Table 11.5 with associated chi-squared values and hypergeometric point probability values

Table	Observed frequencies				Chi-squared	Probability
	O_{11}	O_{12}	O_{21}	O_{22}		
1*	2	0	0	3	18.0000	0.793651×10^{-3}
2*	2	0	0	0	14.0625	0.317460×10^{-2}
3*	0	2	0	2	13.0000	0.238095×10^{-2}
4*	0	0	0	3	11.2500	0.476190×10^{-2}
5	2	0	0	2	10.5625	0.952381×10^{-2}
6	0	2	0	0	9.5625	0.952381×10^{-2}
7	0	0	2	0	9.5625	0.952381×10^{-2}
8	0	2	2	0	9.5625	0.952381×10^{-2}
9	1	0	0	3	9.5625	0.634921×10^{-2}
10	1	1	1	2	9.2500	0.476190×10^{-2}
11	2	0	0	1	9.2500	0.14286
12	1	0	0	0	9.0000	0.634921×10^{-2}
13	0	1	0	0	7.8750	0.952381×10^{-2}
14	0	0	1	0	7.8750	0.952381×10^{-2}
15	0	2	0	1	7.7500	0.014286
16	0	0	2	1	7.7500	0.014286
17	0	0	0	1	7.0000	0.014286
18	0	2	1	1	6.4375	0.019048
19	0	1	2	1	6.4375	0.019048
20	1	1	0	0	6.1875	0.019048
21	1	0	1	0	6.1875	0.019048
22	0	0	0	2	6.0625	0.028571
23	1	1	0	2	5.6875	0.019048
24	1	0	1	2	5.6875	0.019048
25	0	2	1	0	5.6250	0.028571
26	0	1	2	0	5.6250	0.028571
27	0	1	1	2	5.3125	0.019048
28	0	1	0	2	5.1250	0.028571
28	0	0	1	2	5.1250	0.028571
30	1	1	1	0	4.5000	0.028571
31	1	1	1	1	3.8125	0.038952
32	0	1	0	1	3.4375	0.057143
33	0	0	1	1	3.4375	0.057143
34	1	0	0	2	3.2500	0.057143
35	1	0	0	1	3.0625	0.057143
36	1	1	0	1	2.8750	0.057143
37	1	0	1	1	2.8750	0.057143
38	0	1	1	0	2.8125	0.057143
39	0	1	1	1	1.0000	0.114285
Sum						1.000000

For the example data given in Table 11.5, Cohen's measure of effect size is

$$w = \sqrt{\frac{11.2500}{9}} = 1.1180 .$$

11.2.3 An Exact Permutation Analysis

Given the observed marginal frequency totals for the example data, there are only $M = 39$ possible, equally-likely arrangements of cell frequencies in the reference set of all permutations of the $N = 9$ observations given in Table 11.5, making an exact permutation analysis possible. Table 11.6 lists the $M = 39$ arrangements of cell frequencies, the associated chi-squared test statistic values, and the hypergeometric point probability values given by

$$p(O_{11}, \ldots, O_{rc} | R_1, \ldots, R_r, C_1, \ldots, C_c, N) = \frac{\left(\prod_{i=1}^{r} R_i! \right) \left(\prod_{j=1}^{c} C_j! \right)}{N! \prod_{i=1}^{r} \prod_{j=1}^{c} O_{ij}!} .$$

Because the observed marginal frequency totals are fixed, Table 11.6 lists only cell frequencies O_{11}, O_{12}, O_{21}, and O_{22}, as the remaining five cell frequencies can be determined from the observed marginal frequency totals.

Under the Fisher–Pitman permutation model, the exact probability value of $\chi^2 = 11.2500$ is the sum of the hypergeometric point probability values associated with the chi-squared values that are equal to or greater than the observed chi-squared value. For the results listed in Table 11.6, there are four chi-squared test statistic values that are equal to or greater than the observed value of $\chi^2 = 11.2500$: $\chi_1^2 = 18.0000$, $\chi_2^2 = 14.0625$, $\chi_3^2 = 13.0000$, and $\chi_4^2 = 11.2500$, in rows 1, 2, 3, and 4, respectively, and indicated by asterisks. Thus the exact probability value of $\chi^2 = 11.2500$ is

$$0.7937 \times 10^{-3} + 0.3175 \times 10^{-2} + 0.2381 \times 10^{-2} + 0.4762 \times 10^{-2} = 0.0111 .$$

There is a substantial difference between the exact probability value of $P = 0.0111$ and the asymptotic probability value of $P = 0.0239$; that is,

$$\Delta_P = 0.0239 - 0.0111 = 0.0128 .$$

With such sparse data as given in Table 11.5 there are only $M = 39$ possible arrangements of cell frequencies given the marginal frequency totals with only 25 different chi-squared values and it would be unreasonable to expect a continuous

Table 11.7 Example data for Pearson's chi-squared test of independence with $r = 3$ rows, $c = 5$ columns, and $N = 63$ cross-classified observations

		Column				
Row	1	2	3	4	5	Total
1	6	2	5	7	1	21
2	0	8	5	8	4	25
3	1	1	6	6	3	17
Total	7	11	16	21	8	63

mathematical function such as Pearson's χ^2 to fit such a small discrete distribution with any precision.

11.2.4   Example 2

For a second example of a chi-squared analysis of a nominal-nominal contingency table, consider the 3×5 contingency table with cell frequencies given in Table 11.7. Following Eq. (11.2), Pearson's chi-squared test statistic for the frequency data given in Table 11.7 is

$$\chi^2 = N \left(\sum_{i=1}^{r} \sum_{j=1}^{c} \frac{O_{ij}^2}{R_i C_j} - 1 \right)$$

$$= 63 \left[\frac{6^2}{(21)(7)} + \frac{2^2}{(21)(11)} + \cdots + \frac{6^2}{(17)(21)} + \frac{3^2}{(17)(8)} - 1 \right] = 16.6279 .$$

Under the Neyman–Pearson null hypothesis the chi-squared test statistic is asymptotically distributed as Pearson's χ^2 with $(r - 1)(c - 1)$ degrees of freedom. With $(r - 1)(c - 1) = (3 - 1)(5 - 1) = 8$ degrees of freedom, the asymptotic probability value of $\chi^2 = 16.6279$ is $P = 0.0342$, under the assumption of normality.

11.2.5   A Measure of Effect Size

For the frequency data given in Table 11.7, Cramér's measure of effect size is

$$V = \sqrt{\frac{\chi^2}{N[\min(r - 1, c - 1)]}}$$

$$= \sqrt{\frac{16.6279}{63[\min(3 - 1, 5 - 1)]}} = \sqrt{\frac{16.6279}{126.00}} = 0.3633$$

and Cohen's measure of effect size is

$$w = \sqrt{\frac{\chi^2}{N}} = \sqrt{\frac{16.6279}{63}} = 0.2639 \, .$$

11.2.6   An Exact Permutation Analysis

Given the observed marginal frequency totals for the example data, there are $M = 11{,}356{,}797$ possible, equally-likely arrangements of the cell frequencies in the reference set of all permutations of the $N = 63$ observations given in Table 11.7, making an exact permutation analysis possible. Under the Fisher–Pitman permutation model, the exact probability of $\chi^2 = 16.6279$ is the sum of the hypergeometric point probability values associated with the chi-squared values calculated on all M possible arrangements of the cell frequencies, given the observed marginal frequency totals. For the frequency data given in Table 11.7, there are $M = 11{,}356{,}797$ possible, equally-likely arrangements of the cell frequencies given the observed marginal frequency totals, of which 10,559,996 chi-squared test statistic values are equal to or greater than the observed chi-squared value of $\chi^2 = 16.6279$, yielding an exact hypergeometric probability value of $P = 0.0306$. Note that with $M = 11{,}356{,}797$ possible arrangements of the data given in Table 11.7, the asymptotic χ^2 probability value of $P = 0.0342$ closely approximates the exact hypergeometric probability value of $P = 0.0306$.

11.2.7   Goodman–Kruskal's t_a and t_b Measures

While all measures of association based on Pearson's chi-squared are symmetric measures, Goodman and Kruskal's two asymmetric proportional-reduction-in-error measures (t_a and t_b) allow researchers to specify an independent and a dependent variable. Consider two cross-classified, unordered polytomies, A and B, with variable A the dependent variable and variable B the independent variable. Table 11.8

Table 11.8 Notation for the cross-classification of two categorical variables, A_j for $j = 1, \ldots, c$ and B_i for $i = 1, \ldots, r$

	A				
B	a_1	a_2	$\cdots$	a_c	Total
b_1	n_{11}	n_{12}	$\cdots$	n_{1c}	$n_{1.}$
b_2	n_{21}	n_{22}	$\cdots$	n_{2c}	$n_{2.}$
$\vdots$	$\vdots$	$\vdots$	$\ddots$	$\vdots$	$\vdots$
b_r	n_{r1}	n_{r2}	$\cdots$	n_{rc}	$n_{r.}$
Total	$n_{.1}$	$n_{.2}$	$\cdots$	$n_{.c}$	N

provides notation for the cross-classification, where a_j for $j = 1, \ldots, c$ denotes the c categories for dependent variable A, b_i for $i = 1, \ldots, r$ denotes the r categories for independent variable B, N denotes the total of cell frequencies in the table, $n_{i.}$ denotes a marginal frequency total for the ith row, $i = 1, \ldots, r$, summed over all columns, $n_{.j}$ denotes a marginal frequency total for the jth column, $j = 1, \ldots, c$, summed over all rows, and n_{ij} denotes a cell frequency for $i = 1, \ldots, r$ and $j = 1, \ldots, c$.

Goodman and Kruskal's t_a test statistic is a measure of the relative reduction in prediction error where two types of errors are defined. The first type is the error in prediction based solely on knowledge of the distribution of the dependent variable, termed "errors of the first kind" (E_1) and consisting of the expected number of errors when predicting the c dependent variable categories $(a_1, \ldots, a_c)$ from the observed distribution of the marginals of the dependent variable $(n_{.1}, \ldots, n_{.c})$. The second type is the error in prediction based on knowledge of the distributions of both the independent and dependent variables, termed "errors of the second kind" (E_2) and consisting of the expected number or errors when predicting the c dependent variable categories $(a_1, \ldots, a_c)$ from knowledge of the r independent variable categories $(b_1, \ldots, b_r)$.

To illustrate the two error types, consider predicting category a_1 only from knowledge of its marginal distribution, $n_{.1}, \ldots, n_{.c}$. Clearly, $n_{.1}$ out of the N total cases are in category a_1, but exactly which $n_{.1}$ of the N cases is unknown. The probability of incorrectly identifying one of the N cases in category a_1 by chance alone is given by

$$\frac{N - n_{.1}}{N} .$$

Since there are $n_{.1}$ such classifications required, the number of expected incorrect classifications is

$$\frac{n_{.1}(N - n_{.1})}{N}$$

and, for all c categories of variable A, the number of expected errors of the first kind is given by

$$E_1 = \sum_{j=1}^{c} \frac{n_{.j}(N - n_{.j})}{N} .$$

Likewise, to predict $n_{11}, \ldots, n_{1c}$ from the independent category b_1, the probability of incorrectly classifying one of the $n_{1.}$ cases in cell n_{11} by chance alone is

$$\frac{n_{1.} - n_{11}}{n_{1.}} .$$

Since there are n_{11} such classifications required, the number of incorrect classifications is

$$\frac{n_{11}(n_{1.} - n_{11})}{n_{1.}}$$

and, for all cr cells, the number of expected errors of the second kind is given by

$$E_2 = \sum_{j=1}^{c} \sum_{i=1}^{r} \frac{n_{ij}(n_{i.} - n_{ij})}{n_{i.}} .$$

Goodman and Kruskal's t_a statistic can then be defined as

$$t_a = \frac{E_1 - E_2}{E_1} .$$

An efficient computation form for Goodman and Kruskal's t_a test statistic is given by

$$t_a = \frac{N \sum_{i=1}^{r} \sum_{j=1}^{c} \frac{n_{ij}^2}{n_{i.}} - \sum_{j=1}^{c} n_{.j}^2}{N^2 - \sum_{j=1}^{c} n_{.j}^2} . \tag{11.3}$$

A computed value of t_a indicates the proportional reduction in prediction error given knowledge of the distribution of independent variable B over and above knowledge of only the distribution of dependent variable A. As defined, t_a is a point estimator of Goodman and Kruskal's population parameter τ_a for the population from which the sample of N cases was obtained. If variable B is considered the dependent variable and variable A the independent variable, then Goodman and Kruskal's test statistic t_b and associated population parameter τ_b are analogously defined.

11.2.8 An Example Analysis for t_a

To illustrate Goodman and Kruskal's t_a measure of nominal-nominal association, consider the contingency table given in Table 11.9 with $r = 3$ rows, $c = 4$ columns, and $N = 110$ cross-classified ordered observations. Following Eq. (11.3),

Table 11.9 Example data for
Goodman and Kruskal's t_a
and t_b measures of
nominal-nominal association
with $r = 3$ rows, $c = 4$
columns, and $N = 110$
cross-classified observations

	Column (A)				
Row (B)	1	2	3	4	Total
1	24	2	5	6	37
2	0	22	5	8	35
3	1	1	17	19	38
Total	25	25	27	33	110

the observed value of Goodman and Kruskal's t_a test statistic is

$$
t_a = \frac{N \sum_{i=1}^{r} \sum_{j=1}^{c} \frac{n_{ij}^2}{n_{i.}} - \sum_{j=1}^{c} n_{.j}^2}{N^2 - \sum_{j=1}^{c} n_{.j}^2}
$$

$$
= \frac{110 \left(\dfrac{24^2}{37} + \dfrac{2^2}{37} + \cdots + \dfrac{17^2}{38} + \dfrac{19^2}{38} \right) - (25^2 + 25^2 + 27^2 + 33^2)}{110^2 - (25^2 + 25^2 + 27^2 + 33^2)}
$$

$$
= 0.2797 \ .
$$

Under the Neyman–Pearson null hypothesis, H_0: $\tau_a = 0$, $t_a(N - 1)(r - 1)$ is asymptotically distributed as Pearson's χ^2 with $(r - 1)(c - 1)$ degrees of freedom. With $(r - 1)(c - 1) = (3 - 1)(4 - 1) = 6$ degrees of freedom, the asymptotic probability value of $t_a = 0.2797$ is $P = 0.2852 \times 10^{-10}$, under the assumption of normality.

11.2.9 An Exact Permutation Analysis for t_a

Under the Fisher–Pitman permutation model, the exact probability value of an observed value of Goodman and Kruskal's t_a is given by the sum of the hypergeometric point probability values associated with t_a test statistic values that are equal to or greater than the observed value of $t_a = 0.2797$. For the frequency data given in Table 11.9, there are $M = 26{,}371{,}127$ possible, equally-likely arrangements in the reference set of all permutations of cell frequencies given the observed row and column marginal frequency distributions, $\{37, 35, 38\}$ and $\{25, 25, 27, 33\}$, respectively, making an exact permutation analysis possible. There are exactly $1{,}523{,}131$ t_a test statistic values that are equal to or greater than the observed value of $t_a = 0.2797$. The exact probability value of the observed t_a value under the Fisher–Pitman null hypothesis is $P = 0.0578$; that is, the sum of the hypergeometric point probability values associated with values of $t_a = 0.2797$ or greater.

11.2.10   An Example Analysis for t_b

Now consider variable B as the dependent variable. A convenient computing formula for t_b is

$$t_b = \frac{N \sum_{j=1}^{c} \sum_{i=1}^{r} \frac{n_{ij}^2}{n_{.j}} - \sum_{i=1}^{r} n_{i.}^2}{N^2 - \sum_{i=1}^{r} n_{i.}^2}.$$

Thus, for the frequency data given in Table 11.9 the observed value of t_b is

$$t_b = \frac{110 \left(\frac{24^2}{25} + \frac{2^2}{25} + \cdots + \frac{17^2}{27} + \frac{19^2}{33} \right) - (37^2 + 35^2 + 38^2)}{110^2 - (37^2 + 35^2 + 38^2)} = 0.4428 \,.$$

Under the Neyman–Pearson null hypothesis, H_0: $\tau_b = 0$, $t_b(N - 1)(c - 1)$ is asymptotically distributed as Pearson's χ^2 with $(r - 1)(c - 1)$ degrees of freedom. With $(r - 1)(c - 1) = (3 - 1)(4 - 1) = 6$ degrees of freedom, the asymptotic probability value of $t_b = 0.4428$ is $P = 0.9738 \times 10^{-28}$, under the assumption of normality.

11.2.11   An Exact Permutation Analysis for t_b

Under the Fisher–Pitman permutation model, the exact probability value of an observed value of Goodman and Kruskal's t_b is given by the sum of the hypergeometric point probability values associated with t_b test statistic values that are equal to or greater than the observed value of $t_b = 0.4428$. For the frequency data given in Table 11.9, there are $M = 26,371,127$ possible, equally-likely arrangements in the reference set of all permutations of cell frequencies given the observed row and column marginal frequency distributions, {37, 35, 38} and {25, 25, 27, 33}, respectively, making an exact permutation analysis possible. There are exactly 991,488 t_b test statistic values that are equal to or greater than the observed value of $t_b = 0.4428$. The exact probability value of the observed t_b value under the Fisher–Pitman null hypothesis is $P = 0.0376$; that is, the sum of the hypergeometric point probability values associated with values of $t_b = 0.4428$ or greater.

11.2.12 The Relationships Among t_a, t_b, and χ^2

While no general equivalence exists between Goodman and Kruskal's t_a and t_b measures of nominal-nominal association and Pearson's χ^2 test of independence, certain relationships hold among t_a, t_b, and χ^2 under some limited conditions. Four of the relationships can easily be specified.

First, if $n_{i\cdot} = N/r$ for $i = 1, \ldots, r$, then $\chi^2 = N(r-1)t_b$ and $t_b = \chi^2/N(r-1)$. To illustrate the relationship between Goodman and Kruskal's t_b asymmetric measure of nominal-nominal association and Pearson's χ^2 test of independence when $n_{i\cdot} = N/r$ for $i = 1, \ldots, r$, consider the frequency data given in Table 11.10 with $r = 3$ rows, $c = 3$ columns, $N = 30$ cross-classified observations, and $n_{i\cdot} = N/r = 10$ for $i = 1, \ldots, r$. For the frequency data given in Table 11.10 with $N = 30$ observations,

$$
t_b = \frac{N \sum_{j=1}^{c} \sum_{i=1}^{r} \dfrac{n_{ij}^2}{n_{\cdot j}} - \sum_{i=1}^{r} n_{i\cdot}^2}{N^2 - \sum_{i=1}^{r} n_{i\cdot}^2}
$$

$$
= \frac{30 \left(\dfrac{2^2}{5} + \dfrac{3^2}{10} + \cdots + \dfrac{3^2}{10} + \dfrac{6^2}{15} \right) - (10^2 + 10^2 + 10^2)}{36^2 - (10^2 + 10^2 + 10^2)}
$$

$$
= \frac{10}{600} = 0.0167
$$

and

$$
\chi^2 = N \left(\sum_{i=1}^{r} \sum_{j=1}^{c} \frac{n_{ij}^2}{n_{i\cdot} n_{\cdot j}} - 1 \right)
$$

$$
= 30 \left[\frac{2^2}{(10)(5)} + \frac{3^2}{(10)(10)} + \cdots + \frac{3^2}{(10)(10)} + \frac{6^2}{(10)(15)} \right]
$$

$$
= 30 \, (1.0333 - 1) = 1.00 \; .
$$

Table 11.10 Example data for χ^2 and t_b with $r = 3$ rows, $c = 3$ columns, and $N = 30$ cross-classified observations

	Column (A)			
Row (B)	1	2	3	Total
1	2	3	5	10
2	2	4	4	10
3	1	3	6	10
Total	5	10	15	30

Then the observed value of Pearson's χ^2 test statistic with respect to the observed value of Goodman and Kruskal's t_b test statistic is

$$\chi^2 = N(r-1)t_b = 30(3-1)(0.0167) = 1.00$$

and the observed value of Goodman and Kruskal's t_b test statistic with respect to the observed value of Pearson's χ^2 test statistic is

$$t_b = \frac{\chi^2}{N(r-1)} = \frac{1.00}{30(3-1)} = 0.0167 .$$

Second, if $n_{.j} = N/c$ for $j = 1, \ldots, c$, then $\chi^2 = N(c-1)t_a$ and $t_a = \chi^2/N(c-1)$. To illustrate the relationship between Goodman and Kruskal's t_a measure of nominal-nominal association and Pearson's χ^2 test of independence when $n_{.j} = N/c$ for $j = 1, \ldots, c$, consider the frequency data given in Table 11.11 with $r = 2$ rows, $c = 4$ columns, $N = 40$ cross-classified observations, and $n_{.j} = N/c = 10$ for $j = 1, \ldots, c$. For the frequency data given in Table 11.11 with $N = 40$ observations,

$$t_a = \frac{N \sum_{i=1}^{r} \sum_{j=1}^{c} \frac{n_{ij}^2}{n_{i.}} - \sum_{j=1}^{c} n_{.j}^2}{N^2 - \sum_{j=1}^{c} n_{.j}^2}$$

$$= \frac{40 \left(\frac{7^2}{25} + \frac{6^2}{25} + \cdots + \frac{2^2}{15} + \frac{6^2}{15} \right) - (10^2 + 10^2 + 10^2 + 10^2)}{40^2 - (10^2 + 10^2 + 10^2 + 10^2)}$$

$$= \frac{37.3333}{1200} = 0.0311$$

Table 11.11 Example data for χ^2 and t_a with $r = 2$ rows, $c = 4$ columns, and $N = 40$ cross-classified observations

	Column (A)				
Row (B)	1	2	3	4	Total
1	7	6	8	4	25
2	3	4	2	6	15
Total	10	10	10	10	40

and

$$\chi^2 = N \left(\sum_{i=1}^{r} \sum_{j=1}^{c} \frac{n_{ij}^2}{n_{i.}n_{.j}} - 1 \right)$$

$$= 40 \left[\frac{7^2}{(25)(10)} + \frac{6^2}{(25)(10)} + \cdots + \frac{2^2}{(15)(10)} + \frac{6^2}{(10)(15)} \right]$$

$$= 40 (1.0933 - 1) = 3.7333 .$$

Then the observed value of Pearson's χ^2 test statistic with respect to the observed value of Goodman and Kruskal's t_a test statistic is

$$\chi^2 = N(c - 1)t_a = 40(4 - 1)(0.0311) = 3.7333$$

and the observed value of Goodman and Kruskal's t_a test statistic with respect to the observed value of Pearson's χ^2 test statistic is

$$t_a = \frac{\chi^2}{N(c - 1)} = \frac{3.7333}{40(4 - 1)} = 0.0311 .$$

Third, if $r = 2$, then $\chi^2 = Nt_a$ and $t_a = \chi^2/N$, which is Pearson's ϕ^2 coefficient of contingency. Also, if $c = 2$, then $\chi^2 = Nt_b$ and $t_b = \chi^2/N$. Thus, if $r = c = 2$, then $\chi^2 = Nt_a = Nt_b$. To illustrate the relationships between Goodman and Kruskal's t_a and t_b measures of nominal-nominal association and Pearson's χ^2 test of independence with $r = c = 2$, consider the frequency data given in Table 11.12 with $r = 2$ rows, $c = 2$ columns, and $N = 90$ cross-classified observations. For the frequency data given in Table 11.12 with $N = 90$ observations,

$$t_a = \frac{N \sum_{i=1}^{r} \sum_{j=1}^{c} \frac{n_{ij}^2}{n_{i.}} - \sum_{j=1}^{c} n_{.j}^2}{N^2 - \sum_{j=1}^{c} n_{.j}^2}$$

$$= \frac{90 \left(\frac{20^2}{30} + \frac{10^2}{30} + \frac{20^2}{60} + \frac{40^2}{60} \right) - (40^2 + 50^2)}{90^2 - (40^2 + 50^2)}$$

$$= \frac{400}{4000} = 0.10 ,$$

Table 11.12 Example data
for χ^2, t_a, and t_b with $r = 2$
rows, $c = 2$ columns, and
$N = 36$ cross-classified
observations

	Column (A)		
Row (B)	1	2	Total
1	20	10	30
2	20	40	60
Total	40	50	90

$$t_b = \frac{N \sum_{j=1}^{c} \sum_{i=1}^{r} \frac{n_{ij}^2}{n_{\cdot j}} - \sum_{i=1}^{r} n_{i\cdot}^2}{N^2 - \sum_{i=1}^{r} n_{i\cdot}^2}$$

$$= \frac{90 \left(\frac{20^2}{40} + \frac{10^2}{50} + \frac{20^2}{40} + \frac{40^2}{50} \right) - (30^2 + 60^2)}{90^2 - (30^2 + 60^2)}$$

$$= \frac{360}{3600} = 0.10 \,,$$

and

$$\chi^2 = N \left(\sum_{i=1}^{r} \sum_{j=1}^{c} \frac{n_{ij}^2}{n_{i\cdot} n_{\cdot j}} - 1 \right)$$

$$= 90 \left[\frac{20^2}{(30)(40)} + \frac{10^2}{(30)(50)} + \frac{20^2}{(60)(40)} + \frac{40^2}{(60)(50)} \right]$$

$$= 90 \, (1.1000 - 1) = 9.00 \,.$$

Then the observed value of Pearson's χ^2 test statistic with respect to the observed
value of Goodman and Kruskal's t_a test statistic is

$$\chi^2 = N t_a = 90(0.10) = 9.00$$

and the observed value of Goodman and Kruskal's t_a test statistic with respect to
the observed value of Pearson's χ^2 test statistic is

$$t_a = \frac{\chi^2}{N} = \frac{9.00}{90} = 0.10 \,.$$

Also, the observed value of Pearson's χ^2 test statistic with respect to Goodman and Kruskal's t_b test statistic is

$$\chi^2 = N t_b = 90(0.10) = 9.00$$

and the observed value of Goodman and Kruskal's t_b test statistic with respect to the observed value of Pearson's χ^2 test statistic is

$$t_b = \frac{\chi^2}{N} = \frac{9.00}{90} = 0.10 \,.$$

Fourth, if $n_i = N/r$ and $n_{.j} = N/c$ for $i = 1, \ldots, r$ and $j = 1, \ldots, c$, then $\chi^2 = N(c-1)t_a = N(r-1)t_b$. To illustrate the relationships between Goodman and Kruskal's t_a and t_b asymmetric measures of nominal association and Pearson's χ^2 test of independence with $n_i = N/r = 12$ for $i = 1, \ldots, r$ and $n_{.j} = N/c = 9$ for $j = 1, \ldots, c$, consider the frequency data given in Table 11.13 with $r = 3$ rows, $c = 4$ columns, and $N = 36$ cross-classified observations. For the frequency data given in Table 11.13 with $N = 36$ observations,

$$t_a = \frac{N \sum_{i=1}^{r} \sum_{j=1}^{c} \dfrac{n_{ij}^2}{n_{i.}} - \sum_{j=1}^{c} n_{.j}^2}{N^2 - \sum_{j=1}^{c} n_{.j}^2}$$

$$= \frac{36 \left(\dfrac{3^2}{12} + \dfrac{2^2}{12} + \cdots + \dfrac{3^2}{12} + \dfrac{4^2}{12} \right) - (9^2 + 9^2 + 9^2 + 9^2)}{36^2 - (9^2 + 9^2 + 9^2 + 9^2)}$$

$$= \frac{24}{972} = 0.0247 \,,$$

Table 11.13 Example data for χ^2, t_a, and t_b with $r = 3$ rows, $c = 4$ columns, and $N = 36$ cross-classified observations

Row (B)	Column (A)				
	1	2	3	4	Total
1	3	2	4	3	12
2	4	4	2	2	12
3	2	3	3	4	12
Total	9	9	9	9	36

$$t_b = \cfrac{N \displaystyle\sum_{j=1}^{c} \sum_{i=1}^{r} \frac{n_{ij}^2}{n_{\cdot j}} - \sum_{i=1}^{r} n_{i\cdot}^2}{N^2 - \displaystyle\sum_{i=1}^{r} n_{i\cdot}^2}$$

$$= \frac{36 \left(\dfrac{3^2}{9} + \dfrac{2^2}{9} + \cdots + \dfrac{3^2}{9} + \dfrac{4^2}{9} \right) - (12^2 + 12^2 + 12^2)}{36^2 - (12^2 + 12^2 + 12^2)}$$

$$= \frac{32}{864} = 0.0370 \,,$$

and

$$\chi^2 = N \left(\sum_{i=1}^{r} \sum_{j=1}^{c} \frac{n_{ij}^2}{n_{i\cdot} n_{\cdot j}} - 1 \right)$$

$$= 36 \left[\frac{3^2}{(12)(9)} + \frac{2^2}{(12)(9)} + \cdots + \frac{3^2}{(12)(9)} + \frac{4^2}{(12)(9)} \right]$$

$$= 36 \left(\frac{116}{108} - 1 \right) = 2.6667 \,.$$

Then the observed value of Pearson's χ^2 test statistic with respect to the observed value of Goodman and Kruskal's t_a test statistic is

$$\chi^2 = N(c-1)t_a = 36(4-1)(0.0247) = 2.6667$$

and the observed value of Goodman and Kruskal's t_a test statistic with respect to the observed value of Pearson's χ^2 test statistic is

$$t_a = \frac{\chi^2}{N(c-1)} = \frac{2.6667}{36(4-1)} = 0.0247 \,.$$

Also, the observed value of Pearson's χ^2 test statistic with respect to Goodman and Kruskal's t_b test statistic is

$$\chi^2 = N(r-1)t_b = 36(3-1)(0.0370) = 2.6667$$

and the observed value of Goodman and Kruskal's t_b test statistic with respect to the observed value of Pearson's χ^2 test statistic is

$$t_b = \frac{\chi^2}{N(r-1)} = \frac{2.6667}{36(3-1)} = 0.0370 \,.$$

11.2.13   The Relationships Among t_b, δ, and $\Re$

Goodman and Kruskal's t_b measure of nominal-nominal association is directly related to the permutation test statistic δ and, hence, to the permutation-based, chance-corrected $\Re$ measure of effect size. To illustrate the relationships among test statistics t_b, δ, and $\Re$, consider the frequency data given in Table 11.9 on p. 426, replicated in Table 11.14 for convenience. The conventional notation for an $r \times c$ contingency table is given in Table 11.8 on p. 423 where the row marginal frequency totals are denoted by $n_{i.}$ for $i = 1, \ldots, r$, the column marginal frequency totals are denoted by $n_{.j}$ for $j = 1, \ldots, c$, the cell frequencies are denoted by n_{ij} for $i = 1, \ldots, r$ and $j = 1, \ldots, c$, and

$$N = \sum_{i=1}^{r} n_{i.} = \sum_{j=1}^{c} n_{.j} = \sum_{i=1}^{r} \sum_{j=1}^{c} n_{ij} \, .$$

Then for the frequency data given in Table 11.14, Goodman and Kruskal's t_b test statistic is

$$t_b = \frac{N \sum_{j=1}^{c} \sum_{i=1}^{r} \dfrac{n_{ij}^2}{n_{.j}} - \sum_{i=1}^{r} n_{i.}^2}{N^2 - \sum_{i=1}^{r} n_{i.}^2}$$

$$= \frac{110 \left(\dfrac{24^2}{25} + \dfrac{2^2}{25} + \cdots + \dfrac{17^2}{27} + \dfrac{19^2}{33} \right) - (37^2 + 35^2 + 38^2)}{110^2 - (37^2 + 35^2 + 38^2)} = 0.4428 \, .$$

In 1971 Richard Light and Barry Margolin developed test statistic R^2, based on an analysis of variance technique for categorical response variables [6]. Light and Margolin were unaware that R^2 was identical to Goodman and Kruskal's t_b test statistic and that they had asymptotically solved the long-standing problem of testing the null hypothesis that the population parameter corresponding to Goodman and Kruskal's t_b was zero; that is, H_0: $\tau_b = 0$. The identity between R^2 and t_b was first recognized by Särndal in 1974 [9] and later discussed by Margolin and

Table 11.14 Example data for illustrating the relationships among t_b, δ, and $\Re$ with $r = 3$ rows, $c = 4$ columns, and $N = 110$ cross-classified observations

	Column (A)				
Row (B)	1	2	3	4	Total
1	24	2	5	6	37
2	0	22	5	8	35
3	1	1	17	19	38
Total	25	25	27	33	110

Light [7], where they showed that $t_b(N-1)(c-1)$ was distributed as Pearson's chi-squared with $(r-1)(c-1)$ degrees of freedom.

Following Light and Margolin in the context of a completely-randomized analysis of variance for the frequency data given in Table 11.14, the sum-of-squares total is

$$SS_{Total} = \frac{N}{2} - \frac{1}{2N} \sum_{i=1}^{r} n_{i.}^2$$

$$= \frac{110}{2} - \frac{1}{(2)(110)} (37^2 + 35^2 + 38^2) = 36.6455 ,$$

the sum-of-squares between treatments is

$$SS_{Between} = \frac{1}{2} \left(\sum_{i=1}^{r} \sum_{j=1}^{c} \frac{n_{ij}^2}{n_{.j}} \right) - \frac{1}{2N} \sum_{i=1}^{r} n_{i.}^2$$

$$= \frac{1}{2} \left(\frac{24^2}{25} + \frac{2^2}{25} + \cdots + \frac{19^2}{33} \right) - \frac{1}{(2)(110)} (37^2 + 35^2 + 38^2) = 16.2281 ,$$

the sum-of-squares within treatments is

$$SS_{Within} = \sum_{j=1}^{c} \left(\frac{n_{.j}}{2} - \frac{1}{2n_{.j}} \sum_{i=1}^{r} n_{ij^2} \right)$$

$$= \frac{25}{2} - \frac{1}{(2)(25)} (24^2 + 0^2 + 1^2) + \cdots + \frac{33}{2} - \frac{1}{(2)(33)} \left(6^2 + 8^2 + 19^2 \right)$$

$$= 20.4174 ,$$

and Light and Margolin's test statistic is

$$R^2 = \frac{SS_{Between}}{SS_{Total}} = \frac{16.9857}{36.6455} = 0.4428 ,$$

which is identical to Goodman and Kruskal's $t_b = 0.4428$.

The essential factors, sums of squares (SS), degrees of freedom (df), mean squares (MS), and variance-ratio test statistic (F) are summarized in Table 11.15

Table 11.15 Source table for the data listed in Table 11.14

Factor	SS	df	MS	F
Between	16.2281	3	5.4094	28.0835
Within	20.4174	106	0.1926	
Total	36.6455	109		

where $df_{Between} = c - 1 = 4 - 1 = 3$, $df_{Within} = N - c = 110 - 4 = 106$, and $df_{Total} = N - 1 = 110 - 1 = 109$. Under the Neyman–Pearson null hypothesis, H_0: $n_{ij} = n_{i.}/c$ for $i = 1, \ldots, r$ and $j = 1, \ldots, c$, where each of the c treatment groups possesses the same multinomial probability structure, test statistic F is asymptotically distributed as Snedecor's F with $v_1 = r - 1$ and $v_2 = N - r$ degrees of freedom. With $v_1 = r-1 = 4-1 = 3$ and $v_2 = N-r = 110-4 = 106$ degrees of freedom, the asymptotic probability value of $F = 28.0835$ is $P = 0.1917 \times 10^{-12}$, under the assumptions of normality and homogeneity.

For the frequency data given in Table 11.14, the permutation test statistic is

$$\delta = \frac{2SS_{Within}}{N - c} = \frac{2(20.4174)}{110 - 4} = 0.3852 \, ,$$

the exact expected value of test statistic δ under the Fisher–Pitman null hypothesis is

$$\mu_\delta = \frac{2SS_{Total}}{N - 1} = \frac{2(36.6455)}{110 - 1} = 0.6724 \, ,$$

and Mielke and Berry's chance-corrected measure of effect size is

$$\Re = 1 - \frac{\delta}{\mu_\delta} = 1 - \frac{0.3852}{0.6724} = +0.4271 \, ,$$

indicating approximately 43% agreement between variables A and B above what is expected by chance.

Alternatively, in terms of a completely-randomized analysis of variance model the chance-corrected measure of effect size is

$$\Re = 1 - \frac{(N - 1)(SS_{Within})}{(N - c)(SS_{Total})} = 1 - \frac{(110 - 1)(20.4174)}{(110 - 4)(36.6455)} = +0.4271 \, .$$

Then the observed value of test statistic δ with respect to the observed value of Goodman and Kruskal's t_b test statistic is

$$\delta = \frac{2SS_{Between}(1 - t_b)}{t_b(N - c)} = \frac{2(16.2281)(1 - 0.4428)}{(0.4428)(110 - 4)} = 0.3852$$

and the observed value of Goodman and Kruskal's t_b test statistic with respect to the observed value of test statistic δ is

$$t_b = \frac{2SS_{Between}}{\delta(N - c) + 2SS_{Between}} = \frac{2(16.2281)}{(0.3852)(110 - 4) + 2(16.2281)} = 0.4428 \, .$$

The observed value of test statistic δ with respect to the observed value of Fisher's F-ratio test statistic is

$$\delta = \frac{2SS_{\text{Between}}}{F(c-1)} = \frac{2(16.2281)}{(28.0835)(4-1)} = 0.3852$$

and the observed value of Fisher's F-ratio test statistic with respect to the observed value of test statistic δ is

$$F = \frac{2SS_{\text{Between}}}{\delta(c-1)} = \frac{2(16.2281)}{(0.3852)(4-1)} = 28.0835 \ .$$

The observed value of Goodman and Kruskal's t_b test statistic with respect to the observed value of Mielke and Berry's $\mathfrak{R}$ measure of effect size is

$$t_b = \frac{\mathfrak{R}(N-c)+c-1}{N-1} = \frac{(0.4271)(110-4)+4-1}{110-1} = 0.4428$$

and the observed value of Mielke and Berry's $\mathfrak{R}$ measure of effect size with respect to Goodman and Kruskal's t_b test statistic is

$$\mathfrak{R} = 1 - \frac{(N-1)(1-t_b)}{N-c} = 1 - \frac{(110-1)(1-0.4428)}{110-4} = +0.4271 \ .$$

The observed value of Mielke and Berry's $\mathfrak{R}$ measure of effect size with respect to the observed value of Fisher's F-ratio test statistic is

$$\mathfrak{R} = 1 - \frac{(N-1)SS_{\text{Between}}}{F(c-1)SS_{\text{Total}}} = 1 - \frac{(110-1)(16.2281)}{(28.0835)(4-1)(36.6455)} = +0.4271$$

and the observed value of Fisher's F-ratio test statistic with respect to the observed value of Mielke and Berry's $\mathfrak{R}$ measure of effect size is

$$F = \frac{SS_{\text{Between}}(N-1)}{SS_{\text{Total}}(c-1)(1-\mathfrak{R})} = \frac{(16.2281)(110-1)}{(36.6455)(4-1)(1-0.4271)} = 28.0835 \ .$$

11.3 Contingency Measures: Ordinal by Ordinal

There exist numerous measures of association for the cross-classification of two ordinal (ranked) variables. Three popular measures of ordinal-ordinal association are Goodman and Kruskal's symmetric measure of ordinal association denoted by G and two asymmetric measures of ordinal association by Somers denoted by

Table 11.16 Example data for Goodman and Kruskal's G measure of ordinal-ordinal association with $r = 3$ rows, $c = 5$ columns, and $N = 63$ cross-classified observations

	Column (y)					
Row (x)	1	2	3	4	5	Total
1	6	2	5	7	1	21
2	0	8	5	8	4	25
3	1	1	6	6	3	17
Total	7	11	16	21	8	63

Table 11.17 Two sets of $N = 8$ rank scores with no tied scores

	Variable	
Object	x	y
1	1	3
2	3	4
3	2	1
4	4	2
5	5	5
6	7	8
7	8	6
8	6	7

d_{yx} and d_{xy}.[7] These three measures and several others are based on the numbers of concordant and discordant pairs present in the observed contingency table. To illustrate the calculation of concordant and discordant pairs, consider the 3×5 contingency table given in Table 11.16 with $N = 63$ observations.

For any ordered contingency table there are five types of pairs to be considered: concordant pairs (C), discordant pairs (D), pairs that are tied on variable x but not tied on variable y (T_x), pairs tied on variable y but not tied on variable x (T_y), and pairs tied on both variable x and variable y (T_{xy}). Together they sum to the number of possible pairs in the table; that is,

$$C + D + T_x + T_y + T_{xy} = \frac{N(N-1)}{2} .$$

To demonstrate the calculation of concordant (C) and discordant (D) pairs, consider the two sets of rank scores listed in Table 11.17, where there are no tied ranks. Consider the first pair of objects: Objects 1 and 2. For Object 1, $x_1 = 1$ and $y_1 = 3$, and for Object 2, $x_2 = 3$ and $y_2 = 4$. Since $x_1 < x_2$ and $y_1 < y_2$ ($1 < 3$ and $3 < 4$), the pair is considered to be *concordant*. Now consider a second pair of objects: Objects 1 and 3. For Object 1, $x_1 = 1$ and $y_1 = 3$, and for Object 3, $x_3 = 2$ and $y_3 = 1$. Since $x_1 < x_3$ and $y_1 > y_3$ ($1 < 2$ and $3 > 1$), the

---

[7]Goodman and Kruskal's G measure of ordinal association is oftentimes denoted by the lower-case Greek letter γ. In this section γ denotes the population parameter and G denotes the sample test statistic.

Table 11.18 Paired differences: concordant (C) and discordant (D) values for the rank scores listed in Table 11.17

Pair	x_i and x_j	y_i and y_j	Type	Pair	x_i and x_j	y_i and y_j	Type
1	1 < 3	3 < 4	C	15	2 < 5	1 < 5	C
2	1 < 2	3 > 1	D	16	2 < 7	1 < 8	C
3	1 < 4	3 > 2	D	17	2 < 8	1 < 6	C
4	1 < 5	3 < 5	C	18	2 < 6	1 < 7	C
5	1 < 7	3 < 8	C	19	4 < 5	2 < 5	C
6	1 < 8	3 < 6	C	20	4 < 7	2 < 8	C
7	1 < 6	3 < 7	C	21	4 < 8	2 < 6	C
8	3 > 2	4 > 1	C	22	4 < 6	2 < 7	C
9	3 < 4	4 > 2	D	23	5 < 7	5 < 8	C
10	3 < 5	4 < 5	C	24	5 < 8	5 < 6	C
11	3 < 7	4 < 8	C	25	5 < 6	5 < 7	C
12	3 < 8	4 < 6	C	26	7 < 8	8 > 6	D
13	3 < 6	4 < 7	C	27	7 > 6	8 > 7	C
14	2 < 4	1 < 2	C	28	8 > 6	6 < 7	D

Table 11.19 Two sets of rank scores with tied scores

	Variable	
Object	x	y
1	1.5	2
2	1.5	2
3	3.5	4.5
4	5.5	2
5	3.5	4.5
6	5.5	6

pair is considered to be *discordant*. For the untied rank data listed in Table 11.17, the number of concordant pairs is $C = 23$ and the number of concordant pairs is $D = 5$. The

$$\frac{N(N-1)}{2} = \frac{8(8-1)}{2} = 28$$

concordant (C) and discordant (D) pairs for the rank-score data listed in Table 11.17 are listed in Table 11.18.

To illustrate the calculation of the T_x, T_y, and T_{xy} tied pairs, consider the two sets of rank scores listed in Table 11.19, where there are multiple tied rank scores on both variable x and variable y. For the rank scores listed in Table 11.19, $N = 6$, the number of concordant pairs is $C = 8$, the number of discordant pairs is $D = 2$, the number of pairs tied on variable x is $T_x = 1$, the number of pairs tied on variable y is $T_y = 2$, and the number of pairs tied on both variable x and variable y is $T_{xy} = 2$.

Table 11.20 Paired
differences: C, D, T_x, T_y, and
T_{xy} values for the rank scores
listed in Table 11.19

Pair	x_i and x_j	y_i and y_j	Type
1	$1.5 = 1.5$	$2.0 = 2.0$	T_{xy}
2	$1.5 < 3.5$	$2.0 < 4.5$	C
3	$1.5 < 5.5$	$2.0 = 2.0$	T_y
4	$1.5 < 3.5$	$2.0 < 4.5$	C
5	$1.5 < 5.5$	$2.0 < 6.0$	C
6	$1.5 < 3.5$	$2.0 < 4.4$	C
7	$1.5 < 5.5$	$2.0 = 2.0$	T_y
8	$1.5 < 3.5$	$2.0 < 4.5$	C
9	$1.5 < 5.5$	$2.0 < 6.0$	C
10	$3.5 < 5.5$	$4.5 > 2.0$	D
11	$3.5 = 3.5$	$4.5 = 4.5$	T_{xy}
12	$3.5 < 5.5$	$4.5 < 6.0$	C
13	$5.5 > 3.5$	$2.0 < 4.5$	D
14	$5.5 = 5.5$	$2.0 < 6.0$	T_x
15	$3.5 < 5.5$	$4.5 < 6.0$	C

Table 11.20 lists the

$$\frac{N(N-1)}{2} = \frac{6(6-1)}{2} = 15$$

paired differences: concordant pairs (C), discordant pairs (D), pairs tied on variable x (T_x), pairs tied on variable y (T_y), and pairs tied on both variable x and variable y (T_{xy}).

11.3.1   An Example Analysis for G

For the example rank data given in Table 11.16 on p. 438 with $N = 63$ observations, the number of concordant pairs is

$$C = \sum_{i=1}^{r-1} \sum_{j=1}^{c-1} n_{ij} \left(\sum_{k=i+1}^{r} \sum_{l=j+1}^{c} n_{kl} \right)$$

$$= (6)(8+5+8+4+1+6+6+3) + (2)(5+8+4+6+6+3)$$

$$+ \cdots + (5)(6+3) + (8)(3)) = 653 ,$$

the number of discordant pairs is

$$
D = \sum_{i=1}^{r-1} \sum_{j=1}^{c-1} n_{i,c-j+1} \left(\sum_{k=i+1}^{r} \sum_{l=1}^{c-j} n_{kl} \right)
$$

$$
= (1)(0+8+5+8+1+1+6+6) + (7)(0+8+5+1+1+6)
$$

$$
+ \cdots + (5)(1+1) + (8)(1) = 372 \, ,
$$

and Goodman and Kruskal's measure of ordinal-ordinal association is

$$
G = \frac{C - D}{C + D} = \frac{653 - 372}{653 + 372} = +0.2741 \, .
$$

Under the Neyman–Pearson null hypothesis, H_0: $\gamma = 0$, Goodman and Kruskal's G measure of ordinal-ordinal association is asymptotically distributed $N(0, 1)$ as $N \rightarrow \infty$ with a standard error given by

$$
s_G = \sqrt{\frac{N(1 - G^2)}{C + D}} \, .
$$

For the frequency data given in Table 11.16,

$$
z = \frac{G}{\sqrt{\dfrac{N(1 - G^2)}{C + D}}} = \frac{+0.2741}{\sqrt{\dfrac{63[1 - (0.2741)^2]}{653 + 372}}} = +1.1496 \, ,
$$

yielding an asymptotic upper-tail $N(0, 1)$ probability value of $P = 0.1252$, under the assumption of normality.

11.3.2   An Exact Permutation Analysis for G

Under the Fisher–Pitman permutation model, the exact probability value of an observed value of Goodman and Kruskal's G measure of ordinal-ordinal association is given by the sum of the hypergeometric point probability values associated with values of test statistic G that are equal to or greater than the observed value of $G = +0.2741$. For the frequency data given in Table 11.16 with $N = 63$ observations, there are $M = 11{,}356{,}797$ possible, equally-likely arrangements in the reference set of all permutations of cell frequencies given the observed row and column marginal frequency distributions $\{21, 25, 17\}$ and $\{7, 11, 16, 21, 8\}$, respectively, making an exact permutation analysis feasible. The exact probability value of the observed value of test statistic G is $P = 0.0336$; that is, the sum of the hypergeometric point probability values associated with values of $G = +0.2741$ or greater.

11.3.3 The Relationship Between Statistics G and δ

The functional relationships between test statistic δ and Goodman and Kruskal's G measure of ordinal-ordinal association are given by

$$\delta = \frac{N(N-1) - 2G(C+D)}{2N} \quad \text{and} \quad G = \frac{N\left(\dfrac{N-1}{2} - \delta\right)}{C+D}.$$

For the frequency data given in Table 11.16, the observed value of test statistic δ with respect to the observed value of Goodman and Kruskal's G measure of ordinal-ordinal association is

$$\delta = \frac{63(63-1) - 1(+0.2741)(653 + 372)}{(2)(63)} = 26.5404$$

and the observed value of Goodman and Kruskal's G measure of ordinal-ordinal association with respect to the observed value of test statistic δ is

$$G = \frac{63\left(\dfrac{63-1}{2} - 26.5404\right)}{653 + 372} = +0.2741.$$

11.3.4 Somers' d_{yx} and d_{xy} Measures

While Goodman and Kruskal's G measure of ordinal-ordinal association is a symmetric measure, Somers' two asymmetric proportional-reduction-in-error (PRE) measures (d_{yx} and d_{xy}) allow researchers to specify an independent and a dependent variable. For Somers' d_{yx}, the dependent variable is typically the column variable labeled y and for Somers' d_{xy}, the dependent variable is typically the row variable labeled x. The two asymmetric measures are given by

$$d_{yx} = \frac{C-D}{C+D+T_y} \quad \text{and} \quad d_{xy} = \frac{C-D}{C+D-T_x}, \tag{11.4}$$

where C is the number of concordant pairs, D is the number of discordant pairs, T_x is the number of pairs tied on the row variable, and T_y is the number of pairs tied on the column variable. As is evident in Eq. (11.4), Somers included in the denominators of d_{yx} and d_{xy} the number of tied pairs on the dependent variable: T_y for d_{yx} and T_x for d_{xy}. The rationale for including the tied pairs is simply that when variable y is the dependent variable (d_{yx}), then if two values of the independent variable x differ, but the corresponding two values of the dependent variable y do not differ (are tied), there is evidence of a lack of association and the ties on dependent variable y (T_y) should be included in the denominator where they act to decrease the value of d_{yx}. The same rationale holds for Somers' d_{xy} where the ties on dependent variable x (T_x) are included in the denominator.

11.3.5   An Example Analysis for d_{yx}

For the frequency data given in Table 11.16 on p. 438, replicated in Table 11.21 for convenience, the number of concordant pairs is

$$C = \sum_{i=1}^{r-1} \sum_{j=1}^{c-1} n_{ij} \left(\sum_{k=i+1}^{r} \sum_{l=j+1}^{c} n_{kl} \right)$$

$$= (6)(8 + 5 + 8 + 4 + 1 + 6 + 6 + 3) + (2)(5 + 8 + 4 + 6 + 6 + 3)$$

$$+ \cdots + (5)(6 + 3) + (8)(3)) = 653 ,$$

the number of discordant pairs is

$$D = \sum_{i=1}^{r-1} \sum_{j=1}^{c-1} n_{i,c-j+1} \left(\sum_{k=i+1}^{r} \sum_{l=1}^{c-j} n_{kl} \right)$$

$$= (1)(0 + 8 + 5 + 8 + 1 + 1 + 6 + 6) + (7)(0 + 8 + 5 + 1 + 1 + 6)$$

$$+ \cdots + (5)(1 + 1) + (8)(1) = 372 ,$$

Table 11.21 Example data for Somers' d_{yx} and d_{xy} measures of ordinal-ordinal association with $r = 3$ rows, $c = 5$ columns, and $N = 63$ cross-classified observations

	Column (y)					
Row (x)	1	2	3	4	5	Total
1	6	2	5	7	1	21
2	0	8	5	8	4	25
3	1	1	6	6	3	17
Total	7	11	16	21	8	63

the number of pairs tied on variable x is

$$
T_x = \sum_{i=1}^{r} \sum_{j=1}^{c-1} n_{ij} \left(\sum_{k=j+1}^{c} n_{ik} \right)
$$

$$
= (6)(2+5+7+1) + (2)(5+7+1) + (5)(7+1) + (7)(1)
$$

$$
+ \cdots + (1)(6+6+3) + (6)(6+3) + (6)(3) = 494 \,,
$$

the number of pairs tied on dependent variable y is

$$
T_y = \sum_{j=1}^{c} \sum_{i=1}^{r-1} n_{ij} \left(\sum_{k=i+1}^{r} n_{kj} \right)
$$

$$
= (6)(0+1) + (0)(1) + (2)(8+1) + (8)(1)
$$

$$
+ \cdots + (1)(4+3) + (4)(3) = 282 \,,
$$

and Somers' d_{yx} asymmetric measure of ordinal-ordinal association is

$$
d_{yx} = \frac{C-D}{C+D+T_y} = \frac{653 - 372}{653 + 372 + 282} = +0.2150 \,.
$$

For an $r \times c$ contingency table, d_{yx} is asymptotically distributed $N(0, 1)$ under the Neyman–Pearson null hypothesis as $N \to \infty$ with a standard error given by

$$
s_{d_{yx}} = \frac{2}{3r} \sqrt{\frac{(r^2 - 1)(c+1)}{N(c-1)}} \,.
$$

For the frequency data given in Table 11.21,

$$
z = \frac{d_{yx}}{\dfrac{2}{3r} \sqrt{\dfrac{(r^2 - 1)(c+1)}{N(c-1)}}} = \frac{+0.2150}{\dfrac{2}{(3)(3)} \sqrt{\dfrac{(3^2 - 1)(5+1)}{(63)(5-1)}}} = +2.2168 \,,
$$

yielding an asymptotic upper-tail $N(0, 1)$ probability value of $P = 0.0133$, under the assumption of normality.

11.3.6   An Exact Permutation Analysis for d_{yx}

Under the Fisher–Pitman permutation model, the exact probability value of an observed value of Somers' d_{yx} is given by the sum of the hypergeometric point probability values associated with values of test statistic d_{yx} that are equal to or greater than the observed value of $d_{yx} = +0.2150$. For the frequency data given in Table 11.21, there are $M = 11,356,797$ possible, equally-likely arrangements in the reference set of all permutation of cell frequencies given the observed row and column marginal frequency distributions $\{21, 25, 17\}$ and $\{7, 11, 16, 21, 8\}$, respectively, making an exact permutation analysis feasible. The exact probability value of $d_{yx} = +0.2150$ is $P = 0.0331$; that is, the sum of the hypergeometric point probability values associated with values of $d_{yx} = +0.2150$ or greater.

11.3.7   The Relationship Between Statistics d_{yx} and δ

The functional relationships between test statistic δ and Somers' d_{yx} asymmetric measure of ordinal-ordinal association are given by

$$\delta = \frac{N-1}{2} - \frac{d_{yx}(C+D+T_y)}{N} \quad \text{and} \quad d_{yx} = \frac{N\left(\dfrac{N-1}{2} - \delta\right)}{C+D+T_y}.$$

For the frequency data given in Table 11.21, the observed value of test statistic δ with respect to the observed value of Somers' d_{yx} measure of ordinal-ordinal association is

$$\delta = \frac{63-1}{2} - \frac{+0.2150(653+372+282)}{63} = 26.5396$$

and the observed value of Somers' d_{yx} measure of ordinal-ordinal association with respect to the observed value of test statistic δ is

$$d_{yx} = \frac{63\left(\dfrac{63-1}{2} - 26.5396\right)}{653+372+282} = +0.2150.$$

11.3.8   An Example Analysis for d_{xy}

For the frequency data given in Table 11.21, the number of concordant pairs is $C = 653$, the number of discordant pairs is $D = 372$, the number of pairs tied on dependent variable x is $T_x = 494$, and Somers' d_{xy} asymmetric measure of ordinal-ordinal association is

$$d_{xy} = \frac{C-D}{C+D+T_x} = \frac{653-372}{653+372+494} = +0.1850.$$

For an $r \times c$ contingency table, d_{yx} is asymptotically distributed $N(0, 1)$ under the Neyman–Pearson null hypothesis as $N \to \infty$ with a standard error given by

$$s_{d_{yx}} = \frac{2}{3c} \sqrt{\frac{(c^2 - 1)(r + 1)}{N(r - 1)}} \, .$$

For the frequency data given in Table 11.21,

$$z = \frac{d_{yx}}{\dfrac{2}{3c} \sqrt{\dfrac{(c^2 - 1)(r + 1)}{N(r - 1)}}} = \frac{+0.1850}{\dfrac{2}{(3)(5)} \sqrt{\dfrac{(5^2 - 1)(3 + 1)}{(63)(5 - 1)}}} = +2.2480 \, ,$$

yielding an asymptotic upper-tail $N(0, 1)$ probability value of $P = 0.0123$, under the assumption of normality.

11.3.9   An Exact Permutation Analysis for d_{xy}

Under the Fisher–Pitman permutation model, the exact probability value of an observed value of Somers' d_{xy} is given by the sum of the hypergeometric point probability values associated with values of test statistic d_{xy} that are equal to or greater than the observed value of $d_{xy} = +0.1850$. For the frequency data given in Table 11.21, there are $M = 11{,}356{,}797$ possible, equally-likely arrangements in the reference set of all permutation of cell frequencies given the observed row and column marginal frequency distributions $\{21, 25, 17\}$ and $\{7, 11, 16, 21, 8\}$, respectively, making an exact permutation analysis feasible. The exact probability value of $d_{xy} = +0.1850$ is $P = 0.0331$; that is, the sum of the hypergeometric point probability values associated with values of $d_{xy} = +0.1850$ or greater.

11.3.10   The Relationship Between d_{xy} and δ

The functional relationships between test statistic δ and Somers' d_{xy} asymmetric measure of ordinal-ordinal association are given by

$$\delta = \frac{N - 1}{2} - \frac{d_{yx}(C + D + T_x)}{N} \quad \text{and} \quad d_{xy} = \frac{N \left(\dfrac{N - 1}{2} - \delta \right)}{C + D + T_x} \, .$$

For the frequency data given in Table 11.21, the observed value of test statistic δ with respect to the observed value of Somers' d_{xy} measure of ordinal-ordinal association is

$$\delta = \frac{63 - 1}{2} - \frac{+0.1850(653 + 372 + 494)}{63} = 26.5394$$

and the observed value of Somers' d_{xy} measure of ordinal association with respect to the observed value of test statistic δ is

$$d_{xy} = \frac{63 \left(\dfrac{63 - 1}{2} - 26.5394 \right)}{653 + 372 + 494} = +0.1850 \ .$$

11.3.11 Probability Values for d_{yx} and d_{xy}

It may appear inconsistent that while Somers' two measures of effect size differ ($d_{yx} = +0.2150$ and $d_{xy} = 0.1850$), they both yield the same probability value of $P = 0.0331$. It follows from the fact that the denominators of d_{yx} and d_{xy} ($C + D + T_y$ and $C + D + T_x$, respectively) can be computed from just the marginal frequency distributions, which are fixed for all possible arrangements of cell frequencies and are, therefore, invariant under permutation.

It is easily shown that $C + D + T_y$ can be obtained from N and the row marginal frequency distribution. Recall that for the frequency data listed in Table 11.21 on p. 443, the number of concordant pairs is $C = 653$, the number of discordant pairs is $D = 372$, the number of pairs tied on variable y is $T_y = 282$, and $C + D + T_y = 653 + 372 + 282 = 1307$. Then with $N = 63$,

$$C + D + T_y = \frac{1}{2} \left(N^2 - \sum_{i=1}^{r} n_{i.}^2 \right) = \frac{1}{2} \left[63^2 - \left(21^2 + 25^2 + 17^2 \right) \right] = 1307 \ .$$

In such manner $C + D + T_x$ can be obtained from N and the column marginal frequency distribution. For the frequency data listed in Table 11.21, the number of concordant pairs is $C = 653$, the number of discordant pairs is $D = 372$, the number of pairs tied on variable x is $T_x = 494$, and $C + D + T_x = 653 + 372 + 494 = 1519$. Then with $N = 63$,

$$C + D + T_x = \frac{1}{2} \left(N^2 - \sum_{j=1}^{c} n_{.j}^2 \right)$$

$$= \frac{1}{2} \left[63^2 - \left(7^2 + 11^2 + 16^2 + 21^2 + 8^2 \right) \right] = 1519 \ .$$

11.4 Contingency Measures: Nominal by Ordinal

There exist any number of measures of association for which the standard error is unknown. Permutation statistical methods do not rely on knowledge of standard errors and therefore provide much-needed probability values for a number of otherwise very useful measures of association. One measure without a known standard error is Freeman's θ measure of nominal-ordinal association [5, pp. 108–119].

Consider an $r \times c$ contingency table where the r rows are a nominal-level (categorical) independent variable (x) and the c columns are an ordinal-level (ranked) dependent variable (y). For Freeman's θ it is necessary to calculate the absolute sum of the number of concordant pairs and number of discordant pairs for all combinations of the nominal-level independent variable (rows) considered two at a time. Assuming that the column ordered variable (y) is underlying continuous and that ties in ranking result simply from a crude classification of the continuous variable, Freeman's nominal-ordinal measure of association is given by

$$\theta = \frac{\displaystyle\sum_{i=1}^{r-1} \sum_{j=i+1}^{r} |C_{ij} - D_{ij}|}{C + D + T_y}.$$

11.4.1 An Example Analysis for θ

To illustrate the calculation of Freeman's θ measure of nominal-ordinal association, consider the 4×5 contingency table given in Table 11.22 with $N = 40$ observations. For the frequency data given in Table 11.22 with $N = 40$ observations, the number of concordant pairs is

$$C = \sum_{i=1}^{r-1} \sum_{j=1}^{c-1} n_{ij} \left(\sum_{k=i+1}^{r} \sum_{l=j+1}^{c} n_{kl} \right)$$

$$= (1)(5 + 5 + 0 + 0 + 0 + 2 + 2 + 1 + 0 + 0 + 2 + 3)$$

Table 11.22 Example data for Freeman's θ measure of nominal-ordinal association with $r = 4$ rows, $c = 5$ columns, and $N = 40$ cross-classified observations

	Column (y)					
Row (x)	1	2	3	4	5	Total
1	1	2	5	2	0	10
2	10	5	5	0	0	20
3	0	0	2	2	1	5
4	0	0	0	2	3	5
Total	11	7	12	6	4	40

$$+ (2)(5 + 0 + 0 + 2 + 2 + 1 + 0 + 2 + 3)$$

$$+ \cdots + (2)(2 + 3) + (2)(3)) = 304 \ ,$$

the number of discordant pairs is

$$D = \sum_{i=1}^{r-1} \sum_{j=1}^{c-1} n_{i,c-j+1} \left(\sum_{k=i+1}^{r} \sum_{l=1}^{c-j} n_{kl} \right)$$

$$= (0)(10 + 5 + 5 + 0 + 0 + 0 + 2 + 2 + 0 + 0 + 0 + 2)$$

$$+ (2)(10 + 5 + 6 + 0 + 0 + 2 + 0 + 0 + 0)$$

$$+ \cdots + (2)(0 + 0) + (0)(0) = 141 \ ,$$

the number of pairs tied on variable y is

$$T_y = \sum_{j=1}^{c} \sum_{i=1}^{r-1} n_{ij} \left(\sum_{k=i+1}^{r} n_{kj} \right)$$

$$= (1)(10 + 0 + 0) + (10)(0 + 0) + (0)(0)$$

$$+ \cdots + (0)(0 + 1 + 3) + (1)(1 + 3) + (1)(3) = 80 \ ,$$

the concordant and discordant pairs for the $r = 4$ rows considered two at a time are

$$C_{12} = (1)(5 + 5 + 0 + 0) + (2)(5 + 0 + 0) + (5)(0 + 0) + (2)(0) = 20 \ ,$$
$$D_{12} = (0)(10 + 5 + 5 + 0) + (2)(10 + 5 + 5) + (5)(10 + 5) + (2)(10) = 135 \ ,$$

$$C_{13} = (1)(0 + 2 + 2 + 1) + (2)(2 + 2 + 1) + (5)(2 + 1) + (2)(1) = 32 \ ,$$
$$D_{13} = (0)(0 + 0 + 2 + 2) + (2)(0 + 0 + 2) + (5)(0 + 0) + (2)(0) = 4 \ ,$$

$$C_{14} = (1)(0 + 0 + 2 + 3) + (2)(0 + 2 + 3) + (5)(2 + 3) + (2)(3) = 46 \ ,$$
$$D_{14} = (0)(0 + 0 + 0 + 2) + (2)(0 + 0 + 0) + (5)(0 + 0) + (2)(0) = 0 \ ,$$

$$C_{23} = (10)(0 + 2 + 2 + 1) + (5)(2 + 2 + 1) + (5)(2 + 1) + (0)(1) = 90 \ ,$$
$$D_{23} = (0)(0 + 0 + 2 + 2) + (0)(0 + 0 + 2) + (5)(0 + 0) + (5)(0) = 0 \ ,$$

$$C_{24} = (10)(0 + 0 + 2 + 3) + (5)(0 + 2 + 3) + (5)(2 + 3) + (0)(3) = 100 \ .$$
$$D_{24} = (0)(0 + 0 + 0 + 2) + (0)(0 + 0 + 0) + (5)(0 + 0) + (5)(0) = 0 \ ,$$

$$C_{34} = (0)(0 + 0 + 2 + 3) + (0)(0 + 2 + 3) + (2)(2 + 3) + (2)(3) = 16 \ ,$$
$$D_{34} = (1)(0 + 0 + 0 + 2) + (2)(0 + 0 + 0) + (2)(0 + 0) + (0)(0) = 2 \ ,$$

and Freeman's θ is

$$
\theta = \frac{\displaystyle\sum_{i=1}^{r-1}\sum_{j=i+1}^{r} |C_{ij} - D_{ij}|}{C + D + T_y}
$$

$$
= \frac{|20 - 135| + |32 - 4| + |46 - 0| + |90 - 0| + |100 - 0| + |16 - 2|}{304 + 141 + 80}
$$

$$
= 0.7486 .
$$

11.4.2   An Exact Permutation Analysis for θ

Under the Fisher–Pitman permutation model, the exact probability value of an observed value of $\theta = 0.7486$ is given by the sum of the hypergeometric point probability values associated with the values of test statistic θ calculated on all M possible arrangements of the cell frequencies that are equal to or greater than the observed value of $\theta = 0.7486$. For the frequency data given in Table 11.22, there are only $M = 6{,}340{,}588$ possible arrangements in the reference set of all permutations of cell frequencies consistent with the observed row and column marginal frequency distributions, $\{10, 20, 5, 5\}$ and $\{11, 7, 12, 6, 4\}$, respectively, making an exact permutation analysis feasible.

If all M possible arrangements of the observed data occur with equal chance, the exact probability value of Freeman's θ under the Fisher–Pitman null hypothesis is the sum of the hypergeometric point probability values associated with the arrangements of cell frequencies with values of θ that are equal to or greater than the observed value of $\theta = 0.7486$. Based on the underlying hypergeometric probability distribution, the exact probability value of $\theta = 0.7486$ is $P = 0.2105 \times 10^{-10}$.

11.5   Contingency Measures: Nominal by Interval

Pearson's point-biserial correlation coefficient, denoted by r_{pb}, measures the association between a nominal-level (categorical) variable with two categories and an interval-level variable. Pearson's point-biserial correlation coefficient is an important measure in fields such as education and educational psychology where it is typically used to measure the correlation between test questions scored as correct (1) or incorrect (0) and the overall score on the test for N test takers. A low or negative point-biserial correlation coefficient indicates that the test takers with the highest scores on the test answered the question incorrectly and the test takers with the lowest scores on the test answered the question correctly, alerting the instructor to the possibility that the question failed to discriminate properly and may be faulty.

Table 11.23 Example (0, 1) coded data for Pearson's point-biserial correlation coefficient

	Variable			Variable	
Object	x	y	Object	x	y
1	0	99	11	1	86
2	0	99	12	1	90
3	1	98	13	0	97
4	1	98	14	0	95
5	1	97	15	1	92
6	0	89	16	0	98
7	0	95	17	1	86
8	0	94	18	1	85
9	1	92	19	0	94
10	1	60	20	0	96

11.5.1 An Example Analysis for r_{pb}

To illustrate the calculation of Pearson's point-biserial correlation coefficient, consider the dichotomous data listed in Table 11.23 for $N = 20$ observations where variable x is the dichotomous variable and variable y is an unspecified interval-level variable. The point-biserial correlation coefficient is often expressed as

$$r_{pb} = \frac{\bar{y}_0 - \bar{y}_1}{s_y} \sqrt{\frac{n_0 n_1}{N(N-1)}} \, ,$$

where n_0 and n_1 denote the number of y values coded 0 and 1, respectively, $N = n_0 + n_1$, $\bar{y}_0$ and $\bar{y}_1$ denote the means of the y values coded 0 and 1, respectively, and s_y is the sample standard deviation of the y values given by

$$s_y = \sqrt{\frac{1}{N-1} \sum_{i=1}^{N} (y_i - \bar{y})^2} \, .$$

For the data listed in Table 11.23, $n_0 = n_1 = 10$,

$$\bar{y}_0 = \frac{1}{n_0} \sum_{i=1}^{n_0} y_i = \frac{99 + 99 + \cdots + 89}{10} = 88.40 \, ,$$

$$\bar{y}_1 = \frac{1}{n_1} \sum_{i=1}^{n_1} y_i = \frac{98 + 98 + \cdots + 60}{10} = 95.60 \, ,$$

$$s_y = \sqrt{\frac{1}{N-1} \sum_{i=1}^{N} (y_i - \bar{y})^2} = \sqrt{\frac{1456}{20 - 1}} = 8.7539 \, ,$$

and Pearson's point-biserial correlation coefficient is

$$
r_{pb} = \frac{\bar{y}_0 - \bar{y}_1}{s_y} \sqrt{\frac{n_0 n_1}{N(N-1)}} = \frac{88.40 - 95.60}{8.7539} \sqrt{\frac{(10)(10)}{20(20-1)}} = -0.4219 \,.
$$

Alternatively, with

$$
\sum_{i=1}^{N} x_i = 10 \,, \quad \sum_{i=1}^{N} x_i^2 = 10 \,, \quad \sum_{i=1}^{N} y_i = 1840 \,, \quad \sum_{i=1}^{N} y_i^2 = 170{,}736 \,,
$$

$$
\text{and } \sum_{i=1}^{N} x_i y_i = 884 \,,
$$

Pearson's point-biserial correlation coefficient is simply the product-moment correlation between dichotomous variable x and interval-level variable y. Thus,

$$
r_{pb} = \frac{N \sum_{i=1}^{N} x_i y_i - \sum_{i=1}^{N} x_i \sum_{i=1}^{N} y_i}{\sqrt{\left[N \sum_{i=1}^{N} x_i^2 - \left(\sum_{i=1}^{N} x_i \right)^2 \right] \left[N \sum_{i=1}^{N} y_i^2 - \left(\sum_{i=1}^{N} y_i \right)^2 \right]}}
$$

$$
= \frac{(20)(884) - (10)(1840)}{\sqrt{\left[(20)(10) - 10^2 \right] \left[(20)(170{,}736) - 1840^2 \right]}} = -0.4219 \,.
$$

The conventional test of significance for Pearson's point-biserial correlation coefficient is

$$
t = r_{pb} \sqrt{\frac{N-2}{1 - r_{pb}^2}} = -0.4219 \sqrt{\frac{20-2}{1 - (-0.4219)^2}} = -1.9743 \,.
$$

Under the Neyman–Pearson null hypothesis, H_0: $\rho_{pb} = 0$, test statistic t is asymptotically distributed as Student's t with $N - 2$ degrees of freedom. With $N - 2 = 20 - 2 = 18$ degrees of freedom, the asymptotic two-tail probability value of $t = -1.9743$ is $P = 0.0639$, under the assumption of normality. For a critical evaluation of the point-biserial correlation coefficient, see a discussion in *The Measurement of Association* by the authors [2, pp. 417–424].

11.5.2   An Exact Permutation Analysis for r_{pb}

For the bivariate observations listed in Table 11.23, there are only

$$M = \frac{(n_0 + n_1)!}{n_0! \, n_1!} = \frac{(10 + 10)!}{10! \, 10!} = 184{,}756$$

possible, equally-likely arrangements in the reference set of all permutations of the observed scores, making an exact permutation analysis possible. Under the Fisher–Pitman permutation model, the exact probability of an observed value of Pearson's $|r_{pb}|$ is the proportion of $|r_{pb}|$ values calculated on all possible arrangements of the observed data that are equal to or greater than the observed value of $|r_{pb}| = 0.4219$. There are exactly 11,296 $|r_{pb}|$ values that are equal to or greater than the observed value of $|r_{pb}| = 0.4219$. If all arrangements of the $N = 20$ observed scores occur with equal chance, the exact probability value of $|r_{pb}| = 0.4219$ computed on the $M = 184{,}756$ possible arrangements of the observed data with $n_0 = n_1 = 10$ preserved for each arrangement is

$$P(r_{pb} \ge |r_0|) = \frac{\text{number of } r_{pb} \text{ values} \ge |r_0|}{M} = \frac{11{,}296}{184{,}756} = 0.0611 \, ,$$

where $|r_0|$ denotes the observed absolute value of test statistic r_{pb} and M is the number of possible, equally-likely arrangements of the $N = 20$ bivariate observations listed in Table 11.23.

11.6   Contingency Measures: Ordinal by Interval

The best-known and most-widely reported measure of ordinal-by-interval association is Jaspen's multiserial correlation coefficient, which is simply the Pearson product-moment correlation coefficient between an interval-level variable, Y, and a transformation of an ordinal-level variable, X. Given N values on the interval variable and k disjoint, ordered categories on the ordinal variable, the mean standard score of the underlying scale for a given category is given by

$$\bar{Z}_j = \frac{Y_{L_j} - Y_{U_j}}{p_j} \qquad \text{for } j = 1, \ldots, k \, ,$$

where Y_{L_j} and Y_{U_j} are the lower and upper ordinates of the segment of the $N(0, 1)$ distribution corresponding to the jth ordered category, and where p_j is the proportion of cases in the jth of k ordered categories. Given the obtained values of $\bar{Z}_j$, $j = 1, \ldots, k$, and the original N values of the interval-level variable, a standard Pearson product-moment correlation between the Y and $\bar{Z}$ values yields the multiserial correlation coefficient.

11.6.1   An Example Analysis for $r_{Y\bar{Z}}$

To illustrate the calculation of Jaspen's multiserial correlation coefficient, consider the small set of data given in Table 11.24 where $N = 32$ interval-level variables are listed in $k = 4$ disjoint, ordered categories: A, B, C, and D. Table 11.25 illustrates the calculation of Jaspen's multiserial correlation coefficient. The first column, headed X in Table 11.25, lists the $k = 4$ ordered categories of variable X. The second column, headed n, lists the number of observations in each of the k ordered categories. The third column, headed p, lists the proportion of observations in each of the k ordered categories. The fourth column, headed P, lists the cumulative proportion of observations in each of the k ordered categories. The fifth column, headed z, lists the standard score that defines the cumulative proportion from the fourth column under the unit-normal distribution for each of the k ordered categories. For example, for category A the standard score that defines the lowest (left-tail) of the normal distribution with proportion $P = 0.1250$ is $z = -1.1503$. The sixth column, headed Y_L, lists the height of the ordinate at the standard score listed in the fifth column *below* the specified segment of the unit-normal distribution. For example, for category A,

$$Y_{L_A} = \frac{\exp(-z^2/2)}{\sqrt{2\pi}} = \frac{\exp\left[-(-1.1503)^2/2\right]}{\sqrt{2(3.1416)}} = 0.2059 .$$

Table 11.24 Example ordinal-by-interval data for Jaspen's correlation coefficient with $N = 32$ observations

Category			
A	B	C	D
83	91	86	75
78	84	81	58
73	81	80	51
63	78	79	50
	76	77	50
	73	76	48
	69	70	48
	64	64	
	58	63	
	56	59	
		53	

Table 11.25 Calculation of the mean standard scores for the $k = 4$ ordinal categories

X	n	p	P	z	Y_L	Y_U	$\bar{Z}$
A	4	0.1250	0.1250	−1.1503	0.2059	0.0000	+1.6472
B	10	0.3125	0.4375	−0.1573	0.3940	0.2059	+0.6019
C	11	0.3438	0.7813	+0.7766	0.2951	0.3940	−0.2877
D	7	0.2188	1.0000	+1.0000	0.0000	0.2951	−1.3487
Total	32	1.0000					

The seventh column, headed Y_U, lists the height of the ordinate at the standard score listed in the fifth column *above* the specified segment of the unit-normal distribution. For example, for category C,

$$Y_{U_C} = \frac{\exp(-z^2/2)}{\sqrt{2\pi}} = \frac{\exp\left[-(-0.1573)^2/2\right]}{\sqrt{2(3.1416)}} = 0.3940 .$$

The last column, headed $\bar{Z}$, lists the average standard scores for the k ordered categories. For example, for category B,

$$\bar{Z}_B = \frac{Y_{L_B} - Y_{U_B}}{p_B} = \frac{0.3940 - 0.2059}{0.3125} = +0.6019$$

Jaspen's multiserial correlation coefficient is the Pearson product-moment correlation between the Y interval-level values given in Table 11.24 and the transformed $\bar{Z}$ values given in Table 11.25. Table 11.26 lists the Y, $\bar{Z}$, Y^2, $\bar{Z}^2$, and $Y\bar{Z}$ values, along with the corresponding sums.

For the summations given in Table 11.26, the Pearson product-moment correlation between the Y and $\bar{Z}$ values is

$$r_{Y\bar{Z}} = \frac{N\sum_{i=1}^{N} Y_i\bar{Z}_i - \sum_{i=1}^{N} Y_i \sum_{i=1}^{N} \bar{Z}_i}{\sqrt{\left[N\sum_{i=1}^{N} Y_i^2 - \left(\sum_{i=1}^{N} Y_i\right)^2\right]\left[N\sum_{i=1}^{N} \bar{Z}_i^2 - \left(\sum_{i=1}^{N} \bar{Z}_i\right)^2\right]}}$$

$$= \frac{(32)(189.3918) - (2195)(0.0000)}{\sqrt{\left[(32)(155,471) - 2195^2\right]\left[(32)(28.1193) - 0.0000^2\right]}} = +0.5094 .$$

Jaspen's multiserial correlation coefficient is known to be biased. The bias is due to the grouping of the values into k categories. When k is small, the bias can be pronounced. For the example data listed in Table 11.24, the correction for grouping is

$$S_{\bar{Z}} = \left(\frac{1}{N}\sum_{j=1}^{k} n_j\bar{Z}_j^2\right)^{1/2}$$

$$= \left\{\frac{1}{32}\left[(4)(+1.6472)^2 + (10)(+0.6019)^2 + (11)(-0.2877)^2\right.\right.$$

$$\left.\left. + (7)(-1.3487)^2\right]\right\}^{1/2} = 0.9374$$

Table 11.26 Calculation of the sums needed for the Pearson product-moment correlation between variables Y and $\bar{Z}$

Category	Y	$\bar{Z}$	Y^2	$\bar{Z}^2$	$Y\bar{Z}$
A	83	+1.6472	6889	2.7133	+136.7176
	78	+1.6472	6084	2.7133	+128.4816
	73	+1.6472	5329	2.7133	+120.2456
	63	+1.6472	3969	2.7133	+103.7736
B	91	+0.6019	8281	0.3623	+54.7729
	84	+0.6019	7056	0.3623	+50.5596
	81	+0.6019	6561	0.3623	+48.7539
	78	+0.6019	6084	0.3623	+46.9482
	76	+0.6019	5776	0.3623	+45.7444
	73	+0.6019	5329	0.3623	+43.9387
	69	+0.6019	4761	0.3623	+41.5311
	64	+0.6019	4096	0.3623	+38.5216
	58	+0.6019	3364	0.3623	+34.9102
	56	+0.6019	3136	0.3623	+33.7064
C	86	−0.2877	7396	0.0828	−23.8220
	81	−0.2877	6561	0.0828	−22.4370
	80	−0.2877	6400	0.0828	−22.1600
	79	−0.2877	6241	0.0828	−21.8830
	77	−0.2877	5929	0.0828	−21.3290
	76	−0.2877	5776	0.0828	−21.0520
	70	−0.2877	4900	0.0828	−19.3900
	64	−0.2877	4096	0.0828	−17.7280
	63	−0.2877	3969	0.0828	−17.4510
	59	−0.2877	3481	0.0828	−16.3430
	53	−0.2877	2809	0.0828	−14.6810
D	75	−1.3487	5625	1.8190	−101.1525
	58	−1.3487	3364	1.8190	−78.2246
	51	−1.3487	2601	1.8190	−68.7837
	50	−1.3487	2500	1.8190	−67.4350
	50	−1.3487	2500	1.8190	−67.4350
	48	−1.3487	2304	1.8190	−64.7376
	48	−1.3487	2304	1.8190	−64.7376
Sum	2195	0.0000	155,471	28.1193	+189.3918

and the corrected multiserial correlation coefficient is

$$ r_c = \frac{r_{Y\bar{Z}}}{S_{\bar{Z}}} = \frac{+0.5094}{0.9374} = +0.5434 \, . $$

Jaspen's r_c is asymptotically distributed as Student's t under the Neyman–Pearson null hypothesis with $N - 2$ degrees of freedom. If the population parameter,

ρ_c, is assumed to be zero, then for the observed data in Table 11.24,

$$t = \frac{r_c - \rho_c}{\sqrt{\dfrac{1 - r_c^2}{N - 2}}} = \frac{+0.5434 - 0.00}{\sqrt{\dfrac{1 - (0.5434)^2}{32 - 2}}} = +3.5455 \, ,$$

and with $N - 2 = 32 - 2 = 30$ degrees of freedom the asymptotic two-tail probability value of $r_c = +0.5434$ is $P = 0.1308 \times 10^{-2}$, under the assumption of normality.

11.6.2 A Monte Carlo Permutation Analysis for $r_{Y\bar{Z}}$

Because there are

$$M = N! = 32! = 263{,}130{,}836{,}933{,}693{,}530{,}167{,}218{,}012{,}160{,}000{,}000$$

possible, equally-likely arrangements in the reference set of all permutations of the observed values listed in Table 11.24, an exact permutation analysis is not possible and a Monte Carlo analysis is mandated. Let r_o indicate the observed value of r_c. Based on $L = 1{,}000{,}000$ randomly-selected arrangements of the observed data, there are 3069 $|r_c|$ values that are equal to or greater than $|r_o| = 0.5434$, yielding a Monte Carlo probability value of

$$P(|r_c| \geq |r_o|) = \frac{\text{number of } |r_c| \text{ values } \geq |r_o|}{L} = \frac{3069}{1{,}000{,}000} = 0.3069 \times 10^{-2} \, ,$$

where r_o denotes the observed value of r_c and L is the number of randomly-selected, equally-likely arrangements of the ordinal-interval data listed in Table 11.24.

11.7 Summary

Under the Neyman–Pearson model of statistical inference, this chapter examined various measures of nominal-nominal, ordinal-ordinal, nominal-ordinal, nominal-interval, and ordinal-interval association. Asymptotic probability values were provided under either Pearson's χ^2 probability distribution, Student's t distribution, Snedecor's F distribution, or the $N(0, 1)$ probability distribution. Under the Fisher–Pitman permutation model of statistical inference, procedures for both exact and Monte Carlo probability values were developed.

   Six sections provided examples and illustrative analyses of permutation statistical methods for contingency tables. In the first section, goodness-of-fit measures for

k discrete, mutually-exclusive categories were described and permutation methods
were utilized to obtain exact probability values. A measure of effect size for the
chi-squared goodness-of-fit test was presented and illustrated.

The second section illustrated the use of permutation statistical methods for
analyzing contingency tables in which two nominal-level variables have been
cross-classified. Three well-known and widely-used measures of nominal-nominal
association were introduced and analyzed with permutation methods: Cramér's
symmetric V measure, based on Pearson's chi-squared test statistic, and Goodman
and Kruskal's t_a and t_b asymmetric measures, based on the differences between concordant and discordant pairs of observations. The relationships between Pearson's
χ^2 test statistic and Goodman and Kruskal's t_a and t_b measures were described.

The third section illustrated the use of permutation statistical methods for
analyzing contingency tables in which two ordinal-level variables have been cross-
classified. Three popular measures of ordinal-ordinal association were introduced
and analyzed with permutation methods: Goodman and Kruskal's G symmetric
measure of ordinal-ordinal association and Somers' d_{yx} and d_{xy} asymmetric
measures of ordinal-ordinal association.

The fourth section illustrated the use of permutation statistical methods for
analyzing contingency tables in which a nominal-level variable was cross-classified
with an ordinal-level variable. Freeman's θ measure of association for a nominal-
level independent variable and an ordinal-level dependent variable was described
and illustrated with exact permutation statistical methods.

The fifth section illustrated the use of permutation statistical methods for
analyzing contingency tables in which a nominal-level variable was cross-classified
with an interval-level variable. Pearson's point-biserial correlation coefficient for
a dichotomous nominal-level variable and a continuous interval-level variable was
described and analyzed with exact permutation statistical methods.

The sixth section illustrated the use of permutation statistical methods for analyzing contingency tables in which an ordinal-level variable was cross-classified with
an interval-level variable. Jaspen's multi-serial correlation coefficient for ordinal-
interval association was described and analyzed with Monte Carlo permutation
methods.

References

1. Berry, K.J., Johnston, J.E., Mielke, P.W.: Exact goodness-of-fit tests for unordered equiprobable categories. Percept. Motor Skill. **98**, 909–918 (2004)
2. Berry, K.J., Johnston, J.E., Mielke, P.W.: The Measurement of Association: A Permutation Statistical Approach. Springer, Cham (2018)
3. Box, J.F.: R. A. Fisher: The Life of a Scientist. Wiley, New York (1978)
4. Fisher, R.: Has Mendel's work been rediscovered? Ann. Sci. **1**, 115–137 (1936)
5. Freeman, L.C.: Elementary Applied Statistics. Wiley, New York (1965)
6. Light, R.J.: Measures of response agreement for qualitative data: some generalizations and alternatives. Psychol. Bull. **76**, 365–377 (1971)

7. Margolin, B.H., Light, R.J.: An analysis of variance for categorical data, II: small sample comparisons with chi square and other competitors. J. Am. Stat. Assoc. **69**, 755–764 (1974)
8. Mielke, P.W., Berry, K.J.: Exact goodness-of-fit probability tests for analyzing categorical data. Educ. Psychol. Meas. **53**, 707–710 (1993)
9. Särndal, C.E.: A comparative study of association measures. Psychometrika **39**, 165–187 (1974)

Epilogue

The purpose of *A Primer of Permutation Statistical Methods* is to introduce exact and Monte Carlo permutation statistical methods to a new audience of researchers with a limited background in statistics. To this end the book assumes only one course in statistics such as might be taken by an undergraduate student majoring in biology, economics, political science, or psychology. The structure of the book is that of any first-term textbook in statistics and includes measures of central tendency and variability, permutation methods for one-sample tests, tests of two independent samples, matched pairs tests, one-way fully-randomized designs, one-way randomized-blocks designs, simple linear correlation and regression, and the analysis of two-way contingency tables.

Two models of statistical inference are described and compared: the conventional Neyman–Pearson population model that is taught in all introductory courses, and the lesser-known Fisher–Pitman permutation model with which the reader is assumed to be unfamiliar. The Neyman–Pearson population model assumes random sampling from one or more fully specified populations. Under the population model, the level of statistical significance that results from applying a statistical test to the results of an experiment or survey corresponds to the frequency with which the null hypothesis would be rejected in repeated random sampling from a specified population or populations. Because repeated sampling of the specified population(s) is usually impractical, it is assumed that the sampling distribution of test statistics generated under repeated random sampling conforms to an approximating theoretical distribution, such as the normal distribution. The size of a statistical test is the probability under the null hypothesis that repeated outcomes based on random samples of the same size are equal to or more extreme than the observed outcome.

In contrast, the Fisher–Pitman permutation model does not assume random sampling, but is completely data-dependent, relying entirely on the observed data. Thus, a test statistic is computed for the observed data and the observations are then permuted over all possible arrangements of the observed data and the selected

© Springer Nature Switzerland AG 2019
K. J. Berry et al., *A Primer of Permutation Statistical Methods*,
https://doi.org/10.1007/978-3-030-20933-9

test statistic is computed for each arrangement. The proportion of arrangements with test statistic values equal to or more extreme than the observed test statistic yields the exact probability of the observed test statistic value. When the number of possible arrangements of the observed data is very large, exact permutation methods are impractical and Monte Carlo permutation methods become necessary. Monte Carlo permutation methods generate a large random sample of all possible arrangements of the observed data and the Monte Carlo probability is the proportion of arrangements with test statistic values equal to or more extreme than the observed test statistic.

Three main themes characterize the 11 chapters of the book. First, the permutation test statistic, denoted by δ, is introduced and defined. Statistic δ is the fundamental test statistic for permutation statistical methods, serving as a replacement for many conventional test statistics ranging from Student's t test statistic, Fisher's F-ratio test statistic, and Pearson's χ^2 test statistic. Statistic δ is central to the descriptions and analyses presented in Chaps. 5–11 and constitutes a unifying test statistic for many permutation-based analyses.

Second, measures of effect size have become increasingly important in contemporary research with many journals now requiring both tests of significance and measures of effect size. In addition, introductory textbooks routinely include measures of effect size for most statistical tests and measures. Measures of effect size provide information pertaining to the practical or clinical significance of a result, complementing the conventional tests of statistical significance. A relatively new measure of effect size, designated $\Re$, is introduced and described. $\Re$ is a permutation-based, chance-corrected measure of effect size with an interpretation that is easily understood by the average undergraduate. Positive values indicate an effect size that is above what is expected by chance, negative values indicate an effect size that is less than what is expected by chance, and a value of zero indicates an effect size that is equal to what is expected by chance. Effect-size measure $\Re$ is central to the analyses presented in Chaps. 5–11 and constitutes a generalized unifying measure of effect size for many permutation-based analyses.

Third, conventional statistics as taught in every introductory course necessarily assume random sampling, normality, and, where appropriate, homogeneity of variance. Permutation statistical methods are entirely data-dependent and do not assume random sampling, normality, or homogeneity. Moreover, because conventional statistical tests and measures assume normality they rely on squared deviations among sample values. Permutation statistical methods do not assume normality and, therefore, are not limited to squared deviations among values. While almost any positive scaling factor can be used with permutation methods, ordinary Euclidean scaling has proven to be the most justifiable. As such, ordinary Euclidean scaling allows permutation statistical methods to minimize, or in many cases completely eliminate, the influence of extreme values or statistical outliers without resorting to trimming, Winsorizing, or converting raw values to rank scores.

In this introductory book on permutation statistical methods, both exact and Monte Carlo methods are introduced and applied to a wide variety of conventional statistical tests and measures. The permutation methods described provide an alternative approach to conventional statistical methods that is entirely data-dependent, does not depend on the usual assumptions of normality and homogeneity, is ideal for small samples, and is appropriate for both random and nonrandom samples.

Author Index

An "n" following a page number indicates an entry contained within a footnote on that page, an *italic* number indicates an entry in a table or figure heading, and a page number in Roman type indicates a textural reference.

A

Agresti, A., 34, 44
Amonenk, I.S., 49
Andersen, S.L., 5, 26, 27
Armitage, P., 38

B

Babington Smith, B., 20, 23, 178, 349
Barnard, G.A., 156
Bartlett, M.S., 11, 258, 306, 311, 312
Behrens, W.U., 209
Berkson, J., 70
Berry, K.J., 7–10, 12, 13, 33, 36–41, 44–50, 111, 115, 119–122, 166, 167, 169–172, 178, 217, 218, 220–222, 226, 269, 271–277, 294, 327, 331, 336, 344, 386, 392, 436, 437
Biondini, M.E., 39
Blalock, H.M., 123
Box, G.E.P., 5, 26, 27, 130n, 130
Box, J.F., 415
Boyett, J.M., 34, 36, 46
Bradley, R.A., 24, 34
Brooks, E.B., 24
Bross, I.D.J., 47, 70

C

Cade, B.S., 41
Cameron, J., 91

Cochran, W.G., 38
Cohen, B.H., 32
Cohen, J., 2, 3, 7–12, 38, 101, 110, 113, 119–123, 129, 132, 134, 139, 140, 144, 145, 148, 150, 154, 165, 166, 169–174, 177, 178, 180, 184, 189, 191, 196, 198, 202, 204, 207, 217, 218n, 218, 220–222, 225, 226, 228, 235, 240, 241, 245, 246, 252–254, 258, 268, 270n, 270–275, 282, 284, 294, 297, 299, 303, 306, 310, 312, 316, 327, 330–332, 336, 337, 344, 347, 352, 353, 355–358, 419, 421, 423
Cowles, M., 109
Cramér, H., 14, 419, 422, 458
Curran-Everett, D., 48, 59

D

Dabrowska, D.M., 18
D'Andrade, R., 123
Dart, J., 123
David, F.N., 17
Doerfler, T.E., 31
Dudley, H.A.F., 42
Dwass, M., 5, 26, 28

E

Eden, T., 4, 15, 20, 21, 58, 59, 80
Edgington, E.S., 29–31, 35, 69

© Springer Nature Switzerland AG 2019
K. J. Berry et al., *A Primer of Permutation Statistical Methods*,
https://doi.org/10.1007/978-3-030-20933-9

Subject Index

A **bold** page number indicates an important or comprehensive entry on that page and a page number in Roman type indicates a textural reference.

© Springer Nature Switzerland AG 2019
K. J. Berry et al., *A Primer of Permutation Statistical Methods*,
https://doi.org/10.1007/978-3-030-20933-9

CPSIA information can be obtained
at www.ICGtesting.com
Printed in the USA
LVHW081557250820
664082LV00001B/73